Personalizing Asthma Management for the Clinician

Personalizing Asthma Management for the Clinician

STANLEY J. SZEFLER, MD
Director Pediatric Asthma Research Program and Research Medical Director
The Breathing Institute
Children's Hospital Colorado
Professor of Pediatrics
University of Colorado School of Medicine
Aurora, CO, United States

FERNANDO HOLGUIN, MD
Division of Pulmonary Medicine
Department of Medicine
University of Colorado School of Medicine
Aurora, CO, United States

MICHAEL E. WECHSLER, MD, MMSC
Professor of Medicine and Director of the NJH Cohen Family Asthma Institute
Division of Pulmonary
Critical Care & Sleep Medicine
Department of Medicine
National Jewish Health
Denver, CO, United States

ELSEVIER

ELSEVIER

3251 Riverport Lane
St. Louis, Missouri 63043

Content Strategist: Kayla Wolfe
Content Development Manager: Taylor Ball
Content Development Specialist: Alison Swety
Publishing Services Manager: Deepthi Unni
Project Manager: Janish Ashwin Paul
Designer: Gopalakrishnan Venkatraman

Printed in United States of America

Last digit is the print number: 9 8 7 6 5 4 3 2 1

Working together to grow libraries in developing countries

www.elsevier.com • www.bookaid.org

List of Contributors

Leonard B. Bacharier, MD
Robert C. Strunk Endowed Chair for Lung and
   Respiratory Research
Professor of Pediatrics and Medicine
Clinical Director, Division of Pediatric Allergy,
   Immunology, & Pulmonary Medicine
Unit Co-Leader, Patient Oriented Research Unit
Washington University in St. Louis School of
   Medicine
St. Louis Children's Hospital
St. Louis, MO, United States

Nicole Barberis, MD
Division of Allergy and Clinical Immunology
Department of Medicine
National Jewish Health
Denver, CO, United States
Division of Allergy and Clinical Immunology
Department of Internal Medicine
University of Colorado Hospital
Aurora, CO, United States

Gilbert J. Burckart, PharmD
Associate Director for Pediatrics
Office of Clinical Pharmacology
Office of Translational Sciences
Center for Drug Evaluation and Research
US Food and Drug Administration
Silver Spring, MD, United States

William W. Busse, MD
Professor of Medicine, Allergy & Immunology
Division of Allergy, Pulmonary and Critical Care
Department of Medicine
University of Wisconsin School of Medicine and
   Public Health
Madison, WI, United States

Tara F. Carr, MD
Assistant Professor, Medicine and Otolaryngology
Director, Allergy and Immunology
Department of Medicine
University of Arizona
College of Medicine
Tucson, AZ, United States

Mario Castro, MD, MPH
Alan A. and Edith L. Wolff Professor of Pulmonary
   and Critical Care Medicine
Professor of Medicine, Pediatrics, and Radiology
Division of Pulmonary and Critical Care Medicine
Department of Medicine, Pediatrics, and Radiology
Washington University School of Medicine
St. Louis, MO, United States

Kian Fan Chung, MD DSc
Professor of Respiratory Medicine
National Heart & Lung Institute
Imperial College London & Biomedical Research Unit
Royal Brompton and Harefield NHS Foundation Trust
London, United Kingdom

Lisa Cicutto, RN, ACNP(cert), CAE, PhD
Director
Community Outreach and Research
National Jewish Health
Director
Clinical Science Program
University of Colorado Anschutz Medical Campus
Denver, CO, United States

Marc Elie, PhD
Post-doctoral Fellow
Department of Pharmaceutical Sciences
University of Colorado Anschutz Medical Campus
Aurora, CO, United States
School of Pharmacy and Pharmaceutical Sciences
Aurora, CO, United States

Anne M. Fitzpatrick, PhD
Associate Professor and Director
Asthma Clinical Research Program
Department of Pediatrics
Emory University
Atlanta, GA, United States

Monica J. Federico, MD
Breathing Institute
University of Colorado Denver
Children's Hospital Colorado
Aurora, CO, United States

Claudia L. Gaefke, MD
Department of Medicine
University of Arizona, College of Medicine
Tucson, AZ, United States

Dionna Green, MD
Medical Officer, Pediatrics
Policy Lead, Guidance and Policy Team
Office of Clinical Pharmacology | Office of
    Translational Sciences
Center for Drug Evaluation and Research
US Food and Drug Administration
Silver Spring, MD, United States

Tari Haahtela, MD
Professor
Skin and Allergy Hospital
Helsinki University Hospital
Helsinki, Finland

Chase Hall, MD
Division of Pulmonary and Critical Care Medicine
Department of Internal Medicine
Washington University School of Medicine
St. Louis, MO, United States

Heather Hoch, MD, MSCS
Assistant Professor of Pediatrics
Breathing Institute
University of Colorado Denver
Children's Hospital Colorado
Aurora, CO, United States

Fernando Holguin, MD
Division of Pulmonary Medicine
Department of Medicine
University of Colorado School of Medicine
Aurora, CO, United States

Yvonne J. Huang, MD
Division of Pulmonary and Critical Care Medicine
Department of Internal Medicine
University of Michigan Ann Arbor
Anna Arbor, MI, United States

Katherine Johnston, MPH
Children's Hospital Colorado
Aurora, CO, United States

Rohit K. Katial, MD
Professor of Medicine
Division of Allergy and Immunology
Department of Medicine; Associate Vice President
    of Clinical Research and Industry Relationships;
    Co-Director of Cohen Asthma Institute at National
    Jewish Health
Helen Wohlberg and Herman Lambert Chair in
    Pharmacokinetics
National Jewish Health
Professor of Medicine
University of Colorado
Denver, CO, United States
Professor of Medicine
Icahn School of Medicine at Mt. Sinai
New York, NY, United States

Andrew H. Liu, MD
Professor of Pediatrics
Breathing Institute
University of Colorado Denver
Children's Hospital Colorado
Aurora, CO, United States

Jonathan Malka, MD
The Pediatric Associates
North Miami, FL, United States

Yasmeen Nkrumah-Elie, PhD
Postdoctoral Fellow
Skaggs School of Pharmacy and Pharmaceutical
    Sciences
University of Colorado, Anschutz Medical Campus
Aurora, CO, United States

Victor E. Ortega, MD, PhD
Center for Genomics and Personalized Medicine Research
Wake Forest School of Medicine
Medical Center Boulevard
Winston-Salem, NC, United States

Emily J. Pennington, MD
Wake Forest School of Medicine
Medical Center Boulevard
Winston-Salem, NC, United States

Perdita Permaul, MD
Massachusetts General Hospital for Children
Division of Pediatric Allergy and Immunology
Harvard Medical School
Boston, MA, United States

Wanda Phipatanakul, MD, MS
Professor of Pediatrics
Harvard Medical School
Director, Asthma Clinical Research Center
Boston Children's Hospital
Asthma, Allergy and Immunology
Boston, MA, United States

Nichole Reisdorph, PhD, MS
Associate Professor
Department of Pharmaceutical Sciences
School of Pharmacy and Pharmaceutical Sciences
University of Colorado Anschutz Medical Campus
Aurora, CO, United States

Malcolm R. Sears, MB
Professor of Medicine
AstraZeneca Chair in Respiratory Epidemiology
Department of Medicine
McMaster University
Hamilton, ON, Canada
Firestone Institute for Respiratory Health
St. Joseph's Healthcare
Hamilton, ON, Canada

Shweta Sood, MD, MS
Division of Pulmonary and Critical Care Medicine
Department of Internal Medicine
Washington University School of Medicine
St. Louis, MO, United States

Olof Selroos, MD
Professor
Helsinki University
Helsinki, Finland

Joseph D. Spahn, MD
Children's Hospital Colorado
Aurora, CO, United States

Jeffrey R. Stokes, MD
Professor of Pediatrics
Division of Pediatric Allergy, Immunology, &
   Pulmonary Medicine
Washington University in St. Louis School of
   Medicine
St. Louis Children's Hospital
St. Louis, MO, United States

Padmaja Subbarao, MD, MSc
Associate Professor of Pediatrics
Divison of Respiratory Medicine
Department of Pediatrics & Physiology
Hospital for Sick Children and University of Toronto
Toronto, ON, Canada

Stanley J. Szefler, MD
Director Pediatric Asthma Research Program and
   Research Medical Director
The Breathing Institute
Children's Hospital Colorado
Professor of Pediatrics
University of Colorado School of Medicine
Aurora, CO, United States

Eileen Wang, MD, MPH
Assistant Professor of Medicine
Division of Allergy and Clinical Immunology
Department of Medicine
National Jewish Health
Denver, CO, United States

Michael E. Wechsler, MD, MMSc
Professor of Medicine and Director of the NJH Cohen
   Family Asthma Institute
Division of Pulmonary
Critical Care & Sleep Medicine
Department of Medicine
National Jewish Health
Denver, CO, United States

Preface

Like almost everything in my life, this book developed by circumstance, luck, and opportunity. For several years now, I have been fortunate to work with Donald Leung, MD, PhD, as one of the coeditors for *Pediatric Allergy: Principles and Practice* now in its third edition. This book followed *Middleton's, Allergy: Principles and Practice*. Two of the three original editors for that book, the late Elliot Ellis, MD, and the late Elliott Middleton, Jr., MD, were my first mentors while I trained at the State University of New York at Buffalo.

At the Annual Meeting of the American Academy of Allergy, Asthma and Immunology, I usually meet with one of the Elsevier publishing managers to review our *Pediatric Allergy* book. In March 2016, Belinda Kuhn, the Senior Content Strategist at Elsevier, asked me for ideas for a new book. I mentioned that we really need a book on personalized medicine for asthma to integrate and discuss this rapidly evolving literature, especially for clinicians who are busy in practice. She was interested and excited about this idea and she mentioned the new *Hot Topics* series. No sooner did I get back to my office then I had a publishing date, a contract, and an assigned Developmental Editor, Alison Swety. Nothing works better for me than a deadline.

As a pediatrician, I wanted to make sure that I addressed the adult perspective. I contacted my Denver colleagues. First, I invited Michael E. Wechsler, MD, at National Jewish Health, a medical center that built its reputation around asthma, to assist. Then I asked Fernando Holguin, MD, who is leading the development of a new adult asthma program at the University of Colorado, to join us. Both accepted enthusiastically.

Together, we developed a list of chapters to address each of the evolving areas that impact asthma care. We invited authors who could address these challenging topics. They, in turn, invited their young colleagues to assist. I would like to thank Drs. Wechsler and Holguin for assisting me with the development of this book that we entitled *Personalized Asthma Management for the Clinician*. I would also like to thank all of the contributors who took the time out of their very busy schedule. They far exceeded our expectations. Of course, we also thank Belinda and Alison for guiding us through this process, as well as my Administrative Assistant, Lara Webb.

The information around the science of asthma and healthcare is coming so rapidly and in such a volume that guidelines committees cannot keep up with it. Current guidelines tend to speak to the patient with mild to moderate asthma and to the primary care clinician. We hope that we move this newfound information to the next level by speaking to the individualized approach for patients of all ages and severity levels. In this era, we are accustomed to sound bites for communication. Hopefully, this comprehensive set of topics presented in a concise manner will bring you "back to the books."

Stanley J. Szefler, MD
Research Medical Director and Director Pediatric Asthma
Research Program
The Breathing Institute
Children's Hospital Colorado
Aurora, CO, US

Foreword

The past 25 years has witnessed dramatic advances in asthma, including our appreciation of the pathophysiologic and pathogenic basis underlying this airway disease, which affects nearly 10% of our population. First, the prevalence of asthma has escalated like no other chronic disease with an increase in incidence rates beginning nearly 50 years ago. However, the increase in asthma prevalence is not universally distributed but found almost exclusively in westernized areas of the globe. Asthma is a disease of "civilization," and this association has given us clues to its causes and risks. Second, recognition that airway inflammation is a central, and perhaps defining, feature of this chronic disease has been important to improved treatment and the persistent nature of asthma. Airway inflammation directly contributes not only to the pathophysiology of asthma with shortness of breath, wheezing, and airflow obstruction, which is usually variable and intermittent in its intensity, but also to the irreversibility seen in those with more severe disease. Airway inflammation has also become an appropriate target for more effective asthma treatment and treatment directed toward its basic underlying pathology. With this information in mind, a focus on regulating inflammation has led to greater disease control as well as reduced morbidity and mortality. Finally, asthma is now recognized as being not one disease but rather one with "many faces" as reflected in severity, children versus adults, and responsiveness to treatment. Asthma has multiple phenotypes with overlapping features but resulting in unique personalities. Although this very common disease has become more prevalent, an appreciation for the complexity surrounding its eventual expression has greatly expanded. With these changes have come the need for a greater appreciation of its underlying complexities and, perhaps most important, how these changes may translate to earlier recognition and more effective treatment. Common in asthma does not mean simplistic.

The Denver trio of editors for *Personalizing Asthma Management for the Clinician*, Stanley J. Szefler, Fernando Holguin, and Michael E. Wechsler, have brought together key categories of importance to asthma, including biomarkers, phenotypes, prevention of exacerbations, and management and, eventually, prevention, to provide the clinician and student with an updated and integrated view of asthma as seen today, and a knowledge base that will be needed to provide more effective care of this disease. Their comprehensive but analytical and practical approach to the current knowledge of asthma is expected. They are all noted investigators of asthma and are able to translate new concepts to more effective patient care.

Their textbook has identified important topics and advances in asthma that are revolutionizing our approach to this disease. Key chapters include a recognition of current biomarkers in asthma: exhaled nitric oxide (FeNO), eosinophils, both circulating and airway, and emerging discoveries with the use of molecular-based assessments and systems biology analyses. Not only has the identification of biomarkers in asthma been important to improved and earlier disease recognition but also serves as guides to select and apply existing and new interventions to patients and, as a consequence, achieve a greater likelihood of response. It is apparent that treatment of asthma is not a "one-size-fits-all" approach, but rather a more informed and targeted approach that will select the best treatment for individual patients—personalized management. The authors of the various chapters are, like the editors, leaders in asthma and understand the complexities of this disease.

Asthma heterogeneity is seen in many facets and categories—age, sex, and severity. We now know that asthma is different in children and adults, and these differences translate to distinct management approaches. Children are not small adults and their therapeutic needs *and* responsiveness to existing and future treatment are, understandably, age distinct. These topics are front and center in this textbook. Also, as asthma has its beginning in childhood, often early in infancy, a major effort has been made to identify in whom and how these processes begin and progress to become clinically apparent. Early recognition of asthma will reduce disease morbidity. Perhaps more importantly, and close at hand, is the possibility that targeted intervention in high-risk infants can prevent the expression of asthma. These concepts are also part of this text and how these efforts will likely unfold.

Although deaths from asthma have diminished, they still occur and, as most feel, should be preventable. A major contributor to asthma morbidity is exacerbations. In children, asthma exacerbations most frequently follow viral respiratory infections, particularly those due to the common cold virus—rhinovirus. Current treatment with inhaled corticosteroids and long-acting β-agonists reduces the frequency of exacerbations but does not eliminate them. As exacerbations are major factors to asthma morbidity and disease cost, as well as possibly leading to persistent and progressive airway compromises, they need special attention and are given so in this textbook.

The editors also provide the reader with insights into the benefits of "population management" of asthma. The application of principles of public health from basic and applied knowledge of asthma has the potential, and promise, to comprehensively extend knowledge on asthma with population-based approaches. Tari Haahtela and Olof Selroos have provided long-standing informative leadership to asthma management in Finland. Nearly 20 years ago, Finland adopted a nationwide Asthma Program with a goal to decrease the number of days patients were hospitalized with asthma by 50% and to reduce annual costs by a likewise amount, 50%. Their strategy was straightforward: "Asthma is an inflammatory disease and should be treated as such from the very beginning." Their results, with conventional guideline-based treatment, have been extremely impressive and are recounted in their chapter. Their story is a message to all.

The editors cap their textbook with a key contribution, "Future Directions in Asthma Management: Where We Are and Where Are We Going?" Where we are now is at the doorstep of a most exciting period in asthma discovery that will translate to personalized and, consequently, improved treatment. The molecular tools are now readily available and are being applied to well-characterized populations of patients. With this information, it will be possible to bring the endotype, i.e., molecular basis of disease, to the individual patient and specific phenotype. A second step in this quantum leap forward is the application of new treatments that will target pivotal pathways related to individual patient's disease states. Therefore, knowing what specific pathway leads to a patient's asthma can be identified; having the insight to interpret this process, or these processes, holds considerable promise for personalized treatment with greater effectiveness. Perhaps, the same strategy will turn out to be the greatest movement forward—asthma prevention, either secondary or primary. The tools are available and molecular guidance to treatment is rapidly emerging. This is the future; *Personalizing Asthma Management for the Clinician* provides the background and rationale for where we are today and what our next destinations will likely be.

William W. Busse, MD
Professor of Medicine, Allergy & Immunology
Division of Allergy, Pulmonary and Critical Care
Department of Medicine
University of Wisconsin School of Medicine and
Public Health
Madison, WI, US

Introduction

Asthma is a common, chronic respiratory disease affecting 1%–18% of the population in different countries. Based on the definition of asthma derived from the Global Initiative for Asthma (GINA), 2017, asthma is considered to be a heterogeneous disease, usually characterized by chronic airway inflammation. It is defined by the history of respiratory symptoms, such as wheeze, shortness of breath, chest tightness, and cough, that vary over time and in intensity, together with variable expiratory airflow limitation.[1] These variations are often triggered by factors such as exercise, allergen or irritant exposure, change in weather, or viral respiratory infections.

Symptoms and airflow limitation may resolve spontaneously or in response to medication and may sometimes be absent for weeks or months at a time. On the other hand, patients can experience episodic flare-ups (exacerbations) of asthma that may be life-threatening and carry a significant burden to patients and the community. Asthma is usually associated with airway hyperresponsiveness to direct or indirect stimuli and with chronic airway inflammation. These features usually persist, even when symptoms are absent or lung function is normal, but may normalize with treatment.[1] Therefore, the course of asthma may vary among individuals and even within individuals over time. Thus, there is a need for the clinician to personalize or individualize the approach to asthma management.

BACK TO THE BOOKS

Before national asthma guidelines were developed in the early 1980s in New Zealand, clinicians relied on their key opinion leaders, review articles, and books to keep up to date with information. Educational forums were often supported by pharmaceutic firms as new medications were introduced. With the recognition that asthma deaths were increasing in the 1980s, written national, then international, and then worldwide guidelines were developed to gain consensus on asthma management. Updates to these guidelines can vary among the different groups, and long periods of time may pass before an update will occur in a specific country,[2] and in the interim, new treatment strategies and approaches may be developed.

The availability of medications and the cost of care can vary among the various countries and can affect the way different countries emphasize or recommend the use of medications. Recognizing the variability in regulatory status of medications, the GINA has been profiled as an asthma strategy rather than a guideline. GINA is updated on an annual basis with current literature along with periodic full revisions. Even with this conscientious approach to updating GINA with current information, it is difficult to keep up with the rapid evolution of new information. In addition, GINA attempts to meet the needs of developing countries and takes great care to provide management principles that are affordable and accessible. GINA also attempts to meet the needs of primary care physicians. Document size limits the amount of information that can be provided and easily read in the clinical setting.

National guidelines in the United States are being updated in 2017 after a 10-year period; however, only selected topic areas will be updated.[3] Similarly, updates in other countries can vary in time depending on sources of funding to support and disseminate this work as well as the availability of individuals to serve on guidelines committees. This makes it very difficult for countries and panels to keep up with the rapid introduction of new studies pertinent to understanding asthma and potentially impacting management. In some ways, we must now turn "back to the books" to assemble this information and continue to update it rapidly for the practicing clinician. Therefore, we took the opportunity to develop this book on personalized asthma management that could be useful to clinicians who would like a one-stop resource to review up-to-date information on the relevant topics. We assembled a group of authorities to address these key topics important to advancing asthma care.

RAPIDLY DEVELOPING SCIENCE

Over the past 10 years, new scientific information has been introduced that potentially impacts the presentation of asthma in individuals and possibly explains asthma heterogeneity in presentation and treatment response. These areas include genetics, epigenetics, microbiome, environmental assessment, proteomics, and metabolomics, to name a few. In addition, large clinical trials sponsored by government sources as well as pharmaceutic industry have provided new insights on the variability of treatment response, as well as patient characteristics, biomarkers, and genetic markers that may be associated with a favorable response to treatment.

Recently, new treatment strategies and new medications have been introduced, including bronchial thermoplasty, long-acting anticholinergics, biologic response modifiers, and longer-acting inhaled corticosteroids and once daily combination inhaled corticosteroid and long-acting β-adrenergic agonists. There has also been increased emphasis placed on obtaining information that would make these new medications appropriate for use in children, and this has been prompted by the regulatory agencies including the U.S. Food and Drug Administration and the European Medical Agency. There have been ongoing attempts at harmonization in these efforts.

HEALTHCARE CHANGES

Individual countries continue to struggle to find ways to provide optimal medical care for their residents. There is recent emphasis on developing patient-centered care approaches as well as population health and population management strategies. Some countries have even taken a national approach to managing asthma while medical care systems in other countries have developed their own systems of management within a healthcare system. The introduction of the electronic age and computer systems for communication has resulted in the development of electronic medical records. If used appropriately, these records can serve as a source of communication among clinicians supporting individual patients, such as primary care physicians and specialists. Furthermore, they could serve as a resource of information for treatment decisions as they develop. In addition, information from large databases can be evaluated and used to understand the impact of treatment on populations through big data analysis.

Asthma care has advanced with these new tools as well. With the recognition that treatment response can vary among individuals and that biomarkers and patient characteristics could be used to predict treatment response, the opportunities are now enormous for implementing a personalized approach to asthma care. We take the opportunity to now assemble this information to assist clinicians who are specifically interested in keeping up to date on these new areas of science as well as understanding the various factors that are likely to impact asthma care for their patients.

WHAT CAN YOU EXPECT TO LEARN?

We begin the book with a review of a national effort in Finland to improve asthma care (see Chapter 1). The challenges, the strategies, and the accomplishments of this program are summarized for other countries to consider to develop a national effort to improve care. Because individual countries may not have the resources or commitment to approach asthma management on a national basis, we also provide an approach that could be applied within a network of care, such as a pediatric hospital setting (see Chapter 2).

One of the most challenging areas for asthma management is caring for the patient with severe asthma. Many of our new medications are designed to treat this population who are not adequately controlled with our current array of medications. We provide a summary of the unique features of managing severe asthma in adults and children (see Chapters 2, 3, and 4). Because it has been recently recognized that these new medications may be selected by analyzing biomarkers, we provide a detailed discussion of relevant biomarkers, including blood and sputum eosinophils and exhaled nitric oxide, as well as a regulatory perspective on the application of biomarkers in clinical care (see Chapters 5, 6, and 7). In time, new biomarkers will be discovered and applied to clinical care and we provide an overview on the outlook for this area (see Chapter 8). Other areas of development that we address include the application of pharmacogenomics and phenotype assessment for individualizing treatment. Attention has also been directed to the role of the environment on lung health as well as the impact on triggering asthma symptoms (see Chapters 9, 10, and 11).

Meanwhile, new medications are being developed that are designed to regulate inflammatory substances associated with the pathogenesis of asthma, and the current hope is that they will serve to prevent asthma exacerbations as well as the progression of the disease. Indeed, they may eventually serve to halt the onset of the disease. Current opportunities to utilize these strategies to prevent asthma exacerbations are summarized, but one of the weaknesses in the system is patient adherence to currently available medications. This area is also addressed along with new strategies to monitor adherence to treatment (see Chapter 12). Another source of support for children with asthma that is addressed includes school-centered asthma programs (see Chapter 13).

Careful analysis of our successes and failures in treatment will be used to discover pathways of inflammation as well as unmet needs. This area is addressed in a chapter on systems biology (see Chapter 14). We are also beginning to recognize that another aspect of the environment, namely the microbiome, may play a significant role in altering the phenotype of asthma as well as treatment response (see Chapter 15). All of these factors will be needed to understand methods of prevention for the development of asthma as well as the progression of asthma from early, intermittent presentation to severe asthma with irrecoverable loss of lung function over time as described in subsequent chapters (see Chapters 16 and 17). To better understand the individual features of asthma, new imaging techniques are being developed (see Chapter 18). Finally, we end this presentation by projecting what areas could be applied to current medical care that are beyond the current asthma guidelines and what areas are ripe for rapid development in the future (see Chapter 19).

Although this book addresses our current understanding of asthma, we recognize that knowledge about asthma continues to evolve and new therapies and treatment strategies will continue to be developed. If successful in our efforts, we hope to update and add to these topics in future editions of this review of *Personalized Asthma Management for the Clinician.*

Stanley J. Szefler, MD
Fernando Holguin, MD
Michael E. Wechsler, MD, MMSC

REFERENCES

1. Global strategy for asthma management and prevention (updated 2017): Global Initiative for Asthma (GINA). http://www.ginasthma.org.
2. Becker AB, Abrams EM. Asthma guidelines: the global initiative for asthma in relation to national guidelines. *Curr Opin Allergy Clin Immunol.* 2017 Apr;17(2):99–103.
3. *Expert Panel Report 3: Guidelines for the Diagnosis and Management of Asthma.* Bethesda, Maryland: National Institutes of Health, National Asthma Education and Prevention Program; 2007. NIH Publication No. 08–4051. http://www. nhlbi.nih.gov/guidelines/asthma/ asthgdln.pdf.

Contents

1 **A Population Management Model of Asthma and Allergy: Case Finland,** *1*
Tari Haahtela, MD, Olof Selroos, MD

2 **Population Health Management: A Systematic Approach to Asthma Care in a Pediatric Network of Care,** *11*
Monica J. Federico, MD, Katherine Johnston, MPH

3 **Management of Severe Asthma in Adults: New Insights,** *19*
Eileen Wang, MD, MPH, Nicole Barberis, MD, Rohit K. Katial, MD

4 **Management and Prevention of Severe Asthma in Children,** *33*
Anne M. Fitzpatrick, PhD

5 **Exhaled Nitric Oxide as a Biomarker for Asthma Management,** *49*
Joseph D. Spahn, MD, Jonathan Malka, MD

6 **Blood and Sputum Eosinophils as a Biomarker for Selecting and Adjusting Asthma Medication,** *59*
Claudia L. Gaefke, MD, Tara F. Carr, MD

7 **Regulatory Aspects of Pediatric Biomarkers for Assessing Medication Response,** *69*
Gilbert J. Burckart, PharmD, Dionna J. Green, MD

8 **Discovery and Validation of New Biomarkers for Personalizing Asthma Therapy,** *87*
Kian Fan Chung, MD, DSC, FRCP

9 **Pharmacogenomics and Applications to Asthma Management,** *97*
Emily J. Pennington, MD, Michael E. Wechsler, MD, Victor E. Ortega, MD, PhD

10 **Environmental Assessment and Control,** *113*
Perdita Permaul, MD, Wanda Phipatanakul, MD, MS

11 **Phenotype and Genotype Determinants of Asthma Treatments,** *123*
Fernando Holguin, MD, MPH

12 **Predicting and Preventing Asthma Exacerbations,** *129*
Dr. Heather Hoch, MD, MSCS, Dr. Andrew H. Liu, MD

13 **School-Centered Asthma Programs,** *143*
Lisa Cicutto, RN, ACNP(cert), CAE, PhD

14 **Systems Biology Approaches to Asthma Management,** *151*
Yasmeen Nkrumah-Elie, PhD, Marc Elie, PhD, Nichole Reisdorph, PhD, MS

15 **The Microbiome in Asthma: Potential Impact on Phenotype and Medication Response,** *161*
Yvonne J. Huang, MD

16 **Preventing the Development of Asthma: Early Intervention Strategies in Children,** *171*
Jeffrey R. Stokes, MD, Leonard B. Bacharier, MD

17 Identifying and Preventing the Progression of Asthma to Chronic Obstructive Pulmonary Disease, *179*
Padmaja Subbarao, MD, MSc,
Malcolm R. Sears, MB

18 Imaging Procedures and Bronchial Thermoplasty for Asthma Assessment and Intervention, *191*
Shweta Sood, MD, MS, Chase Hall, MD,
Mario Castro, MD, MPH

19 Future Directions in Asthma Management, *207*
Stanley J. Szefler, MD, Fernando Holguin, MD,
Michael E. Wechsler, MD

INDEX, *211*

A Population Management Model of Asthma and Allergy: Case Finland

TARI HAAHTELA, MD • OLOF SELROOS, MD

INTRODUCTION

In Finland (with population 5.5 million), health promotion and prevention of disease has been the main focus of healthcare policies for decades. The comprehensive and integrated healthcare system has been employed in several public health campaigns, e.g., against cardiovascular diseases, diabetes, and obesity. The *Finnish Asthma Program 1994–2004* and *Allergy Program 2008–18* illustrate why public health problems need public health solutions.

FINNISH HEALTHCARE SYSTEM

In Finland, as in all Nordic countries, healthcare sector is mainly publicly funded and financed with general tax revenues.[1] The highest authority is the Ministry of Social Affairs and Health, but the municipalities (local governments) are responsible for providing healthcare to their residents. In addition to general practitioner (GP) services, preventive services have been established for pregnant women, mothers, and infants, as well as school healthcare and dental care for children and young people. Primary healthcare services are provided by about 250 health centers, including at least three times as many maternity and child health clinics and ~1000 units offering occupational health services; one-third of these units are private.

Finland has a well-developed hospital sector (secondary care) with highly advanced specialist treatment. The municipalities also own and operate almost all of the hospitals through cooperation with 21 hospital districts. Finland has five university hospitals (tertiary care) and medical faculties.

The primary care public services are either free for the patient or a small fee is charged. For all public hospital services patient pays a small fee.

Altogether, private sector is much smaller than the public one and complements the public care, especially in larger cities. There are a few private hospitals in the big cities. Patients who use private-sector services pay the cost to the provider, after which they can apply for reimbursement from the Finnish Social Insurance Institution (SII) under the Health Insurance Act. The reimbursement covers nowadays only c.20% of the cost. People can also take private health insurance, which is relatively popular among families with small children. Many pediatricians work in private sector. During the last 5-10 years private sector has enlarged its activities and has become more powerful also in Finland.

Salary or cash allowances are payable to employees during illness. Self-employed people can insure themselves against illness.

INCREASE IN PREVALENCE AND NEED FOR TREATMENT

In most countries the total costs of asthma treatment have gradually increased because of increased asthma prevalence and rapidly growing costs of newer drugs.[2] In Finland the prevalence of asthma in adults was ~6% in the 1990s[3,4] but has increased since then. In the Helsinki capital area, population-based surveys indicated a prevalence of physician-diagnosed asthma of 6.8% in 1996 and 9.4% in 2007.[4] In adults aged 25–64 years, the age-adjusted prevalence of physician-diagnosed asthma increased from 6.1% to 9.5% in men and from 7.8% to 10.8% in women from 1997 to 2012.[5]

In 1987, the Finnish SII listed 83,000 patients with physician-diagnosed asthma who were entitled to special reimbursement for drug costs. They are registered, if their doctor has made a certificate of the need for regular maintenance medication for persistent disease. Six years later, in 1993 the number was 135,000. Twenty-eight years later, in 2015, the figure has tripled to 256,000. During the same period, the population of Finland increased from 4.9 to 5.5 million (11%).

This increase reflected the slow increase in asthma prevalence in the population, but mainly it resulted from earlier and more effective detection and medical intervention (see below).

GETTING STARTED—ASTHMA PROGRAM STRATEGY
Paradigm Change

In the early 1990s asthma was recognized as an *inflammatory condition* with variable airflow limitation.[6,7] The new paradigm emphasized first-line antiinflammatory treatment,[8,9] which was without delay implemented to practice by the *Finnish Asthma Program 1994–2004*. This was a major step to cut disease burden for individual patients as well as for society by improving early diagnostics and medication.[10-12] The program has served a model for others.[13,14]

The Global Asthma Network performed an email survey in 2013–14 in 120 countries (response rate 93%) and reported that 26 countries (23%) had a national asthma strategy plan for children and 24 countries (21%) had for adults.[14] Twenty-two countries (19%) had a strategy for both children and adults. Having asthma strategy plans is apparently a significant first step, but so far little is known about the implementation and results of any strategies.

The Finnish asthma program focused on (1) early diagnosis, (2) active antiinflammatory treatment from the outset, (3) guided self-management, and (4) effective networking with the GPs and pharmacists. Five specific goals were set, for example, decreasing the number hospital days of patients by 50% and reducing annual costs per patient by 50% (Box 1.1). The program comprised both evidence-based management guidelines, which have been available to GPs and nurses via the Internet since 2000, and an action plan with defined tools to achieve the goals. The action plan focused on implementation of new knowledge, especially for primary care. At that time, in the early 1990s the new medical knowledge was: "Asthma is an inflammatory disease and should be treated as such from the very beginning." The key to implementation was an effective network of asthma-responsible professionals and development of an evaluation strategy.

The program was enlarged twice. In 1997 Finnish pharmacies were included in the *Pharmacy Program*, and in 2002 a *Childhood Asthma Mini-Program* was launched. The strategy is outlined in Fig. 1.1.

Early Detection, Timely Treatment

For the patients with asthma, the main improvement was early detection of the disease and its timely treatment: "Hit early and hit hard!" In terms of medication,

---

BOX 1.1
The Finnish Asthma Program 1994–2004: Goals and Main Outcomes in 10 years

1. Patients with early asthma recover
   - The number of children and adults with *new* special reimbursement for drug costs leveled off in 2001 and started even to decrease (need for regular maintenance medication).
2. Quality of life improves, lung function is normal, and working ability corresponds with age
   - Number of patients with severe complications decreased substantially. Disability pensions, allowances for days off work, and the need for rehabilitation decreased by 30–50%.
3. Percentage of patients with severe and moderate asthma is halved from 40% to 20%
   - 20% of patients had severe (uncontrolled) asthma in the early 1990s, 10% in 2001, and 4% in 2010
4. Number of hospital days decreases by 50%
   - Number of hospital days because of asthma fell by 56%, in relation to the number of asthmatics by 70%.
5. Annual costs per patient fall by 50% with early and effective treatment
   - Costs per patient decreased by 36% and related to the increase in gross national product by 50% (compensations for disability, drugs, hospital care, and outpatient doctor visits).

Adapted from Haahtela T, Tuomisto LE, Pietinalho A, et al. A 10 year asthma programme in Finland: major change for the better. *Thorax.* 2006;61:663–670; with permission.

---

the most remarkable change was the increase in the first-line use of inhaled corticosteroids during the early years of the asthma program (1994–99).

Patients with persistent type of asthma have been educated (informed and trained) to employ *guided self-management*, an approach that encourages them to start or increase medication proactively to prevent symptom increase, exacerbations, and asthma attacks. Effective networking of specialists with "local asthma champions," such as GPs (n = 200), asthma nurses (n = 700), and pharmacists (n = 700), has also considerably improved the overall asthma awareness and care in Finland.

Burden Decreased

As a result of the program, the burden of asthma in Finland started to decrease. In 10 years, disability pensions because of asthma almost collapsed by 76% from 1993

Background   **4-step action plan**

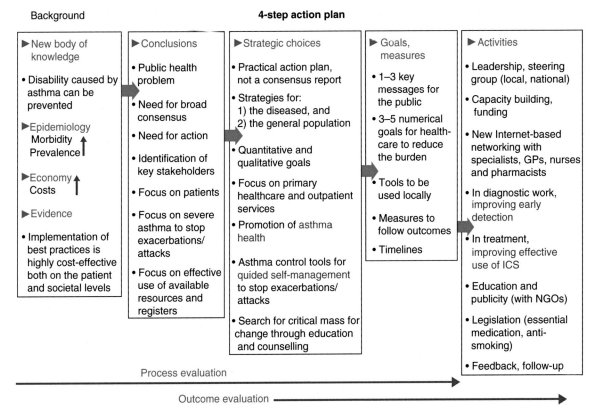

FIG. 1.1 Modified flow chart of the strategic planning, implementation and evaluation of the asthma program 1994–2004. *GP*, general practitioner; *ICS*, inhaled corticosteroid; *NGO*, nongovernmental organization. (From Selroos O, Kupczyk M, Kuna P, et al. National and regional asthma programmes in Europe. *Eur Respir Rev*. 2015;24:474–483; with permission.)

to 2003, and number of hospital days by 56% (70% in relation to the number of asthmatics).[11] This trend has continued, e.g., during the period from 2000 to 2013 the asthma hospital days dropped by 67% (Fig. 1.2).[15, 16] In 2013 around 2300 patients used around 10,000 hospital days with the average stay of 3.7 days. For further reduction, the focus should be more on the risk groups, especially on women over the age of 60 years.[17]

Asthma mortality has been very low: in 2006–13, on average seven annual deaths (range 3–12) under the age of 60 years, and no deaths under the age of 15 years.

Costs Are Down

From 1987 to 2013, the total costs decreased by 14%, from € 222 million to € 191 million (outpatient doctor visits, hospital care, medicines, sickness allowances, disability pensions).[12] During the 6-year period before the asthma program, from 1987 to 1993, the total asthma costs increased from € 222 to € 330 million. The program

was launched in 1994 and in a few years the costs started to level off and then decreased. This happened despite the steady increase (threefold in 1987–2013) in patients with persistent asthma included in the reimbursement register. Costs for primary care visits and medication increased, but overall annual costs per patient decreased by 72%, from € 2656 to € 749. The theoretical total cost savings only for 1 year (2013), comparing actual with predicted costs, were between € 120 and € 475 million, depending on the scenario used (Fig. 1.3).

During the same period, the overall healthcare cost index in Finland increased by 37.5% in real terms. For disease-specific comparison, the costs of breast cancer increased by 140% while the number of patients doubled. From 2000 to 2007, the direct healthcare costs for diabetes increased by 60%, and costs for disability increased by 50%. Against these general trends, total costs for asthma in Finland in 2013 were less than those in 1987.

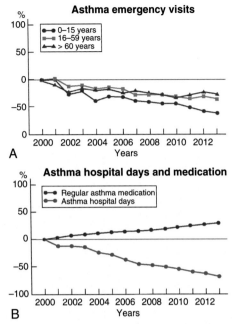

FIG. 1.2 Asthma emergency visits and hospital days in Finland in the 2000s. Numbers are percentage changes after 2000. **(A)** Decrease in asthma emergency visits by 46%, in children by 62%. **(B)** Increase in asthma patients on regular medication. Decrease in asthma hospital days by 67%. (Data from Haahtela T, Valovirta E, Hannuksela M, et al. Finnish nationwide allergy programme at mid-term – change of direction producing results (in Finnish, abstract in English). *The Finn Med J.* 2015;70:2165–2172.)

The extra costs of planning and implementing the program were small, primarily because most of the activities were carried out as part of the routine work of the clinicians and administrators.

The Finnish asthma program resulted in significant cost savings at both the societal and patient levels over the 26-year period. This has been in stark contrast to what was predicted in the early 1990s.

ASTHMA AND ALLERGY EPIDEMIC REMAINED

The main question remained, however, how to stop the "epidemic"? The asthma program reduced markedly the burden but did not have an effect on prevalence. Obviously, true reasons of allergy and asthma increase should be better understood to move from treatment to prevention. The Karelia allergy study, among others, gave some answers.[18] The contrast of prevalence was striking both among children and adults living in Finnish and more rural Russian Karelia. It seemed likely that reasons for allergy increase were not so much the new risk factors, characteristic to modern environment and lifestyle, but *loss of protective factors.*

Noncommunicable diseases, allergy among them, have been on increase everywhere in the urban environments. Human immune system seems to have an adaptation crisis not complying with the fast-changing lifestyle and living conditions. Effective gene-environment interaction is the key issue in tolerance development.[19] Reduced connection to natural environments and, e.g., increased use of processed food may have impoverished human microbiota (dysbiosis), caused immune dysfunction (poor tolerance), and led to inappropriate inflammatory responses. The manifested clinical disease is then largely dependent on individual genetic architecture.

Again, there was a place for a paradigm change. The *Finnish Allergy Programme 2008–18* was introduced to test new thinking in practice and regarded as step 2 to improve allergy health, including asthma.[20, 21]

ALLERGY PROGRAM STRATEGY

The key messages of the program are in Box 1.2. They targeted the general population, patients with allergies and asthma and their families, public-health and patient organizations, and experts and authorities. The more specific goals and indicators for healthcare professionals were quantitative, such as that allergy diets should drop by 50%, and asthma emergency visits should drop by 40% within 10 years. Each of the six goals had its specific tasks, tools, and evaluation methods.[20]

The relevance and acceptance of the messages were tested in 2008 in an email survey among 744 asthma contact persons.[15] The messages were well received. For example, GPs scored *strengthen tolerance* as 9.1 on a scale from 4 to 10; however, allergy management practice left much room for improvement, e.g., availability of *specific immunotherapy* was poor (score 5.4).

An expert nongovernmental organization (NGO), *the Finnish Lung Health Association (Filha)* was responsible for educating healthcare professionals (doctors, nurses, pharmacists, caregivers). The key issue was improving allergen tolerance and simple guidance was provided (Box 1.3). During the years 2008–16 more than 20,000 professionals have participated in the various learning activities.

Lay public has been targeted by three NGOs for (1) allergy and asthma, (2) respiratory health, and (3) skin disorders. Patient organizations arranged regional

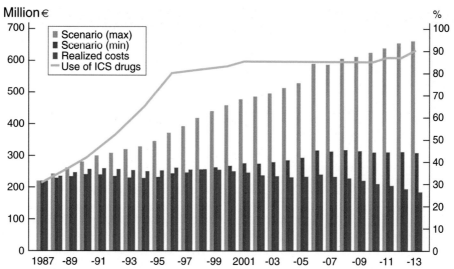

FIG. 1.3 Development of total asthma costs in Finland from 1987 to 2013. The actual (realized) annual expenditures of asthma care (*blue columns*) and the minimum (*red columns*) and maximum scenarios (*gray columns*) of theoretical annual costs. The minimum scenario represents a theoretical annual expenditure, if all of the threefold increase in prevalence was caused by patients with mild asthma. The maximum scenario assumes that the disease severity and standard of care remained at the 1987 level. The *green line* represents the percentage of patients on inhaled corticosteroid (ICS) medication (y-axis on the right). (From Haahtela T, Herse F, Karjalainen J, et al. The Finnish experience to save asthma costs by improving care in 1987–2013. *J Allergy Clin Immunol.* 2017;139:408–414; with permission.)

BOX 1.2
The Finnish Allergy Program 2008–18:
Messages for Both Healthcare Professionals
and Lay Public. Allergy Health is Promoted

Key messages
- Endorse health, not allergy.
- Strengthen tolerance.
- Adopt a new attitude to allergy; avoid allergens only if mandatory.
- Recognize and treat severe allergies early. Prevent exacerbations.
- Improve air quality. Stop smoking.

From Haahtela T, von Hertzen L, Mäkelä M, et al. Finnish Allergy Programme 2008-2018–time to act and change the course. *Allergy.* 2008;63:634–645; with permission.

education for their key personnel and peer workers; this had a major impact on direct patient counseling and distribution of educational material.

Education continued also for the personnel of pharmacies, day care centers, and schools. The Association of Finnish Pharmacies produced material for and ran campaigns concerning allergic rhinitis and atopic eczema during 2009–12. The Association of Kindergarten Teachers in Finland planned a pilot campaign called "Go to nature!" for 2014–15 in southern Karelia, incorporating various outdoor activities into the daycare routine. New guidelines for early childhood education will be introduced to the whole country.

Contact-Person Network

The educational action plan took advantage of the contact-person network created early during the asthma program 1994–2004. At baseline, in 2008, healthcare had about 1500 appointed asthma contact persons (doctors, nurses, pharmacists) originally recruited for the asthma program. This network was reactivated and strengthened for the allergy campaign. The network has been complemented by some 200 nurses in maternity and child health clinics and in schools. Fourteen regional expert allergy groups have begun to coordinate local implementation of new recommendations by educational activities.

Measuring Outcomes

For outcome evaluation, the Finnish healthcare registers provided invaluable data sources: especially, the hospital admission register of National Institute for

BOX 1.3
Practical Advice for Building and Improving Tolerance (Primary Prevention) as Well as Preventing Symptoms and Exacerbations (Secondary and Tertiary Prevention)

Primary prevention
- Support breastfeeding, with solid foods from 4 to 6 months
- No avoidance of environmental allergen exposure (foods, pets), if not proven necessary
- Strengthen immunity by increasing contact with natural environments (e.g., regular physical exercise, healthy diet such as a traditional Mediterranean or Baltic diet, local food)
- Antibiotics only for true need (the majority of microbes are useful and build a healthy immune function)
- Probiotic bacteria in fermented food or other preparations may strengthen the immune function
- No smoking (parental smoking increases the risk of asthma in children)

Secondary and tertiary prevention
- Regular physical exercise is antiinflammatory
- Healthy diets are antiinflammatory (traditional Mediterranean or Baltic diet may improve asthma control)
- Probiotic bacteria in fermented food or other preparations may be antiinflammatory
- Respiratory/skin inflammation treated early and effectively. Maintenance treatment titrated for long-term control
- Allergen-specific immunotherapy promoted for more severe symptoms
  - allergens as such (for foods)
  - sublingual tablets or drops (SLIT) (for pollens)
  - subcutaneous injections (for pollens, pets, mites, insect stings)
- Smoking strictly avoided (asthma and allergy drugs do not have full effect in smokers)

From Haahtela T, Valovirta E, Bousquet J, Mäkelä M, and the Allergy Programme Steering Group. The Finnish Allergy Programme 2008–2018 works. *Eur Respir J*. 2017;49:1–6.

BOX 1.4
The Finnish Allergy Program 2008–18. Six Goals, Indicators, and Main Outcomes at 5 years. The Program Is Still Ongoing

1. Prevent allergy
   - *Indicator*: asthma, rhinitis, and atopic eczema prevalence reduced by 20%.
   - No information yet
2. Improve tolerance
   - *Indicator*: food allergy diets reduced by 50%.
   - Allergy diets in day care—40%
3. Improve allergy diagnostics
   - *Indicator*: patients were skin prick tested in certified testing centers.
   - 30 hospitals and other centers educated, audited, and certified
4. Reduce work-related allergies
   - *Indicator*: occupational allergies reduced by 50%.
   - Occupational allergies—40%
5. Focus on severe allergies and treat in time
   - *Indicator*: good allergy practice works, asthma emergency visits reduced by 40%.
   - Emergency visits—46%, asthma hospital days—67%
6. Reduce allergy and asthma costs
   - *Indicator*: allergy costs reduced by 20%.
   - In the 2000s, total costs—15%, in 2007–13—5%

From Haahtela T, Valovirta E, Hannuksela M, et al. Finnish nationwide allergy programme at mid-term – change of direction producing results (in Finnish, abstract in English). *The Finn Med J*. 2015;70:2165–2172; and Haahtela T, Valovirta E, Bousquet J, Mäkelä M, and the Allergy Programme Steering Group. The Finnish Allergy Programme 2008–2018 works. *Eur Repir J*. 2017, in press; with permission.

Health and Welfare and the drug reimbursement register of the SII. For occupational diseases, Finland has strict legislation, and verified cases are registered by the National Institute of Occupational Health.

The Finnish anaphylaxis register was established in 2000 at the Skin and Allergy Hospital of the Helsinki University Central Hospital.[22] Physicians (mostly allergists) from the whole country voluntarily report cases of severe allergic reactions independent of causative agent. A one-page questionnaire for medical professionals is available on the Internet.

Allergy and asthma costs in 2013 were analyzed from all data sources in collaboration with government officials.

ARE WE ON THE RIGHT TRACK?

The midterm outcome is summarized in Box 1.4. The burden of allergy and asthma has been further reduced since the beginning of the asthma programme.[15,16] In the 2000s, asthma emergency visits decreased by 46% (children 62%) and hospital days decreased by 67%.

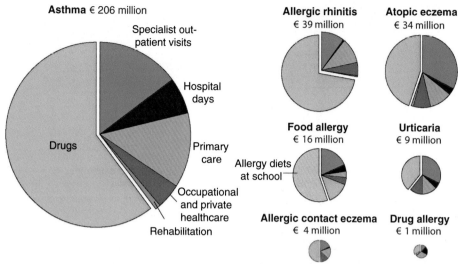

FIG. 1.4 Distribution of direct healthcare costs by main allergic conditions in Finland 2011. Total direct costs were € 319 million. Costs of immunotherapy preparations and unspecified allergic reactions (€ 6 million) are excluded from the figure. Asthma costs were 63% of all costs. (Data from Jantunen J, Kauppi P, Linna M, et al. Asthma and allergy costs in Finland are high but decreasing (in Finnish, abstract in English). *The Finn Med J.* 2014;69:641–646.)

According to a countrywide pharmacy barometer survey, self-reported asthma has become a milder disease or a better controlled disease. At the start of the Finnish asthma program in 1994, it was estimated that 20% of the patients had a severe (or uncontrolled) condition. This figure decreased to 10% in 2001 and to 4% in 2010.[23] The survey has been repeated in 2016, and the percentage of severe condition has again halved to 2.5% (Juha Jantunen, personal communication). In comparison with the 2001 and 2010 cohorts, emergency visits during the previous year had dropped by 86% and hospitalizations by 88%.

In the Helsinki capital region, 40 Finnish day care centers were educated to follow simple pragmatic allergy guidelines.[24] In 2013–15, the prevalence of allergy diets decreased by 43%, from 7.6% to 4.3%. Parent-reported allergies to nuts, fruits, and vegetables decreased among first graders in the first year of elementary schools.[25]

In 2007–13, verified occupational allergies (asthma, allergic rhinitis, allergic contact dermatitis) fell by 40%, registered by the National Institute of Occupational Health. The reduction was not explained by changes in the workforce.

In the first decade of the 2000s, the direct allergy and asthma costs, together with costs for disability pensions, fell by15%.[15,16] Asthma costs decreased by 9%. Distribution of direct healthcare costs by main allergic conditions in Finland 2011 is shown in Fig. 1.4. Asthma comprised 63% of all costs, and drugs were the main cost driver.[26]

LESSONS LEARNED

There are lot of reasons why something cannot be done, and most of them are excuses. Healthcare professionals do not easily change their thinking or the way they practice. They need solid arguments. They have to feel that they are doing something useful for their patients, for themselves, and hopefully for public health. The two keywords are motivate and organize (Fig. 1.5) (Box 1.5).

Some Tips

You can start an asthma program, effort, or plan, whatever you want to call it, in your hospital district, county, province, state or even in an entire country as we did in Finland. Contact your Health Minister or some other high official, and involve patient organizations from the very beginning.

- An asthma program is a marked educational effort. You need some organization that helps in implementing the education and backs you up. We had Filha (expert NGO, Finnish Lung Health Association, former association against tuberculosis).
- Create a small steering group of 7–10 people. Everyone must have a clear motivation and be aware of his/her role and why they participate. They must be active people having an effect on what happens in the grassroot level. With this group you start to create a network of interested people. Keep the organization as simple and flat as possible. You are easily suffocated by the bureaucracy.

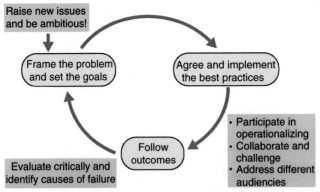

FIG. 1.5 The circle of improvement. (Modified from Mickwitz P. A framework for evaluating environmental policy instruments: context and key concepts. Evaluation 2003;9:415-436.)

BOX 1.5
Arguments for Initiating or not Asthma Program/Plan

ARGUMENTS FOR DOING NOTHING
Lack of
- Money
- Personnel
- Facilities
- Time

NEW
Start-up
- Innovate and bring in new knowledge
- Motivate and make the people enthusiastic!

Remember
- Much of the know-how already exists, but is unemployed
- Resources are there, but not organized for common goals
- Involve main interest groups, especially patient NGOs
- If you know some high authority, bring him/her in to get started

---

- Define a few goals (1–5) with quantitative, numerical indicators (what should be achieved). Define for each goal more specific tasks (what to do), tools (how to do it), and what to measure (outcomes). Find out what already existing registries you can use for follow-up. Make the whole plan as simple as possible[27] (Fig. 1.6).
- In 1 year you do not achieve much, in 5 years a lot, and in 10 years everything changes! Create a follow-up of some cost changes: money talks! Some investment is needed for the educational process, but you start to see the savings already in 2 years. If you find a control area/district, where the actions are not taking place, it helps to convince others.
- You need to spread out the new information. It would be most useful to have a professional media person for that (social media as well).
- In medical practice, focus on more severe forms of asthma, which really cause disability. There you get the best value for money. This also changes the cost-effectiveness of the whole management.
- Start with something familiar and make the first improvements there. Make new simple guidelines and get the process going.
- Create simple *guided self-management* instructions to stop symptom worsening, exacerbations, and attacks. Follow asthma emergency unit visits. You see a drop in a year!
- Collaborate with experts from other fields. Consider mobile applications (eHealth, mHealth), and at least www.pages (in Finland for nine allergic conditions now) to spread out your gospel.
- In allergy, there is no law of escalation, i.e., symptoms would become more severe, if not heavily intervened, treated, and guided. It is often the other way around, especially in childhood, most symptoms disappear or become milder. Mild hypersensitivity reactions can be regarded as part of the normal developmental and immune adaptation process. They are not necessarily DISEASES! Try not to medicalize.
- In Finland, we turned the ideology of allergy prevention around: from avoidance strategy to tolerance strategy, both in terms of immunology and psychology.

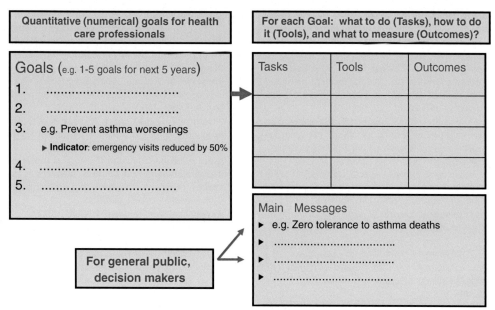

FIG. 1.6 Generic template for a public health program. (From Haahtela T. Evidence for asthma control – zero tolerance to asthma with the Finnish programmes. In: Akdis C, Agache I. eds. *Global Atlas of Asthma*. EAACI; 2013: 135–137; with permission.)

CONCLUSIONS

Finland is the only country, where nationwide, comprehensive public health programs for asthma and allergic disorders have been implemented and results reported. The experience speaks for itself: a systematic and integrated approach with set goals and long-term follow-up has reduced suffering and saved costs. The burden is declining. The campaigns have been based on research and scientific innovations, which have been turned to practical actions. This has been possible in a country where educational level of citizens is relatively high and healthcare is efficiently organized and mainly funded by public money. Integration of the work of primary and secondary care physicians and nurses, pharmacists, and caregivers has been the key for better flow of information, education, and patient care throughout the healthcare system.

There are a lot of asthma patients in Finland and the prevalence is still close to 10%. This population continues to have many problems such as compromised quality of life, underuse and overuse of medication, side effects of drugs, and the need for long-term healthcare. The conventional medication controls the disease in 98% of the asthmatics, if used effectively. The need for new biologic drugs is very small. Nevertheless, individual asthmatics are different, in genotypes and phenotypes, and a good clinician always tailor-makes the treatment details.

In allergy, focusing on the more severe forms of disease and emphasizing health rather than mild problems has encouraged a more efficient use of healthcare resources.

The outcome of the present real-life interventions, including all Finnish citizens without effective controls, is also open for critics. This should not, however, prevent medical communities from taking reasonable action to improve public health, in this case lessening the disability and costs caused by asthma and allergy. Inadequate care of these conditions seems to be a global problem and leads to delays in patient management and poor outcomes.[28]

Revisiting the asthma and allergy paradigms has led to actions relevant to society and healthcare as a whole.

REFERENCES

1. Saltman RB, Teperi J. Health statistics for the nordic countries. *Nord Medico-Statistical Comm.* 2016;104:1–242.
2. Bedouch P, Marra CA, FitzGerald JM, Lynd LD. Trends in asthma-related direct medical costs from 2002 to 2007 in British Columbia, Canada: a population based-cohort study. *PLoS One.* 2012;7:e50949.

3. Pallasaho P, Lundbäck B, Meren M, et al. Prevalence and risk factors for asthma and chronic bronchitis in the capitals Helsinki, Stockholm, and Tallinn. *Respir Med.* 2002;96:759–769.

4. Pallasaho P, Juusela M, Lindqvist A, et al. Allergic rhinoconjunctivitis doubles the risk for incident asthma—results from a population study in Helsinki, Finland. *Respir Med.* 2011;105:1449–1456.

5. Jousilahti P, Haahtela T, Laatikainen T, Mäkelä M, Vartiainen E. Asthma and respiratory allergy prevalence is still increasing among Finnish young adults. *Eur Respir J.* 2015;47:985–987.

6. Laitinen LA, Heino M, Laitinen A, et al. Damage of the airway epithelium and bronchial reactivity in patients with asthma. *Am Rev Respir Dis.* 1985;131:599–606.

7. Bousquet J, Chanez P, Lacoste JY, et al. Eosinophilic inflammation in asthma. *N Engl J Med.* 1990;323:1033–1039.

8. Haahtela T, Järvinen M, Kava T, et al. Comparison of a β_2-agonist, terbutaline, with an inhaled corticosteroid, budesonide, in newly detected asthma. *N Engl J Med.* 1991;325:388–392.

9. Haahtela T, Järvinen M, Kava T, et al. Effects of reducing or discontinuating inhaled budesonide in patients with mild asthma. *N Engl J Med.* 1994;331:700–705.

10. Haahtela T, Klaukka T, Koskela K, et al. Asthma programme in Finland: a community problem needs community solutions. *Thorax.* 2001;56:806–814.

11. Haahtela T, Tuomisto LE, Pietinalho A, et al. A 10 year asthma programme in Finland: major change for the better. *Thorax.* 2006;61:663–670.

12. Haahtela T, Herse F, Karjalainen J, et al. The Finnish experience to save asthma costs by improving care in 1987-2013. *J Allergy Clin Immunol.* 2017;139:408–414.

13. Selroos O, Kupczyk M, Kuna P, et al. National and regional asthma programmes in Europe. *Eur Respir Rev.* 2015;24:474–483.

14. Asher I, Haahtela T, Selroos O, et al. Global Asthma Network Study Group. Global Asthma Network survey suggests more national asthma strategies could reduce burden of asthma. *Allergol Immunopathol (Madr).* 2017;45:105–114. http://dx.doi.org/10.1016/j.aller.2016.10.013.

15. Haahtela T, Valovirta E, Hannuksela M, et al. Finnish nationwide allergy programme at mid-term – change of direction producing results (in Finnish, abstract in English). *Finn Med J.* 2015;70:2165–2172.

16. Haahtela T, Valovirta E, Bousquet J, Mäkelä M. The allergy programme steering group. The Finnish allergy programme 2008-2018 works. *Eur Respir J.* 2017;49:1700470. https://doi.org/10.1183/13993003.00470-2017.

17. Kauppi P, Linna M, Martikainen J, et al. Follow-up of the Finnish Asthma Programme 2000-2010: reduction of hospital burden needs risk group rethinking. *Thorax.* 2013;68:292–293.

18. Haahtela T, Laatikainen T, Alenius H, et al. Hunt for the origin of allergy – comparing the Finnish and Russian Karelia. *Clin Exp Allergy.* 2015;45:891–901.

19. Garn H, Bahn S, Baune BT, et al. Current concepts in chronic inflammatory diseases: interactions between microbes, cellular metabolism, and inflammation. *J Allergy Clin Immunol.* 2016;138:47–56.

20. Haahtela T, von Hertzen L, Mäkelä M, et al. Finnish Allergy Programme 2008-2018–time to act and change the course. *Allergy.* 2008;63:634–645.

21. von Hertzen LC, Savolainen J, Hannuksela M, et al. Scientific rationale for the Finnish Allergy Programme 2008-2018: emphasis on prevention and endorsing tolerance. *Allergy.* 2009;64:678–701.

22. Mäkinen-Kiljunen S, Haahtela T. Eight years of severe allergic reactions in Finland. A register-based report. *WAO J* 2008;1:184–189.

23. Kauppi P, Peura S, Salimäki J, et al. Reduced severity and improved control of self-reported asthma in Finland during 2001-2010. *Asia Pac Allergy.* 2015;5:32–39.

24. Erkkola M, Saloheimo T, Hauta-Alus H, et al. LILLA study group. Burden of allergy diets in Finnish day care reduced by change in practices. *Allergy.* 2016;71:1453–1460.

25. Järvenpää J, Paassilta M, Salmivesi S, et al. Stability of parent reported food allergy in six and 7-year-old children: the first 5 years of the Finnish allergy programme. *Acta Paediatr.* 2014;103:1297–1300.

26. Jantunen J, Kauppi P, Linna M, et al. Asthma and allergy costs in Finland are high but decreasing (in Finnish, abstract in English). *Finn Med J.* 2014;69:641–646.

27. Haahtela T. Evidence for asthma control – zero tolerance to asthma with the Finnish programmes. In: Akdis C, Agache I, eds. *Global Atlas of Asthma.* EAACI; 2013:135–137.

28. Diwakar L, Cummins C, Lilford R, Roberts T. Systematic review of pathways for the delivery of allergy services. *BMJ Open.* 2017;7:e012647. http://dx.doi.org/10.1136/bmjopen-2016-012647.

CHAPTER 2

Population Health Management: A Systematic Approach to Asthma Care in a Pediatric Network of Care

MONICA J. FEDERICO, MD • KATHERINE JOHNSTON, MPH

INTRODUCTION

Population health and population management are not interchangeable terms. Population health programs are aimed at improving the overall health outcomes of a group and may not include coordinated healthcare delivery services or alternative payment models for that care. Population management is "the design, delivery, coordination, and payment of high-quality healthcare services to manage the Triple Aim for a population using the best resources we have available to us within the healthcare system."[1] The Triple Aim refers to improving health by delivering excellent care and decreasing the overall cost of care. A pediatric "network of care" includes the community in the creation of integrated care teams for the patients and families and therefore crosses the lines between population health and population management. The care network may also work with institutions and payers to create alternative methods of payment that may lead to decreased costs.

A healthcare system that aims to improve health and creates a system that integrates community-based caregivers into the redesign of healthcare delivery and the goals of the system is the next era or the "3.0 era of healthcare" per Neil Halfon.[2] A 3.0 Network of Asthma Care (NOAC) creates a safety net for children and families that includes schools and other community-based caregivers such as teachers, coaches, and childcare providers. This work includes initiatives such as education for hospital and community-based medical providers, improved communication between medical providers and community-based providers, education for schools and other caregivers, and building support for children with asthma into the community in which they live (see Fig. 2.1).

The *Finnish Asthma Programme* seen in the chapter by Drs. Tari Haahtela and Olof Selroos is a model that all asthma programs should emulate and learn from.

In the Unites States, the systems of care developed for patients with asthma often vary by the healthcare system, the payer mix and payment structure in the region (fee for service vs. value-based payment), the demographics of the population, the resources available to the system, and other factors. Asthma programs are often the first population-level programs implemented by centers of pediatric care because asthma is the most common chronic disease of childhood and it is the most common chronic reason for expensive inpatient admissions and emergency department (ED) visits for many institutions. Asthma data are also more readily available than data for other complicated chronic diseases of childhood. Finally, community organizations are motivated to address asthma because of the incredible impact asthma has on quality of life. For example, schools focus on asthma because of the impact on school attendance, with over 14 million missed school days per year.[3] This chapter will outline a process for the creation of a NOAC in a country that does not have a national, single-payer health system. Successful NOAC programs in the United States are listed in Table 2.1. Of note, the California Community Asthma Intervention is no longer active due to funding.

MANAGING A POPULATION OF CHILDREN WITH ASTHMA

Define the Priorities and Abilities of the Network of Care Leaders

The first step in establishing a NOAC is understanding the priorities of the organization that will be at the center of the network. There may be an existing asthma strategy plan, as seen in Finland and some states in the United States. Individual health systems that want to establish a NOAC will need to understand what plans and programs are in place. The system will also need to go to

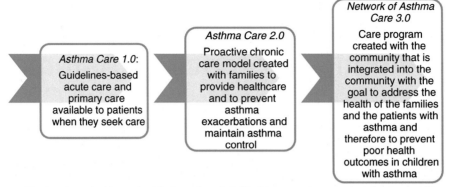

FIG. 2.1 Moving toward a Network of Asthma Care 3.0. Healthcare systems and goals of care will need to evolve into proactive systems that not only prevent disease but also work with communities and families and patients to improve health.

TABLE 2.1
Network of Asthma Care Examples in the United States

Program	Healthcare System/Location	Population	Interventions
Children's Hospital Colorado Asthma Program	Children's Hospital Colorado	Children aged 2 years and older with asthma	1. Clinical care 2. High-risk asthma program 3. Community-based clinics asthma initiative 4. Reach the Peak asthma educator certification course 5. Step Up asthma school program 6. Just Keep Breathing asthma home visit program 7. Community partnerships
King County Asthma Program[4] http://www.kingcounty.gov/depts/health/chronic-diseases/asthma.aspx	Department of Public Health—Seattle and King County	Low-income children and adults with asthma	1. Education for providers, community-based caregivers, and families 2. Asthma home visits 3. Collaboration with health plans
Community Asthma Initiative http://www.childrenshospital.org/centers-and-services/programs/a-_-e/community-asthma-initiative-program/overview	Boston Children's Hospital	Children aged 2–18 years seen in the ED for asthma	1. Clinical care 2. Severe asthma program 2. Asthma home visits 3. Community partnerships
Cincinnati Children's Asthma Center https://www.cincinnatichildrens.org/service/a/asthma	Cincinnati Children's Hospital	Children with asthma	1. Clinical care 2. Severe asthma program 3. Asthma home visits 4. Pharmacy partnership 5. Asthma-free schools 6. Community partnerships
California Community Asthma Intervention[5] https://www.cdph.ca.gov/programs/caphi/Pages/ChildhoodAsthmaInitiative.aspx	Community Health Centers' project performed by University of California San Francisco, California Department of Public Health	Children aged 0–18 years with persistent asthma	1. Provider and clinic staff education and quality improvement 2. Asthma care coordinator for patient navigation and home visits as needed

ED, emergency department.

the community to understand their priorities and current plans or programs that already in place and working work with community organizations to improve the health of children with asthma and their families. Before launching a community integrated NOAC, health systems also need to work within their own clinics and programs to be sure that they are delivering standardized, high-quality, evidence-based care. Studies demonstrate that patient outcomes improve if clinics standardize care with guidelines and education of providers and staff.[6] Further work shows improved outcomes in clinics that take the next step and create a registry of asthma patients, implement recall for higher-risk patients, and follow outcomes.[7] Programs that reach outside of the clinic and integrate or create community-based programming are, for the purpose of this chapter, a NOAC.

Define the Geographic Region of Care

The second step in establishing a NOAC for children with asthma is to identify the region of care. The approach to population-based care requires a thorough understanding of the community in which the patients live, because the community has a significant impact on the healthcare needs of pediatric patients and their families. Children who are poor or who live in communities where stress and violence are more prevalent have worse asthma outcomes and, possibly, more severe disease.[8] Black and Puerto Rican children have increased morbidity and mortality from asthma.[9] Literature also demonstrates that children living in rural settings have decreased access to primary, specialty, and even emergency care in the United States and several countries across the world.

The region of care definition Should be determined by the healthcare system's resources for providing care and supporting or integrating programs into their patients' care. For example, a small, community-based practice may only be able to support a program for children from the local school, while a large academic center may have school-based health clinics, school programs, and a home visit program in several counties. An initial health assessment using data from the local hospital or publicly available data such as census tract data or hospital association discharge data can help identify the gaps in asthma care. In the United States, key payers may also have data. These data can provide a general understanding of the size of the asthma population and the current state of asthma using health outcomes such as healthcare utilization as a marker.

Identify Key Stakeholders and Assess the Needs

The third step is to identify key stakeholders in the care of children with asthma. The evaluation of the region of care will not be complete until the community-based and health system–based stakeholders in asthma, public health and the environment, and pediatric care are involved. Each stakeholder's input will help identify the priorities for asthma care in the NOAC. Community members will help put asthma in context for the providers who may or may not live in that region. They will also be able to identify gaps in asthma care and competing priorities for asthma care programming. Community members will also be able to identify existing programs that could serve as partners in establishing the NOAC. Pediatric care programs should include schools at this stage, because school age children spend most of their time in school and are often more active in school than at home. Therefore, the school may be uniquely positioned to identify poor asthma control and gaps in care. Input from health system providers and staff is also necessary to identify the goals and metrics for asthma care. Providers and staff may be able to identify the gaps in care that they see or hear from patients and families. The overall priorities of the health system will help define the "bandwidth" of the system to support and participate in community-based programs and help program leaders prioritize the needs identified. Family-centered assessment of social determinants of health such as housing, financial, or psychosocial stress will help identify the needs of the population of current patients served by the program and should guide community partnerships.[10]

Identify the Target Population

Key stakeholder interviews and information gathered from the needs assessment will help the NOAC leaders begin to narrow the focus onto a specific population of children with asthma. The host and leaders of the NOAC will need to further define the population to those patients to whom they have access or on whom they feel they may have the greatest impact. Finances may limit the number of children who are eligible. Some funders or healthcare systems may require that the program decreases costs.[11] Programs that have shown significant return on investment focus on patients who are at high risk for future health care utilization such as emergency department or hospital admission. Children at the highest risk for severe exacerbations and incurring significant costs due to healthcare utilization are those who have been seen in the ED or hospital before.[12]

Set Priorities

Using the data collected in the needs assessment and input from key stakeholders, program leaders must decide on one or more interventions to implement.

These are most often evidence-based programs shown to be effective in similar settings or with a similar population. It is important to note that these programs may need significant adaptation or even an entirely innovative approach to be successful in a different setting. Once the NOAC program leaders and key stakeholders have a plan in place, the next step in setting priorities is establishing which programs can be accomplished with no funding, which will need funding and should be prioritized, and which will need long-term investment. With each program development, a plan for sustaining the program or integrating the work with other, funded programs is essential to program implementation. Each program will need a clear problem statement and plan and each implementation cycle of a program will require a Specific, Measurable, Attainable and agreed upon, Realistic, and Time-limited goal (SMART). Each cycle will also require baseline data to inform Plan, Do, Study, Act cycles.

Build a Team and a Steering Committee

The team members of the NOAC will depend on the scope of the project. Clinical expertise and front-line caregivers are key to the success of the team. However, the backbone of the team is often the program manager, the patient support team (educators, navigators, community health workers), and the analysis team. The make up of the patient support team staff may vary by initiative and by location in the United States or around the world. The choice of staff varies by the scope of the program, the community the program is serving, and the sustainability model for the program. For example, clinic-based programs may require patient navigators to help patients get to appointments and navigate schools and pharmacies. School programs, such as the Step Up asthma program[13] and those described in Cicutto's chapter of this text,[14] School-centered asthma programs, have been successful with educators who may also help the families communicate with their clinical providers. Home visit programs have been successful with community health workers and nurses. Program sustainability will vary by the funding mechanisms available. A NOAC in a closed or capitated system must rely on decreased overall cost of care through decreased utilization to fund community health workers. In other areas of the United States, incentive payments for high-quality care and decreased cost may support the program.

A steering committee made up of key stakeholders in the community, family members of patients, and other experts in program development will help with program development. and evaluation while also providing the perspective of program participants. The steering committee should be aware of the current NOAC activities and outcomes. The steering committee should also be consulted before there are significant changes made or as expansion is considered.

Collect Baseline Health Data

Data that characterize patients, the process of asthma care, and the outcomes of care are necessary to develop program goals and the impact of the program over time. Baseline data is essential to data review over time. Iterative review of data evaluating the processes and health outcomes of the NOAC team and programs will inform quality improvement evaluations over time.

Some baseline data collection will occur during the needs assessment, but other data needs will likely be identified as projects are prioritized. Baseline patient data not only characterize the patient population but may also allow for risk stratification of patients. Risk stratification of patients can be used to direct resources to patients at high risk for poor health outcomes and poor asthma control.

Understanding the spectrum of asthma severity can also help guide and prioritize asthma programming at a community level. For example, school-based asthma outreach programs may choose to target communities with a high concentration of patients with barriers to attending specialty care clinics. Baseline asthma care process data can be used to direct asthma education for clinical providers and staff and should be linked to outcome data such as healthcare utilization (ED visits and hospitalizations) across the population.

Data collection for baseline data will also help the program leaders and key stakeholders understand what data are readily available. For example, administrative data such as claims data are often available through healthcare system data and office management systems. Primary care and health system collaboration can also help estimate the size of a population the NOAC will be caring for using coded visits and claims. Claims data in a closed system can also be used to evaluate process of care through pharmacy billing charges. Administrative data are most useful when the providers, coders, and practice managers agree on the definition of asthma and which codes should be used. Patients seen and coded as "wheeze" or "reactive airway disease" may not be included in the population. Table 2.2 provides a list of key data elements for establishing an asthma program.

The most difficult aspect of asthma care to characterize using data is process of care data. Process data

TABLE 2.2
Key Metrics for Asthma Care

Measure	Definition
Patient Panel size	• The number of patients with asthma included in the program
Population demographics (*note: some demographic markers such as income level are hard to obtain without patient interview. Insurance is often used as a proxy of income and of poverty*)	• Age, sex, race, ethnicity, parental primary language, income level, insurance, address/zip code
Asthma care data	• Asthma severity • Asthma control (ideally measured objectively using a survey tool) • Treatment step or asthma medications • Pulmonary function testing • Asthma education (asthma action plan creation can be a surrogate marker) • Number of visits or contacts in 12 months • Medication adherence (*patient report [less reliable] and pharmacy refill data are common methods of collecting adherence data if claims data are not available*)
Asthma outcome data	• Days missed from school and work • Symptom-free days • Oral steroid use over 12 months • Emergency department visits in 12 months • Hospitalizations in 12 months
Cost of asthma care	• Hospital utilization and outpatient visits • Program costs • Medications • Days missed from work/school

such as how the asthma diagnosis is made by providers, asthma severity, and asthma control are not documented in a consistent way across providers, practices, and often, within health systems. Process data documented as discrete data (data that are always collected from the same place and have a defined unit, such as heart rate) can be collected from an electronic health record (EHR) if the EHR is set up to gather the data in a standard way. For example, asthma severity can be captured as a flowsheet row in many EHRs if the flowsheet is set up and providers and staff can work its use into their workflow. Medication lists can also be discrete data if they are regularly updated. Unfortunately, if a system, clinic, or school has never collected or followed data, it is possible that data are being entered in variable ways into several fields. Therefore, baseline data collection will help the NOAC program understand what data are readily available and what data collection will require new provider or staff workflows.

Team Education

All members of the team should understand the mission and goals of the NOAC. The overall goal of extending the care of asthma beyond the clinic visit is to improve health. Improving health requires understanding the disease, working with providers, and adhering to the treatment plan. Therefore, education about asthma, appropriate for the learner, and a standard approach to asthma care and patient education are essential to every member of the NOAC, from the program leaders providers, nurses, staff, and to community-based caregivers. Training in motivational interviewing and a standardized approach to adherence will also help align the work on the NOAC. An understanding of chronic disease management[15] and quality improvement will facilitate the implementation of change over time and will help the NOAC team members respond to data about the process and health outcomes of the program.

IMPLEMENTATION EXAMPLE: CHILDREN'S HOSPITAL COLORADO

In Denver, the Children's Hospital Colorado Asthma Program was first organized to identify, treat, and improve outcomes for children with asthma at the highest risk for severe exacerbations (Fig. 2.2). Children with frequent, severe exacerbations are poorly

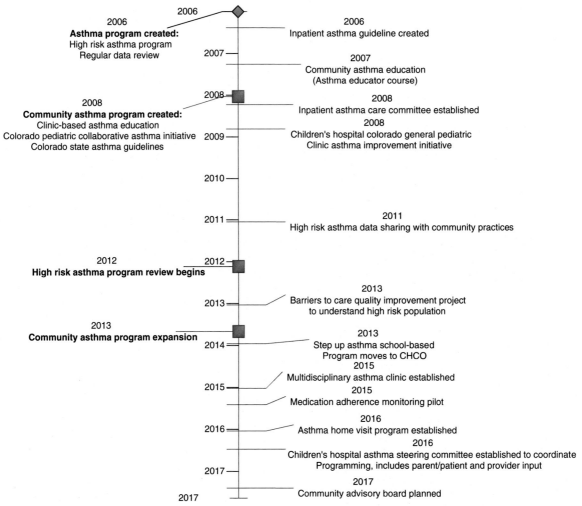

2006

2006
Asthma program created:
High risk asthma program
Regular data review

2006
Inpatient asthma guideline created

2007

2007
Community asthma education
(Asthma educator course)

2008

2008
Community asthma program created:
Clinic-based asthma education
Colorado pediatric collaborative asthma initiative
Colorado state asthma guidelines

2008
Inpatient asthma care committee established
2008
Children's hospital colorado general pediatric
Clinic asthma improvement initiative

2009

2010

2011

2011
High risk asthma data sharing with community practices

2012
High risk asthma program review begins

2012

2013
Barriers to care quality improvement project
to understand high risk population

2013

2013
Community asthma program expansion

2014

2013
Step up asthma school-based
Program moves to CHCO
2015
Multidisciplinary asthma clinic established
2015
Medication adherence monitoring pilot

2015

2016

2016
Asthma home visit program established
2016
Children's hospital asthma steering committee established to coordinate
Programming, includes parent/patient and provider input

2017

2017
Community advisory board planned

2017

FIG. 2.2 Timeline of the creation of the Children's Hospital Colorado Network (CHCO) of Asthma Care.

controlled, are at high risk for future exacerbations, incur high healthcare costs, and may have baseline severe asthma that requires an alternative approach to asthma care. Most children with asthma do not have high risk or severe asthma and are at low risk for medication side effects. These patients usually seek care in their primary medical home with their primary care provider.

Baseline data at Children's Hospital Colorado (CHCO) in 2006 indicated that more than half of the children seen in the ED or hospital were coming back to the ED or hospital in the following 12 months. Hospital-based providers and community-based providers identified gaps in care for those high-risk patients in the initial needs assessment, including identification

of patients and the need for a standard approach to asthma care. There were 300 outpatient specialty visits per year for asthma and an inpatient asthma pathway had recently been implemented.

The first 6 years were dedicated to creating the infrastructure needed to support the program, including regular data reporting, community partnerships, and statewide guidelines for asthma care. By 2012, there were over 3000 outpatient asthma specialty visits per year in the asthma program and over 75 education sessions had been completed for community-based providers and staff at their clinics. An asthma educator certification course was also established for nurses, respiratory therapists, community-based medical office staff, school-based nurses, and other asthma caregivers. Several regional asthma educational sessions were completed for medical providers.

In 2012, program staff began a 2-year community needs assessment and a quality improvement project, both aimed at better understanding the high-risk population and the barriers to receiving clinic-based care these patients and families faced. The results confirmed what previous data indicated: the high-risk population seen at CHCO is 76% Medicaid, 52% Latino, and 24% Spanish speaking; the African-American population is low, reflecting the demographics of Denver. Barrier questions highlighted the impact of chaotic situations often encountered by low-income families, including the caregivers' inability to miss additional work after a child's hospitalization. In 2014, these results, statewide asthma data, CHCO data, and key stakeholder input all informed the creation of a CHCO Asthma Strategic Plan. This plan led to rapid expansion of asthma clinical and translational research to inform clinical programming, focused expansion of CHCO's asthma program into the community, and an expansion and coordination of services for the highest-risk patients. Expanded programming includes the following:

1. A multidisciplinary asthma clinic was established and modeled after several existing programs, including Cincinnati Children's Hospital. Children who have been seen in intensive care, hospitalized more than twice in 12 months, or who are poorly controlled on high-dose asthma medications are seen in the clinic by allergy, pulmonary, social work, and, as needed, speech therapy and nutrition

2. An established school-based asthma education and case management program, Step Up, moved to CHCO in 2014. Based on previous experience, the CHCO high-risk program evaluation, and the CHCO Asthma Strategic Plan, the Step Up program obtained funding for expansion. The SMART goal of this program was to expand to include other counties with high concentrations of high-risk asthma patients, including a train the trainer program for school nurses, within 2 years.

3. An evening clinic targeting high-risk patients was established to facilitate asthma management in families who are unable to miss school or work to attend appointments during normal clinic hours.

4. A clinical trials program was established to advance principles of clinical research and translation to clinical care. Examples include a trial of adherence monitoring technology and evaluation of new medications and treatment strategies.

5. A new home visit program, Just Keep Breathing, was created with a goal to extend high-risk care into the home. The SMART goal of that program was to create a community health worker program in 1 year and to enroll 50 families and complete at least one visit over 2 years.

6. A CHCO asthma steering committee was established to standardize data definitions, coordinate current programming, and work with parents and providers to evaluate and expand future work.

7. A CHCO community asthma board will meet by the end of 2017 to evaluate ongoing programming and guide our expansion.

Fig. 2.2 shows the evolution of the CHCO asthma program from a hospital-based asthma program to a NOAC.

KEYS TO SUCCESS
Summary

As healthcare financing moves away from a fee-for-service model toward innovative payment models, including capitation, a healthcare system's success will rest on its ability to proactively manage the health of its patient population. Coordinating with other local stakeholders by creating a pediatric care network is an effective way to address population health. In the example provided above from Denver, there were several keys to success. These include having (1) an organized asthma team with clear goals and defined program leadership roles; (2) regular and accurate data reports to review processes and health outcomes; (3) well-defined initiatives and goals; and (4) continuous funding from multiple sources. An active NOAC will enable care teams in multiple settings to provide coordinated, high-quality asthma care to their pediatric patients.

REFERENCES

1. Stiefel M, Nolan K. *A Guide to Measuring the Triple Aim: Population Health, Experience of Care, and Per Capita Cost*IHI Innovation Series white paper Cambridge, Massachusetts: Institute for Healthcare Improvement; 2012. Available at: http://www.ihi.org/communities/blogs/_layouts/15/ihi/community/blog/itemview.aspx?List=81ca4a47-4ccd-4e9e-89d9-14d88ec59e8d&ID=50.

2. Halfon N, et al. Applying a 3.0 transformation framework to guide large-scale health system reform. *Health Aff.* 2014;33(11):2003–2011.

3. *Asthma's Impact on the Nation: Data From the CDC National Asthma Control Program.* Available at: https://www.cdc.gov/asthma/impacts_nation/asthmafactsheet.pdf.

4. Campbell JD, et al. Community health worker home visits for Medicaid-enrolled children with asthma: effects on asthma outcomes and costs. *Am J Pub Health.* 2015;105:2366–2372.

5. Lob SH, et al. Promoting best-care practices in childhood asthma: quality improvement in community health centers. *Pediatrics.* 2011;128(1):20–26.

6. Halterman JS, et al. Improved preventive care for asthma. *Arch Pediatr Adolesc Med.* 2006;160:1018–1025.

7. Bunik M, et al. Quality improvement for asthma care within a hospital-based teaching clinic. *Acad Pediatr.* 2011;11(1):58–65.

8. Keet CA, et al. Urban residence, neighborhood poverty, race/ethnicity, and asthma morbidity among children in Medicaid. *J Asthma Clin Immunol.* 2017. http://dx.doi.org/10.1016/j.jaci.2017.01.036. [epub ahead of print].

9. Akinbami LJ, et al. Trends in racial disparities for asthma outcomes among children 0 to 17 years, 2001-2010. *J Asthma Clin Immunol.* 2014;134(3):547–553.

10. Henize AW, et al. A road map to address the social determinants of health through community collaboration. *Pediatrics.* 2015;136(4):e993–e1001.

11. Bhaumik U. A cost analysis for a community-based case management intervention program for pediatric asthma. *Journal of Asthma.* 2013;50(3):310–317.

12. Bloomberg GR, et al. Hospital readmissions for childhood asthma: a 10-year metropolitan study. *Am J Resp Crit Care Med.* 2003;167(8):1068–1076.

13. Liptzin DR, Gleason MC, Cicutto L, et al. Developing, implementing and evaluating a school-centered asthma program: Step-Up Asthma Program. *J Allergy Clin Immunol Pract.* 2016;4:972–979.

14. Cicutto L. *School-Centered Asthma Programs.* [Chapter 13]. [this issue].

15. Norris SL, Glasgow RE, Engelgau MM, Os'Connor PJ, McCulloch D. Chronic disease management. *Dis Manag Health Outcomes.* 2003;11(8):477–488.

Management of Severe Asthma in Adults: New Insights

EILEEN WANG, MD, MPH • NICOLE BARBERIS, MD • ROHIT K. KATIAL, MD

INTRODUCTION

Asthma is a chronic disease broadly characterized by airway hyperresponsiveness, luminal obstruction, and airway inflammation. However, this definition lacks specificity and does not delineate the heterogeneity of asthma that is now well appreciated. Despite this, the American Thoracic Society (ATS),[1] National Heart, Lung, and Blood Institute (NHLBI),[2] and Global Initiative for Asthma (GINA)[3] all have, in their respective ways, further stratified asthma by varying levels of severity and disease burden based on clinical criteria. However, there remains a lack of consensus on disease definitions, best diagnostic assessment tools, and markers of therapeutic response despite the development of new targeted therapies. In this chapter, we will discuss new insights and definitions in the assessment and management of severe asthma in the adult population. Please refer to Chapter 4 entitled "Management of Severe Asthma in Children: Management and Prevention" for a thorough discussion on severe asthma in children.

DEFINITION OF SEVERE ASTHMA

Over the years, the definition of severe asthma has evolved, reflecting our changing understanding of the complexities of asthma pathogenesis and management. These attempts to define asthma severity are integral to developing uniform diagnostic and management approaches for both clinical and research purposes.

In 2007, the NHLBI published the Expert Panel Report 3 (EPR-3) guidelines that categorized asthma as intermittent or mild, moderate, or severe persistent based in part on Forced Expiratory Volume in 1 Second (FEV1) and symptoms.[2] However, this construct did not adequately reflect the disease burden and heterogeneity in response to medications in the severe asthma group.

Thus, in 2010, the World Health Organization (WHO) Consultation on Severe Asthma expanded categorization of asthma severity to include not only level of current control, treatment prescribed, and risk of exacerbations but also responsiveness to treatment. Additionally, the WHO Consultation further classified severe asthma into three distinct groups: untreated, difficult-to-treat, and treatment-resistant or refractory. Difficult-to-treat asthma included those with inadequate response to treatment secondary to poor adherence, poor medication technique, and/or uncontrolled aggravating or masquerading comorbidities such as gastroesophageal reflux disease; obesity; obstructive sleep apnea; nicotine dependence; chronic rhinosinusitis; aspiration, chronic infection, aspirin exacerbated respiratory disease; and chronic obstructive pulmonary disease. In contrast, refractory asthma encompassed disease that remained uncontrolled despite addressing comorbidities and adherence.[4]

As the understanding of asthma phenotypes/endotypes began to be better appreciated along with the need to specifically study severe asthmatics given their high healthcare utilization, a need for a better definition of severe asthma was developed in 2014 by the International European Respiratory Society and American Thoracic Society (ERS/ATS). This classification scheme further defined severe asthma as specifically "asthma that requires treatment with high-dose inhaled corticosteroids (ICSs) plus a second controller (for the previous year) or systemic corticosteroids (for 50% or more of the previous year) to prevent it from becoming 'uncontrolled' or that remains 'uncontrolled' despite high intensity therapy."[1]

These evolving definitions moved away from previous severity classifications—which were composite assessments weighing heavily on particular characteristics of the disease, such as lung function and symptoms—while highlighting medication burden and comorbidities. While there is still a lack of consensus on how best to define asthma severity and control, there remains a need for standardization in defining the heterogeneity of asthma both for clinical and research purposes.

EPIDEMIOLOGY OF SEVERE ASTHMA

According to the 2014 Centers for Disease Control and Prevention National Health Interview Survey data, 7.4% of the adult population in the United States carried a diagnosis of asthma. Of those, 50% were uncontrolled and 65% had persistent asthma.[5] It was estimated that 5%–10% of asthmatics were classified with severe asthma; however, a precise figure was difficult to determine given the heterogeneity of the disease, lack of clear classification guidelines, and incomplete reporting.[1,6] In 2015, data from a Dutch cohort estimated the prevalence of refractory asthma despite good adherence and inhalation technique at 3.6% of all adult asthmatics prescribed ICS/long-acting β-agonist (LABA) maintenance controller therapy.[6] Prevalence based on cellular phenotyping suggested that 50% of patients with varying degrees of severity had eosinophilic involvement based on sputum or biopsy.[7–9] As many of these studies included asthmatics on inhaled and/or systemic corticosteroids, estimates may have underreported the true prevalence of eosinophilic asthma because of the corticosteroid-responsive nature of eosinophils.

KEY FEATURES OF THE ASSESSMENT AND PATHOPHYSIOLOGY OF ASTHMA

The assessment of asthma—particularly uncontrolled, severe, or refractory—requires understanding of the nuances of the complex mechanisms behind airway inflammation, bronchial tone, and their relationship to one another. For instance, as previously noted, the predominant means of classifying asthma severity had been based on lung function testing and reversibility with administration of a short-acting bronchodilator. Therefore, FEV1 had been viewed as a clinical surrogate of underlying airway inflammation, often leading to increases in antiinflammatory therapies when FEV1 is reduced.[10] However, in a study of mild to moderately severe allergic asthmatics, Crimi et al. found weak relationships between baseline FEV1 and airway inflammation as defined by sputum or bronchoalveolar lavage (BAL) eosinophils. They also demonstrated poor correlation between airway hyperresponsiveness to methacholine and airway eosinophilic inflammation based on sputum or BAL.[11]

Not only lung function seems to be a weak correlate of airway inflammation, but also, largely arising from studies of novel therapies, our conceptualization of a direct concordance between FEV1 and systemic corticosteroid-requiring exacerbations may not be completely accurate. Pavord and colleagues determined that subjects who had the greatest improvement in exacerbations after antiinterleukin (anti-IL)-5 therapy were those with less than 50 mL change in FEV1 after receiving salbutamol rather than those with 50–150 mL and greater than 150 mL change. Thus, the authors noted that the underpinnings of asthma exacerbations may differ from those pathways driving bronchial tone.[12] Specifically, anti-IL-5 worked best in those who had symptoms and airflow limitation resulting from corticosteroid-responsive inflammation rather than smooth muscle contraction.[13] Furthermore, in a study comparing asthmatics during periods of poor control and exacerbations, Reddel et al. discovered that during exacerbations, postbronchodilator peak expiratory flow rates (PEFRs) were not significantly different from prebronchodilator values. In contrast, during periods of poor control, defined as the week before the onset of an exacerbation, PEFR significantly improved with bronchodilator therapy. The authors noted that while exacerbations caused by reductions in ICS dosage or increased allergen exposure resulted in similar lability of PEFR, the sustained airway obstruction seen in presumed viral exacerbations supports the notion of uncoupling bronchial tone from airway inflammation–driving exacerbations.[14] Additionally, tumor necrosis factor (TNF)-inhibitor studies in asthma demonstrated a similar discordance between lung function and asthma exacerbations. Blockade of TNF-α in severe asthma improved FEV1, bronchial hyperresponsiveness to methacholine,[15,16] and quality of life but did not reduce exacerbations, suggesting mechanistic differences behind exacerbations as opposed to lung function.[17] Finally, mechanical interventions such as bronchial thermoplasty (BT) did not demonstrate a robust response in improving FEV1 but showed a positive effect on exacerbations.[18–20]

These examples elucidate how symptoms, lung function, exacerbations, bronchial reactivity, cellular profiles, and inflammation reflect the complex and diverse pathogenesis of asthma and represent different elements of the airway axis. Therefore, better understanding of the interrelationship of these measures may provide guidance on truly personalizing management.[21]

TREATMENT

Classic management of asthma includes short-acting β-agonists (SABA) and ICSs with or without long-acting β-agonists. Traditional add-on medications and therapies include short-acting antimuscarinics, antileukotrienes,

TABLE 3.1
Traditional Asthma Therapies

Medication/Class	EPR-3 Recommendation
ICS	Low dose recommended in Step 2. Medium dose indicated in Steps 3 and 4
ICS/LABA	Low-dose ICS/LABA recommended in Step 3 Medium-dose ICS/LABA recommended in Step 4 High-dose ICS/LABA recommended in Steps 5 and 6
SAMA	No recommendations
LTRA	Alternative in Step 2. Add-on therapy in Steps 3, 4, and 5
Theophylline	Alternative in Step 2. Add-on therapy in Steps 3, 4, and 5
Allergen immunotherapy	Consider in patients with allergic asthma in Steps 2, 3, and 4
Oral corticosteroids	Two-week course to confirm reversibility. Indicated in Step 6

Data from medication package inserts and Chung KF, Wenzel SE, Brozek JL, et al. International ERS/ATS guidelines on definition, evaluation and treatment of severe asthma. *Eur Respir J.* 2014;43:343–373; Expert Panel report 3 (EPR-3): guidelines for the diagnosis and management of asthma-summary report 2007. *J Allergy Clin Immunol.* 2007;120:S94–S138; *Global Strategy for Asthma Management and Prevention.* Global Initiative for Asthma (GINA); 2015.

theophylline, allergen immunotherapy, and systemic corticosteroids, which are outlined in Table 3.1. However, understanding of novel therapeutics (Table 3.2) to include anticholinergics, biologics, BT, and macrolide antibiotics will be the focus in this chapter.

Anticholinergics

In September 2015, the U.S. Food and Drug Administration (FDA) approved Spiriva Respimat (tiotropium), a long-acting muscarinic antagonist, for use in asthma. In the asthmatic patient who remained poorly controlled on high-dose ICS/LABA, ERS/ATS suggested that tiotropium should be used in the setting of intolerance to β-agonists,[1] and GINA suggested the same in Steps 3 to 4.[3] The addition of tiotropium was studied in various asthmatic populations on different levels of controller therapy. In 2010, a three-way, double-blind, triple-dummy, crossover study of 210 adult asthmatic patients uncontrolled on low-dose ICS compared doubling the dose of ICS, addition of salmeterol, versus addition of tiotropium. Tiotropium was found to be superior to a doubling dose of ICS and noninferior to addition of a LABA as measured by improvement in PEFR, FEV1, and asthma control as assessed by the Asthma Control Questionnaire (ACQ).[22] Furthermore, a study in more severe asthmatics on medium-dose ICS found tiotropium to be noninferior to salmeterol as add-on therapy in terms of FEV1 and asthma control as assessed by ACQ.

TABLE 3.2
Advanced, New, and Emerging Asthma Therapies

Therapy	Target/Mechanism	Status	Ages for Which the Therapy Is Approved
Tiotropium	Long-acting muscarinic antagonist	FDA approved in 2015 for long-term, once-daily, maintenance treatment	12 years and older
Omalizumab	Anti-IgE	FDA approved in 2003 for moderate-to-severe allergic asthmatics aged 12 years and older and later in 2016 to include those ages 6–11 years of age	12 years and older (2003 approval) 6–11 years of age (2016 approval)
Mepolizumab	Anti-IL-5	FDA approved in 2015 for severe asthmatics with eosinophilic phenotype	12 years and older
Reslizumab	Anti-IL-5	FDA approved in 2016 for severe asthmatics with eosinophilic phenotype	18 years and older
Benralizumab	Anti-IL-5Rα	Not yet approved	N/A
Lebrikizumab	Anti-IL-13	Not yet approved (asthma program on hold)	N/A
Tralokinumab	Anti-IL-13	Not yet approved	N/A

Continued

TABLE 3.2
Advanced, New, and Emerging Asthma Therapies—cont'd

Therapy	Target/Mechanism	Status	Ages for Which the Therapy Is Approved
Dupilumab	Anti-IL-4Rα	Not yet approved for asthma FDA approved for moderate-to-severe atopic dermatitis	N/A
CRTh2 antagonists	Antagonism of CRTh2 pathway	Not yet approved	N/A
Bronchial thermo-plasty	Radiofrequency thermal energy at 65°C, delivered in a series of three bronchoscopies, to target airway smooth muscle	FDA approved in 2010 for severe persistent asthmatics not well controlled with ICS/LABA	18 years and older
Macrolide antibiotics	Protein synthesis inhibition via binding to 50S ribosomal subunit	Not yet approved for asthma	N/A

FDA, U.S. Food and Drug Administration; *IgE*, immunoglobulin E; *IL*, interleukin; *N/A*, not applicable.

This study was not powered for assessment on differences in exacerbation rates or time to first exacerbation.[23] Two replicate, randomized, placebo-controlled trials with a total of 912 poorly controlled asthmatics on combination ICS/LABA therapy found significantly increased time to first exacerbation, decreased risk of severe exacerbations, and increased baseline FEV1 with the addition of tiotropium. The mean degrees of improvement in FEV1 after 24 weeks in these studies were 86 mL in trial 1 and 154 mL in trial 2. Although the magnitude of these changes does not appear to be large, one must realize this was in addition to a LABA, thus magnifying the clinical significance of the noted changes. Additionally, not only were there lung function improvements as expected for a bronchodilator, but also improvements in exacerbations.[24]

Anti-IgE
Omalizumab
Omalizumab is a recombinant, DNA-derived, humanized IgG1κ monoclonal anti-IgE antibody that binds to the Fc region of IgE, thereby preventing IgE from binding to the FcεR1 receptor on mast cells and basophils and inhibiting release of inflammatory mediators.[25] Omalizumab was approved by the FDA in 2003 for use in moderate-to-severe allergic asthmatics aged 12 years and older and later in 2016 to include those aged 6–11 years.

Numerous studies have supported the role of omalizumab therapy in allergic asthmatics. In 2001, Busse et al. demonstrated that allergic asthmatics who remained symptomatic on any dose ICS had significantly fewer exacerbations (rates of 0.28 per patient in omalizumab group vs. 0.54 per patient in placebo group) in addition to improvement in asthma symptoms, FEV1, morning PEFR, and reduction in rescue medication use.[26] In asthmatics on high-dose ICS/LABA with or without other controllers, Hanania et al. found that omalizumab significantly decreased exacerbation rates by 25%. Furthermore, Asthma Quality-of-Life Questionnaire (AQLQ) scores and need for rescue inhaler improved.[27] Finally, a metaanalysis of 3429 children and adults with moderate-to-severe asthma yielded reductions in the rate of exacerbations (38 per 100 patient-years with omalizumab as compared with 70 in placebo, RR = 0.57), use of rescue medications (0.5 fewer puffs per day), and improvements in AQLQ scores. There was no significant difference in FEV1 or PEFR.[28]

In 2013, with the purpose of exploring Th2 inflammatory biomarkers as potential predictors of response to omalizumab, Hanania et al. analyzed biomarkers of FeNO, peripheral blood eosinophil count, and serum periostin using prespecified and post hoc analyses in severe allergic asthmatics inadequately controlled with high-dose ICS/LABA. For each of the three biomarkers, those with higher levels had greater reductions in exacerbations compared with those with lower levels: FeNO 53% versus 16%, peripheral eosinophils 32% versus 9%, periostin 30% versus 3%, respectively. Of note, the confidence intervals were wide and additional studies are needed to prospectively verify these findings.[29] Ledford et al. conducted an omalizumab withdrawal study, the Xolair Persistency of Response After Long-Term Therapy (XPORT), in patients with moderate-to-severe asthma with the primary outcome of time-to-severe asthma exacerbations. Continuation of omalizumab up to 52 weeks showed benefits in terms of symptom control and rate of exacerbations compared with those withdrawn to placebo. Therefore, these results seem to argue against disease-modifying effects of omalizumab in allergic asthma. However, because the baseline exacerbation rates and Asthma Control Test/ACQ scores before omalizumab initiation were unknown for the subjects, the authors were unable to definitively determine the extent to which benefits may persist after omalizumab withdrawal.[30]

The most common adverse events associated with omalizumab treatment were nasopharyngitis, headache, sinusitis, and upper respiratory tract infections. Pooled data from patients aged 12–75 years did not reveal increased adverse events when compared with placebo.[31-33] Anaphylaxis was reported as 0.14% with omalizumab therapy and 0.07% in controls.[32] A variety of malignancies were reported in omalizumab-treated patients (0.5%) versus control patients (0.2%) in 2003 pooled data,[32,33] which raised concern for increased risk of malignancy with treatment. With significant growth of the trial database, another pooled analysis was done in 2010 that included 11,459 patients, 7789 of whom were treated with omalizumab. Omalizumab-treated patients were found to have a malignancy incidence rate of 4.14 per 1000 patient-years of observation as compared with 4.45 for the control group and there were no cluster of malignancies identified.[34] Similarly, a postmarketing trial enrolled 7857 patients (5007 omalizumab treated and 2829 control) from 2004 to 2006 and followed them over 5 years. Crude malignancy rates were similar between the two groups: 16 per 1000 patient-years in the omalizumab group versus 19.1 in the control group.[35]

EOSINOPHILIC ASTHMA AND THE BIOLOGICS

Approximately 50% of all asthmatics based on the Belgian registry[9] had evidence of eosinophilia in peripheral blood and/or sputum. FeNO values are typically increased in many of the patients with allergic and eosinophilic airway inflammation, whereas levels are normal or low in neutrophil-predominant phenotypes. FeNO values have been touted as a surrogate measure of eosinophilic airway inflammation because they correlate mildly to moderately (r = 0.26–0.6) with sputum eosinophil counts.[36-38] Much of the focus on biomarkers in eosinophilic asthma has been on FeNO and peripheral eosinophilia because they are practical measures in terms of their reliability and reproducibility, relatively low cost, and ease of obtainment. However, the development of newer targeted medications—mepolizumab (anti-IL-5), reslizumab (anti-IL-5), benralizumab (anti-IL-5Rα), lebrikizumab (anti-IL-13), tralokinumab (anti-IL-13), and dupilumab (anti-IL-4Rα)—delineated the underlying drivers to both increased eosinophils and exhaled nitric oxide. For example, mepolizumab did not lower FeNO levels but resulted in the reduction of peripheral and sputum eosinophil counts through its action on IL-5.[12,39] In contrast, dupilumab and lebrikizumab did not significantly affect peripheral eosinophilia but lowered FeNO levels, which are now known to be driven by IL-4 and IL-13.[40-43] These drugs have helped us understand the complexity of asthma immunopathogenesis, while clarifying the operative pathways for the various biomarkers of interest.

Anti-Interleukin-5
Mepolizumab
Mepolizumab is a humanized, monoclonal, IgG1κ antibody that inhibits IL-5 from binding to its receptor on the eosinophil surface and inhibits eosinophil recruitment, growth, differentiation, and activation. It was approved by the FDA in November 2015 for the treatment of severe asthmatics aged 12 years and older with an eosinophilic phenotype. Administration is 100 mg every 4 weeks subcutaneously. Preclinical trials of mepolizumab showed reduction in blood and sputum eosinophilia by 80%–100%.[44] This was later supported by a double-blind, placebo-controlled trial by Menzies-Gow et al. suggesting that anti-IL-5 therapy may induce partial arrest of maturation of the eosinophil lineage in the bone marrow, and IL-5 may be involved in local tissue eosinophilopoiesis. In this study, mepolizumab decreased mature eosinophil numbers in the bone marrow by 70% and significantly decreased bronchial mucosa eosinophil progenitors.[45]

Initial mepolizumab studies did not demonstrate benefit in terms of airway hyperresponsiveness,[46] FEV1, rescue medication use, AQLQ scores, or asthma symptoms scores,[47] thus diminishing interest to develop targeted treatments to eosinophils. Unfortunately, patients were not stratified by eosinophil counts.[47]

However, the 2012 Mepolizumab for Severe Eosinophilic Asthma (DREAM) trial, a double-blind, placebo-controlled trial at 81 centers in 13 countries, isolated asthmatic patients with evidence of eosinophilic inflammation. Patients were randomly assigned to receive mepolizumab (75, 250, or 750 mg intravenous) or placebo. The primary measured outcome was the rate of clinically significant asthma exacerbations. Recruited patients met ATS criteria for refractory asthma and had evidence of eosinophilic inflammation based on sputum eosinophilia >3%, FeNO >50 parts per billion (ppb), peripheral eosinophil counts ≥ 300 cells/μL, and/or loss of asthma control after a 25% or less reduction in regular maintenance inhaled or oral corticosteroids. The analyses showed that compared with placebo, all doses of mepolizumab significantly reduced the number of exacerbations per patient per year: 48% for 75 mg, 39% for 250 mg, and 52% for 750 mg. The differences in effect between doses were not significant. Furthermore, efficacy was found to be greater with increased baseline eosinophil counts and number of exacerbations in the previous year. Interestingly, the efficacy of mepolizumab was not significantly greater in atopic individuals. Furthermore, traditional markers of asthma such as FEV1 were not related to the efficacy of mepolizumab.[12] This again illustrates discordance between FEV1 and corticosteroid-responsive inflammation underlying the mechanisms for exacerbation.

Mepolizumab has also been shown to have oral corticosteroid (OCS)-sparing effects. In a study with severe eosinophilic asthmatics on daily OCSs, Bel et al. found a 50% median reduction in baseline OCS doses in the mepolizumab group compared with placebo. In addition, despite reductions in the dose of OCSs, mepolizumab reduced exacerbations and improved control and quality of life.[39,48]

Regarding safety, overall, the frequency of adverse events was similar across treatment groups and was found to be low.[12] Hypersensitivity reactions were rare and generally occurred within hours of administration. In initial trials, there were two serious adverse reactions of herpes zoster. Ongoing open-label extension studies of 998 patients have reported additional cases of herpes zoster; however, the number of additional cases remains unavailable at this time. Therefore, it is the authors' opinion that at a minimum, patients in whom the varicella vaccination is indicated should receive the vaccine before initiation of mepolizumab. Several adverse events occurred with an incidence of 3% or greater and more common than placebo including headache, injection-site reaction, back pain, fatigue, influenza, urinary tract infection, abdominal pain, pruritus, eczema, and muscle spasms. No serious life-threatening anaphylactic reactions were reported

during the clinical trials. However, there have been reports in postmarketing data, thus leading to a label change.[49]

Reslizumab

Reslizumab is a humanized, IgG4κ monoclonal antibody that inhibits IL-5 binding to the α-subunit of the IL-5 receptor complex on the eosinophil. In contrast to mepolizumab, reslizumab is dosed on weight and administered intravenously (IV) every 4 weeks. Reslizumab was approved in 2016 for severe eosinophilic asthmatics aged 18 years and older.

In two duplicate, multicenter, double-blind, parallel-group, randomized, placebo-controlled phase 3 trials in 2015, Castro et al. evaluated the effect of reslizumab in inadequately controlled asthmatics on medium-dose to high-dose ICS who had peripheral eosinophilia ≥400 cells/μL and ≥1 exacerbations in the previous year. Subjects were randomly assigned to receive reslizumab 3.0 mg/kg IV or placebo every 4 weeks for 52 weeks. The primary endpoint was the frequency of clinical asthma exacerbations, defined as worsening asthma requiring the use of systemic corticosteroids, twofold increase in ICS and/or systemic corticosteroids for ≥3 days, or emergency care. Secondary endpoints included change in baseline FEV1, rescue medication use, peripheral eosinophil counts, ACQ scores, and AQLQ scores. Compared with placebo, those on reslizumab were found to have a statistically significant decreased rate of clinical asthma exacerbations (pooled data rate ratio 0.46) and peripheral eosinophilia, along with increased baseline FEV1, ACQ scores, and AQLQ scores. In addition, subgroup analyses revealed that reslizumab resulted in greater reductions in asthma exacerbation rates in those with a history of more frequent exacerbations. Change in rescue medication use did not differ between groups.[50]

In contrast to the previous study that selected patients based on an eosinophilic phenotype, in 2016, Corren et al. conducted a phase 3 randomized, double-blind, placebo-controlled trial in subjects with inadequately controlled asthma on at least medium-dose ICS irrespective of peripheral eosinophil counts. Subjects were randomly assigned to reslizumab 3.0 mg/kg IV or placebo every 4 weeks for 16 weeks. There was no statistically significant difference in baseline FEV1, the primary endpoint. However, although the study was not powered to determine the efficacy of reslizumab across various subgroups based on peripheral eosinophil levels, in subjects with eosinophil counts ≥400 cells/μL, there was a statistically significant improvement in FEV1 and trends toward improvement in ACQ scores and rescue medication use.[51] Of note, however, the change in FEV1 in the placebo group in those with eosinophils ≥400 cells/μL was lower than the other subgroups and thus amplified the treatment effect in the highest eosinophil group.

In another phase 3 randomized, placebo-controlled study, Bjermer et al. further evaluated the efficacy of reslizumab (0.3 or 3.0 mg/kg IV every 4 weeks for 16 weeks) in asthmatics with peripheral eosinophil counts ≥ 400 cells/μL inadequately controlled by at least a medium-dose ICS. Compared with placebo, the reslizumab groups had significant improvements in the primary endpoint of prebronchodilator FEV1 (115 mL in reslizumab 0.3 mg/kg group and 160 mL in reslizumab 3.0 mg/kg group) and secondary endpoints of rescue medication use, ACQ scores, and peripheral eosinophil levels. Because of the limited 16-week duration, the study was not designed to assess the impact on asthma exacerbations.[52] Weight-based dosing could potentially be advantageous in treatment of obese patients when compared with other anti-IL-5 therapies, but this has not been studied to date.

In terms of safety data, anaphylaxis during or within 20 min after reslizumab infusion was observed at 0.3% in placebo-controlled trials and was seen as early as the second infusion. There were no reports of anaphylaxis in the placebo group. In pooled data, there was an increase in malignancy (0.6% in treatment group vs. 0.3% in controls) without clustering of any particular type. Transient elevations of creatinine phosphokinase were observed more frequently in the treatment group (20%) versus the placebo group (18%) but were not treatment-limiting. Myalgias were reported in 1% of the treatment group and 0.5% of the placebo group. Oropharyngeal pain was described at greater than 2% incidence and more common than placebo.[53]

Benralizumab

Benralizumab, currently in phase 3 development, is a humanized, afucosylated, recombinant IgG1κ monoclonal antibody that not only binds the α-subunit of the IL-5 receptor, thereby inhibiting activation and proliferation of eosinophils, but also binds the Fc receptor FcγRIIα on natural killer cells. This results in eosinophil apoptosis via antibody-dependent cell-mediated cytotoxicity and decreased eosinophilia.[54,55]

In a dose-ranging phase 2b study, benralizumab (20 and 100 mg subcutaneous every 4 weeks for the first three doses, then every 8 weeks) reduced exacerbations rates by 57% and 43%, respectively, in adults with uncontrolled asthma on medium-dose to high-dose ICS/LABAs with two to six exacerbations in the year prior to enrollment and peripheral eosinophils ≥ 300 cells/μL. There was no

statistically significant difference in exacerbation rates in noneosinophilic patients.[56] Furthermore, in a phase 2, randomized, placebo-controlled study, a single infusion of IV benralizumab (0.3 or 1 mg/kg) given during an asthma exacerbation decreased asthma exacerbation rates in the following 12 weeks by 49% and exacerbations requiring hospitalization by 60%.[57]

Two double-blind, randomized, parallel-group, placebo-controlled, phase 3 trials, CALIMA and SIROCCO, compared benralizumab as add-on therapy to ICS/LABA, dosed 30 mg subcutaneous (SC) every 4 weeks (Q4W) and 30 mg SC every 8 weeks (Q8W), to placebo. Both studies included asthmatics with two or more exacerbations in the past year on high-dose ICS/LABAs and CALIMA also included patients on medium-dose ICS/LABAs. Subjects were included regardless of eosinophil counts but stratified based on a cutoff of 300 cells/μL. Compared with placebo, for both dosing regimens of benralizumab, there were statistically significant reductions in the exacerbation rates in CALIMA for the high eosinophil group (rate ratios Q4W 0.64, Q8W 0.72) and for the low eosinophil group (rate ratios Q4W 0.64, Q8W 0.60). SIROCCO also supported this finding for the high eosinophil group (rate ratios Q4W 0.55, Q8W 0.49), but only for the Q4W dosing for the low eosinophil group (rate ratio Q4W 0.70). In contrast, in both studies, prebronchodilator FEV1 was significantly improved only for the high eosinophil groups. This finding was observed for both dosing regimens of benralizumab. Interestingly, asthma symptom scores improved in the Q8W benralizumab dosing groups but not the Q4W groups for the CALIMA high eosinophil group and the SIROCCO high and low eosinophil group. Neither dosing regimen in the CALIMA low eosinophil group had statistically significant changes in asthma symptoms scores. One explanation for the difference in exacerbation rates between the two studies may be the level of asthma severity of the subjects. As noted, CALIMA enrolled patients on medium-dose to high-dose ICS/LABAs, whereas SIROCCO enrolled only those on high-dose ICS/LABA.[58,59]

Regarding safety, in a phase 2b trial, most adverse events were described as mild to moderate. Adverse events with incidences 5% or greater in the benralizumab group when compared with placebo were nasopharyngitis and injection-site reactions.[55] In the two phase 3 trials, adverse events were less with benralizumab when compared with placebo, with the most common adverse event being nasopharyngitis. Worsening of asthma was noted in 4%–8% of the placebo group.[58,59] Serious adverse events related to study treatment were <1%. In CALIMA, three patients had serious events: one had an urticarial eruption, two had worsening of asthma and herpes zoster infection.[58] In SIROCCO, there were three serious adverse events related to treatment: allergic granulomatous angiitis, panic attack, and paresthesias.[59]

Anti-Interleukin-4 and Anti-Interleukin-13
Lebrikizumab

Lebrikizumab is a humanized, monoclonal antibody blocking IL-13. IL-4 and IL-13 functionally overlap in that they both signal through TL-4Rα.[60] IL-4 can promote isotype switching to IgE, expression of VCAM-1, transmigration of eosinophils across the endothelium, and production of chemokines by the airway epithelium.[61,62] IL-13, more so than IL-4, acts on the airway epithelium to promote goblet cell hyperplasia, mucin overproduction, and induction of airway hyperresponsiveness. IL-13 also facilitates production of TGF-β, which promotes airway remodeling.[60]

Two replicate, randomized, double-blind, placebo-controlled phase 2b studies (LUTE and VERSE) were done in patients with uncontrolled asthma despite medium-dose to high-dose ICS plus a second controller. No exacerbation history was required for entry into the study, and 52% of subjects did not have an exacerbation in the previous year. Baseline serum periostin levels were used for stratification. Pooled data showed lower exacerbation rates in the lebrikizumab treatment group compared with placebo, and this finding was more marked in the periostin-high group (60% reduction; 95% CI 18%–80%) versus periostin-low group (5%; 95% CI 81%–47%). Additionally, there was an improvement in FEV1 in periostin-high patients. However, the wide confidence intervals should be noted.[63]

Then, two phase 3 trials, LAVOLTA I and LAVOLTA II, assessed the efficacy and safety of lebrikizumab in uncontrolled asthmatics stratified by biomarkers of periostin and peripheral eosinophils. Biomarker-high patients (periostin ≥50 ng/mL or peripheral eosinophils ≥ 300 cells/μL) were found to have a statistically significant reduction in exacerbations (rate ratio 0.49 in the lebrikizumab 37.5 mg dosing group and 0.70 in the lebrikizumab 125 mg dosing group) in LAVOLTA I. However, LAVOLTA II failed to yield statistically significant results.[64] The reason for these inconsistent results is not clearly understood, but as a result, further research into and development of lebrikizumab for asthma are currently on hold.

Tralokinumab

Tralokinumab is a recombinant human monoclonal antibody against IL-13. A randomized, double-blind, placebo-controlled, muticenter phase 2b study in adult severe asthmatics, all on high-dose ICS/LABAs with two to six exacerbations in the previous year, found significant improvements in prebronchodilator FEV1 of 7.3% (CI 2.6–12, P = .003) for every 2-week dosing compared with placebo, but not for every 4-week dosing. There was no significant improvement in asthma exacerbation rates with tralokinumab. However, in a post hoc subgroup analysis, patients not on long-term OCSs with baseline FEV1 reversibility ≥12% in the every 2-week dosing group demonstrated a nonsignificant reduction in exacerbations. There are currently ongoing phase 3 trials investigating these effects along with periostin and dipeptidyl peptidase-4 as potential biomarkers.[65]

Dupilumab

Dupilumab is a fully human monoclonal antibody against the IL-4 receptor α-subunit (IL-4Rα), which is activated by both IL-4 and IL-13. As a result, binding of IL-4Rα results in blockade of both IL-4 and IL-13.[40] The roles of IL-4 and IL-13 in asthma have been discussed in the previous section. At the time of publication of this chapter, the antibody has not obtained approval for asthma but was approved for moderate-to-severe atopic dermatitis.[66,67]

In terms of the efficacy of dupilumab in asthma, Wenzel et al. conducted a randomized, double-blind, placebo-controlled, parallel-group, multicenter study in moderate-to-severe eosinophilic asthmatics based on elevated peripheral eosinophilia or elevated sputum eosinophil level. The treatment group received dupilumab 300 mg SC weekly. Compared with placebo, the dupilumab group had a significant reduction in exacerbations of 87%. Interestingly, although biomarkers associated with Th2 inflammation—such as FeNO, eotaxin-3, IgE, thymus and activation-regulated chemokine—were reduced and FEV1 improved, there was no clear pattern with serum eosinophils.[42] Similar reductions in exacerbations were seen in a 2016 randomized, double-blind, placebo-controlled, dose-ranging trial in adult patients on medium-dose to high-dose ICS/LABAs. Subjects were randomized to receive dupilumab 200 mg every 2 or 4 weeks with a loading dose of 400 mg, 300 mg SC every 2 or 4 weeks with a loading dose of 600 mg, or placebo. The primary measured outcome was change from baseline FEV1. After 24 weeks of treatment, the greatest changes in baseline FEV1 were noted in eosinophilic asthmatics, defined as having peripheral eosinophils >300 cells/μL, with both the 200 and 300 mg SC dosing every 2 weeks (mean change of 0.38 L or 22.9% and 0.38 L or 24.9%, respectively). In comparison with placebo, these groups also had the greatest reduction in annual exacerbation rates of

71.2% and 80.7%. However, importantly, these significant effects were noted in the overall population and noneosinophilic groups who received the dosing every 2 weeks.[41] Based on the results of this study, an upcoming phase 3 trial will utilize a 2-week dosing regimen.

In terms of safety, the side effect profile included injection-site reactions with an apparent dose-response relationship, nasopharyngitis, upper respiratory tract infections, nausea, and headaches.[41,42] In patients with baseline peripheral eosinophil counts ≥300 cells/μL, there was an observed transient increase in eosinophilia that resolved with withdrawal of treatment.[41]

Additionally, dupilumab had shown promise in chronic sinusitis with nasal polyposis, a condition frequently complicating severe eosinophilic asthma. Adults with chronic sinusitis with nasal polyposis refractory to intranasal corticosteroids were randomized to intranasal steroids plus dupilumab versus intranasal steroids alone. Notably, approximately half of the patients in this study had asthma. The group treated with dupilumab plus intranasal steroids showed improvement in endoscopic polyp burden during the 16-week treatment period in addition to Lund-Mackay CT score and sense of smell.[68]

Others
CRTh2 antagonists

Chemoattractant Receptor-homologous molecule expressed on T-Helper type 2 cells (CRTh2) is a prostaglandin D2 (PGD2) receptor. Mast cell involvement has been implicated in severe asthma, and activated mast cells generate PGD2. PGD2 acts through the thromboxane receptor to promote smooth muscle constriction and platelet aggregation, which could contribute to bronchoconstriction.[69] PGD2 can induce not only bronchoconstriction but also allergic airway inflammation as shown in animal models. Inhibition of PGD2 may also lead to reduced Th2 cytokine levels, particularly IL-4, IL-5, and IL-13.[70]

Two phase 2 randomized, placebo-controlled, parallel-group trials examined the effects of CRTh2 receptor antagonism on lung function and asthma control in patients with or without ICS. In study 1, patients had stable asthma (FEV1 65%–110%) and were withdrawn from ICS. Four weeks of treatment with the CRTh2 receptor antagonist resulted in nonsignificant effects on mean morning PEFR, rescue medication use, asthma symptoms, symptom-free days, and asthma control days. In study 2, patients had uncontrolled asthma (FEV1 40%–85%) despite high-dose ICS and were randomized to either one of the three dosing regimens of the study drug or placebo. Treatment with any of the three dosing regimens of the CRTh2 receptor

antagonist yielded significant improvement in ACQ-5. Otherwise, there were no significant changes in PEFR, rescue medication use, asthma symptoms, symptom-free days, or asthma control days.[71] In a randomized, double-blind, placebo-controlled, double-dummy trial, efficacy and safety of a CRTh2 antagonist versus placebo and montelukast were studied with the primary endpoint as changes in trough FEV1. Study patients were symptomatic asthmatics with prebronchodilator FEV1 60%–85% on fluticasone propionate 88 mcg twice daily. Compared with placebo, the CRTh2 antagonist treatment group had a 3.87% change in baseline FEV1 (P = .005), whereas the montelukast treatment group had a 2.37% change (P < .06) but the difference between the two groups was not statistically significant.[72] Further work is needed to determine whether this molecule will ultimately bring about a significant reduction in exacerbation rates.

Bronchial thermoplasty

In asthma, a well-known component of the underlying pathophysiology is airway remodeling, which in part is characterized by epithelial denudation, smooth muscle hypertrophy, and hyperplasia.[73–75] Not only do the smooth muscle changes contribute to bronchoconstriction, but there is also evidence that smooth muscle cells can be proinflammatory through the release of cytokines and chemokines.[76] Therefore, in theory, targeting smooth muscle could result in improvement in underlying airway physiology. As a result, BT was developed as a mechanical approach to treatment. The FDA approved BT for severe refractory asthma in 2010. This procedure uses radiofrequency thermal energy at 65°C, delivered in a series of three bronchoscopies to target airway smooth muscle. Therefore, BT may be most beneficial in asthmatics in whom bronchial tone, as measured by increased bronchial reactivity, is a primary driver of their poor control. However, the treatment was not studied with this degree of patient characterization.

Three pivotal studies have evaluated the efficacy and safety of BT in asthma. These are the Asthma Intervention Research (AIR) in 2007, Research in Severe Asthma (RISA) in 2007, and AIR-2 in 2010.[18–20]

AIR was a randomized controlled study of 112 moderate-to-severe persistent adult asthmatics who had been controlled on ICS/LABA but lost control with withdrawal of LABA. At 12-month follow-up, those who had undergone BT had improvements in the frequency of mild exacerbations. Mild exacerbations were defined as a minimum of one of the following on 2 consecutive days: reduction in morning PEFRs of >20% from baseline, need for >3 additional puffs of rescue medication above baseline use, or nocturnal awakening due to asthma symptoms. The BT treatment group was also found to have improvements in the secondary endpoints of symptom-free days, symptom scores, ACQ scores, AQLQ scores, PEFRs, and rescue medication use. However, there was no significant difference in prebronchodilator FEV1 or airway hyperresponsiveness to methacholine.[20]

Importantly, of these three studies, RISA was the only one to include asthmatics dependent on chronic OCSs. RISA was a randomized controlled trial of 32 severe persistent adult asthmatics comparing BT to a control group during a 16-week steroid-stable phase followed by a 14-week steroid-wean phase, during which baseline OCS or ICS doses were reduced. The BT group had improvements in ACQ and AQLQ scores, along with decreased SABA use. Prebronchodilator FEV1 improved only during the steroid-stable phase but not during the steroid-wean phase. There was no significant difference noted in symptom-free days, PEFR, or airway hyperresponsiveness to methacholine. During the steroid-wean phase, four of eight BT subjects were able to completely wean off of OCSs through to the end of the 52-week study as compared with only one of seven control subjects. Although there was a trend toward greater reduction in OCS and ICS doses in the BT group compared with controls, the difference did not reach statistical significance. Exacerbations were not specifically studied. However, in the posttreatment period, hospitalization rates were similar in both groups.[19]

Lastly, AIR-2, a study of 288 severe persistent adult asthmatics, was the only BT study that was blinded and included a sham control. In this 2010 study, both the BT and sham control groups had improvements in the primary endpoint and AQLQ score, and as a result there was not a statistically significant difference between the two groups in terms of changes in AQLQ scores. In terms of secondary endpoint measures, the BT group had statistically significant decreases in the rate of severe exacerbations, emergency department visits, and number of days lost from work/school but no statistically significant differences in morning PEFR, FEV1, symptom-free days, symptom scores, ACQ scores, rescue medication use, or rate of hospitalizations.[18] However, because AIR-2 excluded those with FEV1 ≤ 60% of predicted, four or more OCS bursts for asthma, or three or more asthma hospitalizations in the prior year, these results may not apply to many severe asthmatics for whom BT would be considered. For the interpretation and application of these data clinically, it is important to note that these trials did not enroll based on a particular phenotype but rather on level of asthma severity.

In summary, these trials showed consistent effects on various control measures, quality of life, and mild exacerbation improvement but not a significant impact on lung function.

Regarding safety, for the BT groups, although all three of these studies had increased frequency of hospitalizations and adverse events during the treatment period, these effects did not appear to persist in the follow-up periods.[18–20] In addition, AIR, RISA, and AIR-2 had long-term safety data up to 5 years that revealed stable lung function and imaging.[77–79]

Macrolide antibiotics

Although not currently approved by the FDA for use in asthma, macrolide antibiotics have been studied for nearly 15 years in uncontrolled asthma with mixed results. Kraft et al. studied clarithromycin treatment in asthmatics with M. pneumoniae or C. pneumoniae, and found an increase in FEV1 of 200 cc, indicating possible benefit in patients with chronic infection. The subjects in this study had asthma defined by a decrease in FEV1 by 20% with <8 mg/mL of methacholine and an improvement in FEV1 ≥12% after bronchodilator but were not classified further by severity.[80] Sutherland et al. studied clarithromycin in asthmatics on ICS separated by whether they were polymerase chain reaction (PCR) positive or negative for *Mycoplasma pneumoniae* or *Chlamydophila pneumoniae* from endobronchial biopsies. Irrespective of PCR status, there was a significant improvement in bronchial hyperresponsiveness in both groups, whereas bronchodilator responsiveness, AQLQ scores, asthma control based on ACQ scores, and fractional exhaled nitric oxide (FeNO) were not significantly changed.[81] Simpson et al. studied a more severe cohort of patients poorly controlled on ICS or ICS/LABA. Treatment with clarithromycin resulted in a significant decrease in IL-8 and sputum neutrophilia and improvement in quality of life. These results were most marked in patients with noneosinophilic asthma.[82] None of these studies specifically reported effects on exacerbations.

Johnston et al. studied patients in the midst of an acute asthma exacerbation in the Telithromycin, Chlamydophila, and Asthma trial (TELICAST). Adult asthmatics with increased wheeze, PEFR <80% predicted, and no overt evidence of a bacterial infection were enrolled in this double-blind, parallel-group, randomized, placebo-controlled, multinational study and treated with telithromycin (800 mg daily for 10 days) or placebo. There was a significant improvement in asthma symptoms but no significant effect on change in morning PEFR.[83]

Azithromycin for Prevention of Exacerbations in Severe Asthma Trial (AZISAST) in 2013 studied 250 mg of azithromycin daily as add-on therapy to ICS/LABA therapy for 6 months in exacerbation-prone asthmatic patients irrespective of cellular phenotyping in a double-blind, placebo-controlled fashion. The primary endpoint was defined as the rate of severe exacerbations (requiring hospitalization, emergency room visit, and/or systemic corticosteroids for at least 3 days) and/or lower respiratory tract infections (LRTIs) requiring antibiotic treatment. Compared with placebo, those treated with azithromycin did not have differences in the rate of the primary endpoint. However, in the subgroup analyses, patients with noneosinophilic asthma (as defined by blood eosinophilia <200 cells/μL) treated with azithromycin had statistically significantly lower rates of both the primary endpoint (severe exacerbations and/or LRTIs requiring antibiotics) and severe exacerbations.[84] This leads us to a point of cautious optimism in the potential role of macrolide antibiotics in asthma, especially in the setting of personalized medicine with directed therapeutics based on a Type 2 low clinical phenotype. However, this approach needs further study.

SUMMARY AND FUTURE CONSIDERATIONS

Severe asthma is a heterogeneous disease with numerous phenotypes. The emergence of several new biologic therapies challenges us to both redefine severe asthma and reshape our paradigm for personalized and targeted medicine. Biologic therapies improve our understanding of disease heterogeneity and help us create case definitions for severe asthma while delineating disease pathogenesis and determining responder profiles for the broad array of therapeutics.

In this chapter, we have summarized emerging treatments for severe asthma beyond the traditional therapies. We have discussed new insights into stratifying patients by phenotype and endotype to drive decision-making regarding treatment. Most of our current therapies are targeting subjects with elevated Type 2 inflammatory markers. Less is known about Type 2 low marker phenotypes. Hopefully, in the future, reliable and accessible biomarkers will be available to help guide which therapies to choose and may even provide a route to monitor disease control and guide duration of therapy. We may benefit from developing an algorithm or protocol to standardize care, but this is still in premature phases. As we have discussed in this chapter, careful patient selection will enrich response to a particular drug because each targeted therapy is not expected to be equally efficacious for all patient populations. As these therapies are new, we need to support ongoing research to determine value in associated diseases, such as rhinosinusitis, and efficacy and safety of combining biologic therapies.

REFERENCES

1. Chung KF, Wenzel SE, Brozek JL, et al. International ERS/ATS guidelines on definition, evaluation and treatment of severe asthma. *Eur Respir J.* 2014;43:343–373.
2. Expert Panel report 3 (EPR-3): guidelines for the diagnosis and management of asthma-summary report 2007. *J Allergy Clin Immunol.* 2007;120:S94–S138.
3. *Global Strategy for Asthma Management and Prevention.* Global Initiative for Asthma (GINA); 2015.
4. Bousquet J, Mantzouranis E, Cruz AA, et al. Uniform definition of asthma severity, control, and exacerbations: document presented for the World Health Organization Consultation on Severe Asthma. *J Allergy Clin Immunol.* 2010;126:926–938.
5. Center for Disease Control Data, Statistics, and Surveillance. https://www.cdc.gov/asthma/asthmadata.htm.
6. Hekking PP, Wener RR, Amelink M, Zwinderman AH, Bouvy ML, Bel EH. The prevalence of severe refractory asthma. *J Allergy Clin Immunol.* 2015;135:896–902.
7. Wenzel SE. Asthma: defining of the persistent adult phenotypes. *Lancet.* 2006;368:804–813.
8. Wenzel SE. Asthma phenotypes: the evolution from clinical to molecular approaches. *Nat Med.* 2012;18:716–725.
9. Schleich F, Brusselle G, Louis R, et al. Heterogeneity of phenotypes in severe asthmatics. The Belgian Severe Asthma Registry (BSAR). *Respir Med.* 2014;108:1723–1732.
10. Reddel HK, Taylor DR, Bateman ED, et al. An official American Thoracic Society/European Respiratory Society statement: asthma control and exacerbations: standardizing endpoints for clinical asthma trials and clinical practice. *Am J Respir Crit Care Med.* 2009;180:59–99.
11. Crimi E, Spanevello A, Neri M, Ind PW, Rossi GA, Brusasco V. Dissociation between airway inflammation and airway hyperresponsiveness in allergic asthma. *Am J Respir Crit Care Med.* 1998;157:4–9.
12. Pavord ID, Korn S, Howarth P, et al. Mepolizumab for severe eosinophilic asthma (DREAM): a multicentre, double-blind, placebo-controlled trial. *Lancet.* 2012;380:651–659.
13. Pavord ID, Haldar P, Bradding P, Wardlaw AJ. Mepolizumab in refractory eosinophilic asthma. *Thorax.* 2010;65:370.
14. Reddel H, Ware S, Marks G, Salome C, Jenkins C, Woolcock A. Differences between asthma exacerbations and poor asthma control. *Lancet.* 1999;353:364–369.
15. Obase Y, Shimoda T, Mitsuta K, Matsuo N, Matsuse H, Kohno S. Correlation between airway hyperresponsiveness and airway inflammation in a young adult population: eosinophil, ECP, and cytokine levels in induced sputum. *Ann Allergy Asthma Immunol.* 2001;86:304–310.

16. Thomas PS, Yates DH, Barnes PJ. Tumor necrosis factor-alpha increases airway responsiveness and sputum neutrophilia in normal human subjects. *Am J Respir Crit Care Med.* 1995;152:76–80.

17. Matera MG, Calzetta L, Cazzola M. TNF-alpha inhibitors in asthma and COPD: we must not throw the baby out with the bath water. *Pulm Pharmacol Ther.* 2010;23:121–128.

18. Castro M, Rubin AS, Laviolette M, et al. Effectiveness and safety of bronchial thermoplasty in the treatment of severe asthma: a multicenter, randomized, double-blind, sham-controlled clinical trial. *Am J Respir Crit Care Med.* 2010;181:116–124.

19. Pavord ID, Cox G, Thomson NC, et al. Safety and efficacy of bronchial thermoplasty in symptomatic, severe asthma. *Am J Respir Crit Care Med.* 2007;176:1185–1191.

20. Cox G, Thomson NC, Rubin AS, et al. Asthma control during the year after bronchial thermoplasty. *N. Engl J Med.* 2007;356:1327–1337.

21. Chipps BE, Corren J, Israel E, et al. Asthma Yardstick: practical recommendations for a sustained step-up in asthma therapy for poorly controlled asthma. *Ann Allergy Asthma Immunol.* 2017;118:133–142.e3.

22. Peters SP, Kunselman SJ, Icitovic N, et al. Tiotropium bromide step-up therapy for adults with uncontrolled asthma. *N. Engl J Med.* 2010;363:1715–1726.

23. Kerstjens HA, Casale TB, Bleecker ER, et al. Tiotropium or salmeterol as add-on therapy to inhaled corticosteroids for patients with moderate symptomatic asthma: two replicate, double-blind, placebo-controlled, parallel-group, active-comparator, randomised trials. *Lancet Respir Med.* 2015;3:367–376.

24. Kerstjens HA, Engel M, Dahl R, et al. Tiotropium in asthma poorly controlled with standard combination therapy. *N. Engl J Med.* 2012;367:1198–1207.

25. Strunk RC, Bloomberg GR. Omalizumab for asthma. *N. Engl J Med.* 2006;354:2689–2695.

26. Busse W, Corren J, Lanier BQ, et al. Omalizumab, anti-IgE recombinant humanized monoclonal antibody, for the treatment of severe allergic asthma. *J Allergy Clin Immunol.* 2001;108:184–190.

27. Hanania NA, Alpan O, Hamilos DL, et al. Omalizumab in severe allergic asthma inadequately controlled with standard therapy: a randomized trial. *Ann Intern Med.* 2011;154:573–582.

28. Rodrigo GJ, Neffen H, Castro-Rodriguez JA. Efficacy and safety of subcutaneous omalizumab vs placebo as add-on therapy to corticosteroids for children and adults with asthma: a systematic review. *Chest.* 2011;139:28–35.

29. Hanania NA, Wenzel S, Rosen K, et al. Exploring the effects of omalizumab in allergic asthma: an analysis of biomarkers in the EXTRA study. *Am J Respir Crit Care Med.* 2013;187:804–811.

30. Ledford D, Busse W, Trzaskoma B, et al. A randomized multicenter study evaluating Xolair persistence of response after long-term therapy. *J Allergy Clin Immunol.* 2016;140(1).

31. Humbert M, Busse W, Hanania NA, et al. Omalizumab in asthma: an update on recent developments. *J Allergy Clin Immunol Pract.* 2014;2:525–536.e1.

32. Corren J, Casale TB, Lanier B, Buhl R, Holgate S, Jimenez P. Safety and tolerability of omalizumab. *Clin Exp Allergy.* 2009;39:788–797.

33. Genentech. *Omalizumab Prescribing Information;* July 2016.

34. Busse W, Buhl R, Fernandez Vidaurre C, et al. Omalizumab and the risk of malignancy: results from a pooled analysis. *J Allergy Clin Immunol.* 2012;129:983–989.e6.

35. Long A, Rahmaoui A, Rothman KJ, et al. Incidence of malignancy in patients with moderate-to-severe asthma treated with or without omalizumab. *J Allergy Clin Immunol.* 2014;134:560–567.e4.

36. Silkoff PE, Lent AM, Busacker AA, et al. Exhaled nitric oxide identifies the persistent eosinophilic phenotype in severe refractory asthma. *J Allergy Clin Immunol.* 2005;116:1249–1255.

37. Spahn JD, Malka J, Szefler SJ. Current application of exhaled nitric oxide in clinical practice. *J Allergy Clin Immunol.* 2016;138:1296–1298.

38. Dweik RA, Boggs PB, Erzurum SC, et al. An official ATS clinical practice guideline: interpretation of exhaled nitric oxide levels (FENO) for clinical applications. *Am J Respir Crit Care Med.* 2011;184:602–615.

39. Ortega HG, Liu MC, Pavord ID, et al. Mepolizumab treatment in patients with severe eosinophilic asthma. *N. Engl J Med.* 2014;371:1198–1207.

40. Simpson EL, Bieber T, Guttman-Yassky E, et al. Two phase 3 trials of dupilumab versus placebo in atopic dermatitis. *N Engl J Med.* 2016;375:2335–2348.

41. Wenzel S, Castro M, Corren J, et al. Dupilumab efficacy and safety in adults with uncontrolled persistent asthma despite use of medium-to-high-dose inhaled corticosteroids plus a long-acting β2 agonist: a randomised double-blind placebo-controlled pivotal phase 2b dose-ranging trial. *Lancet.* 2016;388:31–44.

42. Wenzel S, Ford L, Pearlman D, et al. Dupilumab in persistent asthma with elevated eosinophil levels. *N. Engl J Med.* 2013;368:2455–2466.

43. Corren J, Lemanske RF, Hanania NA, et al. Lebrikizumab treatment in adults with asthma. *N. Engl J Med.* 2011;365:1088–1098.

44. Hart TK, Cook RM, Zia-Amirhosseini P, et al. Preclinical efficacy and safety of mepolizumab (SB-240563), a humanized monoclonal antibody to IL-5, in cynomolgus monkeys. *J Allergy Clin Immunol.* 2001;108:250–257.

45. Menzies-Gow A, Flood-Page P, Sehmi R, et al. Anti-IL-5 (mepolizumab) therapy induces bone marrow eosinophil maturational arrest and decreases eosinophil progenitors in the bronchial mucosa of atopic asthmatics. *J Allergy Clin Immunol.* 2003;111:714–719.

46. Leckie MJ, ten Brinke A, Khan J, et al. Effects of an interleukin-5 blocking monoclonal antibody on eosinophils, airway hyper-responsiveness, and the late asthmatic response. *Lancet.* 2000;356:2144–2148.

47. Flood-Page P, Swenson C, Faiferman I, et al. A study to evaluate safety and efficacy of mepolizumab in patients with moderate persistent asthma. *Am J Respir Crit Care Med.* 2007;176:1062–1071.

48. Bel EH, Wenzel SE, Thompson PJ, et al. Oral glucocorticoid-sparing effect of mepolizumab in eosinophilic asthma. *N. Engl J Med.* 2014;371:1189–1197.

49. GlaskoSmithKline. *Mepolizumab Product Monograph Including Patient Medication Information;* August 2016.

50. Castro M, Zangrilli J, Wechsler ME, et al. Reslizumab for inadequately controlled asthma with elevated blood eosinophil counts: results from two multicentre, parallel, double-blind, randomised, placebo-controlled, phase 3 trials. *Lancet Respir Med.* 2015;3:355–366.

51. Corren J, Weinstein S, Janka L, Zangrilli J, Garin M. Phase 3 study of reslizumab in patients with poorly controlled asthma: effects across a broad range of eosinophil counts. *Chest.* 2016;150:799–810.

52. Bjermer L, Lemiere C, Maspero J, Weiss S, Zangrilli J, Germinaro M. Reslizumab for inadequately controlled asthma with elevated blood eosinophil levels: a randomized phase 3 study. *Chest.* 2016;150:789–798.

53. Teva. *Reslizumab Prescribing Information;* March 2016.

54. Busse WW, Katial R, Gossage D, et al. Safety profile, pharmacokinetics, and biologic activity of MEDI-563, an anti-IL-5 receptor alpha antibody, in a phase I study of subjects with mild asthma. *J Allergy Clin Immunol.* 2010;125:1237–1244.e2.

55. Laviolette M, Gossage DL, Gauvreau G, et al. Effects of benralizumab on airway eosinophils in asthmatic patients with sputum eosinophilia. *J Allergy Clin Immunol.* 2013;132:1086–1096.e5.

56. Castro M, Wenzel SE, Bleecker ER, et al. Benralizumab, an anti-interleukin 5 receptor alpha monoclonal antibody, versus placebo for uncontrolled eosinophilic asthma: a phase 2b randomised dose-ranging study. *Lancet Respir Med.* 2014;2:879–890.

57. Nowak RM, Parker JM, Silverman RA, et al. A randomized trial of benralizumab, an antiinterleukin 5 receptor alpha monoclonal antibody, after acute asthma. *Am J Emerg Med.* 2015;33:14–20.

58. FitzGerald JM, Bleecker ER, Nair P, et al. Benralizumab, an anti-interleukin-5 receptor alpha monoclonal antibody, as add-on treatment for patients with severe, uncontrolled, eosinophilic asthma (CALIMA): a randomised, double-blind, placebo-controlled phase 3 trial. *Lancet.* 2016;388:2128–2141.

59. Bleecker ER, FitzGerald JM, Chanez P, et al. Efficacy and safety of benralizumab for patients with severe asthma uncontrolled with high-dosage inhaled corticosteroids and long-acting beta2-agonists (SIROCCO): a randomised, multicentre, placebo-controlled phase 3 trial. *Lancet.* 2016;388:2115–2127.

60. Chatila TA. Interleukin-4 receptor signaling pathways in asthma pathogenesis. *Trends Mol Med.* 2004;10:493–499.

61. Steinke JW, Borish L. Th2 cytokines and asthma. Interleukin-4: its role in the pathogenesis of asthma, and targeting it for asthma treatment with interleukin-4 receptor antagonists. *Respir Res.* 2001;2:66–70.

62. de Groot JC, Ten Brinke A, Bel EH. Management of the patient with eosinophilic asthma: a new era begins. *ERJ Open Res.* 2015;1.

63. Hanania NA, Noonan M, Corren J, et al. Lebrikizumab in moderate-to-severe asthma: pooled data from two randomised placebo-controlled studies. *Thorax.* 2015;70:748–756.

64. Hanania NA, Korenblat P, Chapman KR, et al. Efficacy and safety of lebrikizumab in patients with uncontrolled asthma (LAVOLTA I and LAVOLTA II): replicate, phase 3, randomised, double-blind, placebo-controlled trials. *Lancet Respir Med.* 2016;4:781–796.

65. Brightling CE, Chanez P, Leigh R, et al. Efficacy and safety of tralokinumab in patients with severe uncontrolled asthma: a randomised, double-blind, placebo-controlled, phase 2b trial. *Lancet Respir Med.* 2015;3:692–701.

66. Regeneron. *Dupilimab Prescribing Information;* March 2017. Revised.

67. FDA. *Approved New Eczema Drug Dupixent;* March 28, 2017.

68. Bachert C, Mannent L, Naclerio RM, et al. Effect of subcutaneous dupilumab on nasal polyp burden in patients with chronic sinusitis and nasal polyposis: a randomized clinical trial. *JAMA.* 2016;315:469–479.

69. Fajt ML, Gelhaus SL, Freeman B, et al. Prostaglandin D(2) pathway upregulation: relation to asthma severity, control, and TH2 inflammation. *J Allergy Clin Immunol.* 2013;131:1504–1512.

70. Miller D, Wood C, Bateman E, et al. A randomized study of BI 671800, a CRTH2 antagonist, as add-on therapy in poorly controlled asthma. *Allergy Asthma Proc.* 2017;38:157–164.

71. Kuna P, Bjermer L, Tornling G. Two Phase II randomized trials on the CRTh2 antagonist AZD1981 in adults with asthma. *Drug Des Devel Ther.* 2016;10:2759–2770.

72. Hall IP, Fowler AV, Gupta A, et al. Efficacy of BI 671800, an oral CRTH2 antagonist, in poorly controlled asthma as sole controller and in the presence of inhaled corticosteroid treatment. *Pulm Pharmacol Ther.* 2015;32:37–44.

73. Nair P, Martin JG, Cockcroft DC, et al. Airway hyperresponsiveness in asthma: measurement and clinical relevance. *J Allergy Clin Immunol Pract.* 2017;5(3).

74. James A, Mauad T, Abramson M, Green F. Airway smooth muscle hypertrophy and hyperplasia in asthma. *Am J Respir Crit Care Med.* 2012;186:568. author reply 9.

75. Hirota N, Martin JG. Mechanisms of airway remodeling. *Chest.* 2013;144:1026–1032.

76. Panettieri Jr RA. Airway smooth muscle: immunomodulatory cells? *Allergy Asthma Proc.* 2004;25:381–386.

77. Thomson NC, Rubin AS, Niven RM, et al. Long-term (5 year) safety of bronchial thermoplasty: asthma Intervention Research (AIR) trial. *BMC Pulm Med.* 2011;11:8.

78. Pavord ID, Thomson NC, Niven RM, et al. Safety of bronchial thermoplasty in patients with severe refractory asthma. *Ann Allergy Asthma Immunol.* 2013;111:402–407.

79. Wechsler ME, Laviolette M, Rubin AS, et al. Bronchial thermoplasty: long-term safety and effectiveness in patients with severe persistent asthma. *J Allergy Clin Immunol.* 2013;132:1295–1302.

80. Kraft M, Cassell GH, Pak J, Martin RJ. Mycoplasma pneumoniae and Chlamydia pneumoniae in asthma: effect of clarithromycin. *Chest.* 2002;121:1782–1788.

81. Sutherland ER, King TS, Icitovic N, et al. A trial of clarithromycin for the treatment of suboptimally controlled asthma. *J Allergy Clin Immunol.* 2010;126:747–753.

82. Simpson JL, Powell H, Boyle MJ, Scott RJ, Gibson PG. Clarithromycin targets neutrophilic airway inflammation in refractory asthma. *Am J Respir Crit Care Med.* 2008;177:148–155.

83. Johnston SL, Blasi F, Black PN, Martin RJ, Farrell DJ, Nieman RB. The effect of telithromycin in acute exacerbations of asthma. *N. Engl J Med.* 2006;354:1589–1600.

84. Brusselle GG, Vanderstichele C, Jordens P, et al. Azithromycin for prevention of exacerbations in severe asthma (AZISAST): a multicentre randomised double-blind placebo-controlled trial. *Thorax.* 2013;68:322–329.

CHAPTER 4

Management and Prevention of Severe Asthma in Children

ANNE M. FITZPATRICK, PHD

ABBREVIATIONS

ACQ   Asthma Control Questionnaire
ACT   Asthma Control Test
ATS   American Thoracic Society
CACT   Childhood Asthma Control Test
CFC   Chlorofluorocarbon
CRTH2   Chemoattractant receptor-homologous molecule expressed on T-helper type 2 cells
ERS   European Respiratory Society
FEV$_1$ Forced expiratory volume in 1 s
FVC   Forced vital capacity
HFA   Hydrofluoroalkane
ICS   Inhaled corticosteroid
LABA   Long-acting β-agonist
LTRA   Leukotriene receptor antagonist
PDE$_4$ Phosphodiesterase 4
TRACK   Test for Respiratory and Asthma Control in Kids
WHO   World Health Organization

INTRODUCTION

Despite advances in asthma knowledge and care since the early 2000s, asthma control remains suboptimal in a large number of affected patients. In the United States, nearly 50% of patients with asthma experience an exacerbation each year, with a slightly higher exacerbation prevalence in children less than 18 years as compared with adults.[1,2] Although death rates from asthma have steadily declined, morbidity from asthma remains significant.[1] Episodes of wheezing, breathlessness, chest tightness, and coughing are common despite the use of preventative controller medications for asthma and result in disproportionate healthcare utilization and costs, particularly in children.[3–5] Similar trends have also been observed globally. Nearly 14% of the world's children experience asthma symptoms; despite reductions in mortality with improved availability of asthma medications, affected children continue to have substantial disability, which also impacts the ability of their parents to work.[6,7]

The factors responsible for poor asthma control in children are complex (Fig. 4.1). Limited access to asthma care and poor adherence to evidence-based asthma medication are clearly major causes of preventable disease burden in children, even in developed countries.[8] Exposure to aeroallergens and tobacco smoke and comorbid conditions such as obesity also contribute to asthma risk and poorer outcomes in children.[9–12] Nonetheless, there is a relatively small subset of children with "severe" or "refractory" asthma who have ongoing symptoms and airway inflammation despite appropriate treatment,[13] which is likely due to altered underlying biologic and physiologic mechanisms that regulate inflammation and glucocorticoid receptor signaling.[14–16] While the exact prevalence of severe asthma in children is unknown, it is thought to be somewhat rare in countries with good asthma medication access[17] and likely affects less than 5% of children with asthma.[13] However, these children with severe asthma may account for a large proportion of all pediatric-related asthma healthcare encounters[18–20] and may be at increased risk for long-term medication-related side effects[21] and life-threatening exacerbations that impair quality of life and promote absenteeism from school and work.[11,22]

Severe asthma in children is difficult to treat, and novel or alternative methods to promote asthma control in these children are clearly needed. There is growing recognition that severe asthma in children is a highly heterogeneous condition associated with a variety of "phenotypes" (i.e., clinical characteristics), necessitating a more "personalized" as opposed to a "one-size-fits-all" approach.[23] However, the evidence base for severe asthma care in children remains quite limited.[13] This chapter outlines strategies for the definition and diagnosis of severe asthma in children and reviews phenotype-directed treatment strategies. Unique aspects of children with severe asthma, as well as future directions for application of precision medicine, are also discussed.

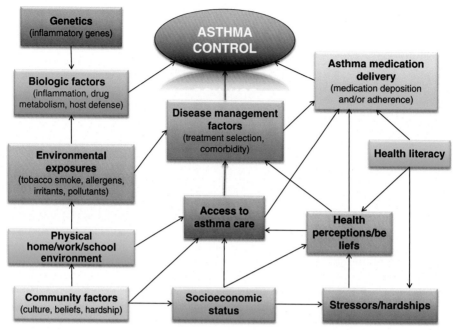

FIG. 4.1 Factors associated with asthma control in children. The *arrows* represent hypothesized variable relationships.

DEFINITION OF SEVERE ASTHMA IN CHILDREN AND ADOLESCENTS

A major challenge that remains in the field is the definition of severe asthma. Historically, the term "severe asthma" was used in the context of exacerbations and frequently described patients with hospitalizations or life-threatening exacerbations irrespective of medication use and other factors, which are critical in the management of the disorder (Fig. 4.1). An important advance in the field came from the recognition that asthma "severity" and asthma "control" are related but not interchangeable concepts. Whereas asthma "control" refers to the extent to which asthma symptoms are observed in a patient (or are reduced by treatment), asthma "severity" refers to the difficulty in controlling asthma with treatment (i.e., the biological activity of the underlying disease state).[24] Thus, although a patient may have asthma that is not controlled, he/she may not necessarily have severe asthma.

There are some limitations to this view of asthma severity. First, it differs from severity definitions used in other chronic disease states such as diabetes and hypertension, which grade the severity of the illness according to the presence of other disease-related complications (i.e., diabetes-associated retinopathy or neuropathy) or diagnostic biomarkers (i.e., systolic

blood pressure above 180 mm Hg). Second, this view of asthma severity implies that all patients with asthma are appropriately treated with asthma medications and does not account for overprescription of therapy or lack of dosing step-down. Third, this view of asthma severity may not generalize well to global areas (or areas in affluent nations) where asthma is highly prevalent, yet it is underdiagnosed and/or undertreated because of limited accessibility of medical professionals, limited availability of essential asthma controller medications, and the absence guideline-based care.[6] To this end, the World Health Organization (WHO) drafted a uniform definition of severe asthma for global application during a workshop in 2009, which defined severe asthma as "uncontrolled asthma which can result in risk of frequent severe exacerbations (or death) and/or adverse reactions to medications and/or chronic morbidity (including impaired lung function or reduced lung growth in children)."[25] The WHO report also identified three groups of severe asthma: (1) untreated severe asthma, (2) difficult-to-treat severe asthma from external factors (i.e., comorbidity or exposures), and (3) treatment-resistant severe asthma. The intent of this definition was to permit more meaningful estimates of the prevalence of severe asthma worldwide and to promote healthcare planning and policy for public health

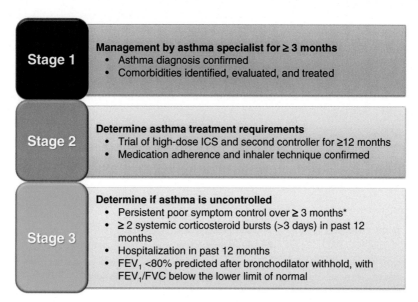

*ACQ score >1.5, ACT or CACT score <20, or "not well controlled" by guidelines

FIG. 4.2 Recommended three-stage approach to the diagnosis of severe asthma in children. *ACQ,* Asthma Control Questionnaire; *ACT,* Asthma Control Test; *CACT,* Childhood Asthma Control Test; *FEV₁,* forced expiratory volume in one second; *FVC,* forced vital capacity; *ICS,* inhaled corticosteroid.

purposes but was not intended to facilitate pathophysiologic study of disease mechanisms across the world because those may vary markedly between regions and the three groups of patients proposed.[26]

Given the global focus of the WHO's report on severe asthma, the European Respiratory Society (**ERS**) and the American Thoracic Society (**ATS**) convened a Task Force workshop in 2011 with a twofold purpose: (1) to develop a consensus definition of severe asthma for children and adults aged 6 years and older and (2) to provide evidence-based care approaches for countries with reasonable access to asthma medication and asthma specialty providers.[13] The Task Force proposed that the definition of severe asthma (in a patient ≥6 years who presents with asthma that is challenging to treat) occurs in stages (Fig. 4.2). Stage 1 is to confirm the diagnosis of asthma with spirometry and bronchodilator reversibility testing (and airway hyperresponsiveness testing if necessary) and to have the asthma managed by an asthma specialist for at least 3 months. Key information obtained from the clinical examination include growth and nutrition, chest deformity, chest auscultation before and after forced coughing, assessment of atopic disease, upper airway pathology, finger clubbing, abnormal cardiovascular signs, and treatment-related side effects. In this stage, comorbidities are also identified and managed Patients with

"difficult-to-treat" asthma resulting from obesity, sinus disease, or other medical factors that improve with treatment are excluded from the severe asthma diagnosis. Management of environmental triggers, including aeroallergens and tobacco smoke exposure, should also be attempted in this stage. In some cases, chest radiographs, computed tomography, swallow evaluations, and bronchoscopy with endobronchial biopsy may be required to rule out other disorders that mimic asthma in children (Table 4.1).

Stage 2 of the diagnosis is to determine the treatment requirements of the patient, with severe asthma defined as "asthma that requires treatment with high-dose inhaled corticosteroids (**ICSs**) and a second controller (and/or systemic corticosteroids) to prevent it from becoming uncontrolled, or which remains uncontrolled despite this therapy." In children, "Gold Standard/International Guidelines treatment" was further defined by the ERS/ATS as high-dose ICS plus a long-acting β-agonist (**LABA**), a leukotriene modifier (namely a leukotriene receptor antagonist [**LTRA**] in children), or theophylline and/or continuous or near-continuous systemic corticosteroids.[13] Thresholds of high-dose ICS are age-dependent (see Table 4.2) and correspond to Global Initiative for Asthma Steps 4–5 care.[27] Because chlorofluorocarbon ICS preparations have been removed from the market and replaced with

TABLE 4.1
Disorders That May Mimic Asthma in Children

Disorder	Common Symptoms in Children
Aspiration during swallowing or secondary to gastroesophageal reflux	Noisy breathing, wheezing, coughing/gagging during feeds, stridor, chest discomfort
Bronchiectasis	Recurrent infections, productive cough
Cardiac disease	Cardiac murmurs, syncope, shortness of breath or fatigue with activity
Chronic lung disease of prematurity	Preterm delivery with symptoms since birth, wheezing, coughing with decreased activity tolerance
Chronic upper airway cough syndrome	Sneezing, itching, blocked nose, throat clearing
Congenital malformation of the lung or airways	Difficulty breathing, infections, wheezing, shortness of breath, pneumonia
Cystic fibrosis	Excessive cough and mucous production, gastrointestinal symptoms, infections
Extrabronchial obstruction (vascular rings, mediastinal cysts or tumors)	Stridor, wheezing, cough, difficulty swallowing, respiratory distress, respiratory infections
Foreign body inhalation or ingestion (acute or retained)	Sudden onset of coughing or choking, persistent or recurrent cough or wheeze, pneumonia, focal bronchiectasis
Hyperventilation or dysfunctional breathing	Dizziness, paresthesia, sighing
Primary ciliary dyskinesia	Recurrent infections, productive cough, sinusitis
Supraglottic obstruction (tonsillar/adenoid hypertrophy)	Hoarseness, difficulty breathing, airway obstruction
Vocal cord dysfunction	Difficulty breathing, inspiratory wheezing, stridor

TABLE 4.2
Definition of High-Dose Inhaled Corticosteroid Treatment for Children

Inhaled Corticosteroid	Inhaler Type	How Supplied (US Brand Name)	Age 6–11 years (mcg)	Age ≥ 12 years (mcg)
Beclomethasone dipropionate	HFA	QVAR®	320	640
Budesonide	DPI	Pulmicort Flexhaler®	720	1440
Budesonide	nebules	Pulmicort Respules®	2000	4000
Budesonide/formoterol	HFA	Symbicort®	320	640
Ciclesonide	HFA	Alvesco®	320	640
Flunisolide hemihydrate	HFA	Aerospan®	1250	2500
Fluticasone furoate	DPI	Arnuity® Ellipta®	100	200
Fluticasone furoate/vilanterol	DPI	Breo® Ellipta®	100	200
Fluticasone propionate	DPI	Flovent® Diskus®	500	1000
Fluticasone propionate/salmeterol	DPI	Advair Diskus®	500	1000
Fluticasone propionate	HFA	Flovent®	440	880
Fluticasone propionate/salmeterol	HFA	Advair®	460	920
Mometasone furoate	DPI	Asmanex® Twisthaler®	440	880
Mometasone furoate	HFA	Asmanex®	400	800
Mometasone furoate/formoterol	HFA	Dulera®	400	800

Values are shown as the lower total daily dose threshold, in micrograms (mcg), for dry powder inhaler (DPI) and hydrofluoroalkane (HFA) preparations available in the United States. Many of the medications listed are not approved by the U.S. Food and Drug Administration for use in children but may be used off-label for the treatment of asthma.

hydrofluoroalkane (HFA) preparations, exact bioequiv-alency and glucocorticoid receptor binding affinity of the newer HFA products have not been thoroughly studied. The guidelines in Table 4.2 are based largely on expert opinion from the ERS/ATS Task Force and available product formulations approved by the United States Food and Drug Administration and European Medicines Agency for routine use. In this diagnostic stage, patients are also expected to receive an adequate trial of these therapies for at least 1 year (or at least 6 months for systemic corticosteroids) and to dem-onstrate acceptable medication adherence. This is an important consideration because adherence to ICS is generally quite poor, and most children with asthma receive less than 80% of prescribed ICS doses.[28] Evalu-ation of pharmacy claims data or other measures may be required, because patient self-reports and objective assessments of ICS adherence rarely agree.[28] Inhaled medication technique is another consideration because improper technique can result in decreased particle deposition in the airways and poorer asthma control.[29] Repeated demonstration and patient self-demonstra-tion is necessary because fewer than 25% of children with asthma and their caregivers administer inhaled medications properly.[30,31]

Stage 3 of the diagnosis is to determine whether patients meeting criteria for severe asthma have asthma that is controlled or uncontrolled. The Task Force defined uncontrolled asthma as any one of the fol-lowing: (1) poor symptom control, (2) two or more systemic corticosteroid bursts (>3 days each) in the previous year, (3) hospitalization in the previous year, or (4) airflow limitation. Poor symptom control was further defined as an Asthma Control Questionnaire (ACQ) score consistently above 1.5,[32,33] an Asthma Control Test[34] or Childhood Asthma Control Test (CACT)[35] score consistently below 20, or consistent "not-well-controlled" status as defined by asthma treat-ment guidelines from the National Asthma Education and Prevention Program[36] or the Global Initiative for Asthma[27] over the 3 months of asthma specialist evalu-ation. Airflow limitation was further defined as forced expiratory volume in one second (FEV$_1$) below 80% of predicted norms in the presence of FEV$_1$/forced vital capacity below the lower limit of normal following a short-acting and long-acting bronchodilator withhold (typically at least 4 and 12 h, respectively). Specific reference equations for lung function testing were not explicitly recommended by the Task Force but should be selected according to the age, race, and ethnicity of the patient evaluated. For example, the 2012 reference equations from the Global Lung Function Initiative are

commonly used in the United States and Europe and were derived from 97,759 records from healthy, non-smoking Caucasians, African-Americans, and North and South East Asians 3–95 years of age.[37]

KEY FEATURES OF SEVERE ASTHMA IN CHILDREN

As a group, children with severe asthma tend to be char-acterized by ongoing symptoms and recurrent exac-erbations that significantly impair quality of life.[38–40] Although not all children with severe asthma are atopic, the majority of children with ERS/ATS-defined severe asthma (>80%) have multitrigger wheezing with sensitization to aeroallergens, in contrast to adults with severe asthma.[39–42] Airflow limitation and air trapping with incomplete reversal after bronchodilator admin-istration are other prominent features.[38–40,43,44] These patterns of obstructed lung function persist well into the adult years[45] and place children with severe asthma at significantly higher risk (i.e., 32 times higher than nonsevere asthma) of developing chronic obstructive pulmonary disease even in the absence of smoking.[46]

Despite these similarities, it is increasingly recognized that severe asthma in children is a complex and hetero-geneous disorder with multiple clinical "phenotypes," defined for the purpose of this review as observable char-acteristics that may (or may not) relate to an underlying disease mechanism (defined as an "endotype"). Statistical cluster analyses have been performed on children across the severity spectrum in attempts to identify these phe-notypes, which differ according to allergic sensitization, race, asthma duration, pulmonary function measures, medication utilization, exacerbations, and inflamma-tory biomarkers.[47–50] For example, a cluster analysis of children aged 6–17 years enrolled in the National Heart, Lung and Blood Institute's Severe Asthma Research Program was performed using 12 clinically accessible characteristics including demographics, lung function and exhaled nitric oxide values, medication use, symp-tom frequency, healthcare utilization, and aeroallergen sensitization.[48] This analysis yielded four "clusters" or phenotypes of asthma (Fig. 4.3). Cluster 1 (30% of chil-dren) was characterized by a later age of symptom onset, normal lung function, and relatively mild disease with less atopy and fewer medication requirements. Cluster 2 (32% of children) was characterized by an early age of onset, slightly lower (yet still normal) lung function and increased allergic sensitization, asthma symptoms, and medication use. Children in Cluster 3 (20% of chil-dren) had an early age of asthma onset, atopic features, the highest prevalence of comorbidity, increased airway

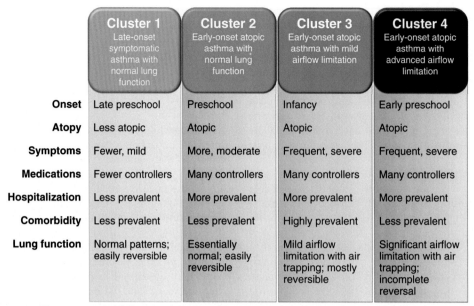

	Cluster 1 Late-onset symptomatic asthma with normal lung function	Cluster 2 Early-onset atopic asthma with normal lung function	Cluster 3 Early-onset atopic asthma with mild airflow limitation	Cluster 4 Early-onset atopic asthma with advanced airflow limitation
Onset	Late preschool	Preschool	Infancy	Early preschool
Atopy	Less atopic	Atopic	Atopic	Atopic
Symptoms	Fewer, mild	More, moderate	Frequent, severe	Frequent, severe
Medications	Fewer controllers	Many controllers	Many controllers	Many controllers
Hospitalization	Less prevalent	More prevalent	More prevalent	More prevalent
Comorbidity	Less prevalent	Less prevalent	Highly prevalent	Less prevalent
Lung function	Normal patterns; easily reversible	Essentially normal; easily reversible	Mild airflow limitation with air trapping; mostly reversible	Significant airflow limitation with air trapping; incomplete reversal

FIG. 4.3 Phenotypes of childhood asthma identified by cluster analysis of children enrolled in the National Heart, Lung and Blood Institute Severe Asthma Research Program.

hyperresponsiveness to methacholine, and airflow limitation. Children in Cluster 4 (18% of children) had the most advanced disease, with an early age of symptom onset accompanied by atopic features, partially reversible and more advanced airflow obstruction, and the greatest burden of symptoms and associated medication use.[48] Although Clusters 3 and 4 were not associated with accepted definitions of asthma severity, replication in a separate pediatric asthma population demonstrated that they were associated with differential and limited response to asthma therapies.[51] However, association of these phenotypes with biologic endotypes remains unclear, and continued replication and longitudinal validation of clustering approaches is needed.

EARLY IDENTIFICATION OF SEVERE ASTHMA IN YOUNGER CHILDREN

Although the definition of severe asthma proposed by the ERS/ATS is intended for use in children aged 6 years and older, it stands to reason that severe asthma may also be present in younger children. Many school-age children with severe asthma report an early onset of symptoms, often before 2 years of age.[39,48] Indeed, the burden of wheezing in preschool children is significant and is associated with recurrent exacerbations necessitating healthcare utilization and impaired caregiver quality of life.[40] Lung function abnormalities have

also been identified in 3-day-old infants[52] and 2- to 3-month-old infants[53] and predict asthma and reduced lung function in childhood and adulthood, even after adjustment for smoking status, allergic sensitization, parental asthma, and other potential confounders. Ventilation defects, including diffuse small defects and large focal defects, are also prominent in children with asthma as young as 3 years of age and correlate with other features of asthma severity.[54] However, classical hallmarks of type 2 inflammation, such as airway eosinophilia and reticular basement membrane thickening that are commonly found in older children with asthma, may not be identifiable in symptomatic infants 12–24 months of age.[55] Although airway eosinophilia and reticular basement membrane thickening are present in some preschool children after 24 months,[56] airway markers of remodeling and inflammation are unrelated in this age group.[57] Preschool children, compared with older children, also have lower airway smooth muscle area and higher vascularity and mucous gland area.[57] Preschool children may also have more neutrophilic versus eosinophilic patterns of airway inflammation[58–60] and less prevalent allergic sensitization (i.e., 30%–50% with a positive aeroallergen test) as compared with older children,[40] perhaps due to an increased burden of respiratory viral infection.

The diagnosis of asthma in children less than 6 years can be challenging in the routine clinical setting because not all wheezing in this age group indicates asthma. Viral infections may trigger wheezing, particularly in the case of respiratory syncytial virus or rhinovirus; therefore it is often difficult (or impossible) to distinguish viral bronchiolitis from an initial asthma presentation. Spirometry is also not feasible in this age group, and there are no available and easily obtained biomarkers, aside from systemic markers of type 2 inflammation, namely blood eosinophils and aeroallergen sensitization.[61] Treatment guidelines from the National Asthma Education and Prevention Panel (2007) proposed a definition of severe asthma in preschool children with near-continuous symptoms during the day, nighttime awakenings more than once weekly, use of rescue bronchodilators several times per day, and extremely limited daily activities.[36] However, this definition has not been validated by clinical studies. More recent guidelines from the Global Initiative for Asthma (2017) do not address a definition of asthma severity in young children but instead recommend assessment of asthma control, including current symptom control over the past 4 weeks and future risk for poor asthma outcomes.[27] Although a working schema for assessing asthma control in young children was provided in that report,[27] it was based on expert opinion given the limited number of validated questionnaires for the assessment of asthma control in young children. Because the ACQ and CACT questionnaires recommended by the ERS/ATS are validated only to age 6 and 4 years, respectively,[32,35] the Test for Respiratory and Asthma Control in Kids (**TRACK**) was recently developed and validated for children less than 5 years of age, which assesses key components of asthma impairment and risk through five caregiver-completed questions.[62] The TRACK instrument is responsive to changes in asthma control,[63] with a clinically meaningful change of 10 or more points indicating a need for reassessment.[64]

The diagnostic approach to the young child with presumed severe asthma might therefore involve (1) asthma specialist management for at least 3 months with the asthma diagnosis confirmed and comorbidity managed, (2) a trial of ICS and a second controller medication for at least 12 months with confirmation of medication adherence and technique, and (3) determination whether the asthma is uncontrolled despite best therapy attempts, with poor control defined by a TRACK score <80, at least two systemic corticosteroid bursts in the past 12 months, or hospitalization in the past 12 months despite best therapy attempts. Thresholds of high-dose ICS in this age group are not well established and the use of high-dose ICS is controversial given the potential risks of adrenal suppression

TABLE 4.3
Definition of Low-Dose Inhaled Corticosteroid Treatment for Children 5 years of Age and Younger

Inhaled Corticosteroid	How Supplied (US Brand Name)	Age ≤5 years (mcg)
Beclomethasone dipropionate	QVAR®	80
Budesonide (nebules)	Pulmicort Respules®	500
Budesonide/formoterol	Symbicort®	160
Fluticasone propionate	Flovent®	88
Fluticasone propionate/salmeterol	Advair®	90

Values are shown as the total daily dose, in micrograms (mcg). Doses were modified from the Global Initiative for Asthma guidelines[27] for available US formulations. Not all of the medications listed are approved by the U.S. Food and Drug Administration for use in young children but may be used off-label for the treatment of asthma.

and growth suppression, particularly in younger children.[65,66] A reasonable guideline for ICS initiation and dosing escalation in young children is provided in the recent Global Initiative for Asthma report, which recommends the following: Step 1, intermittent bronchodilator use; Step 2, daily low-dose ICS; Step 3, doubling of the daily low-dose ICS; and Step 4, continued therapy plus addition of an LTRA, or alternatively, referral to an asthma specialist.[27] Low doses of ICS for young children are listed in Table 4.3.

ESTABLISHED MEDICATIONS FOR THE TREATMENT OF SEVERE ASTHMA IN CHILDREN

Although the treatment of children with severe asthma is based largely on extrapolated data from adult studies, corticosteroids remain the cornerstone of therapy given the inflammatory features associated with the disorder. In children, "Gold Standard/International Guidelines treatment" is defined as high-dose ICS plus a second controller medication (either a LABA, LTRA, theophylline, and/or continuous or near-continuous systemic corticosteroids).[13] The recommendation for intensive corticosteroid treatment is based on observations of relative corticosteroid insensitivity in patients with severe asthma, which can be highly variable and associated with numerous underlying mechanisms.[67] Corticosteroid insensitivity has not been well studied in children with severe asthma, but in one report, only 11% of children with severe asthma had a "complete" response to systemic corticosteroids, evidenced by improvements in symptoms, FEV_1, FEV_1 bronchodilator reversibility, and exhaled nitric oxide concentrations.[68] Separate yet similar studies of children with severe asthma have further highlighted discordance between asthma symptoms, lung function parameters, exhaled nitric oxide concentrations, and blood and sputum eosinophil counts after corticosteroid administration,[14,15,69] highlighting the complexity of the corticosteroid response in children and the need for comprehensive assessment of multiple disease domains in the clinical setting. Close monitoring of side effects in severe asthma treated with high-dose ICS and repeated or continuous systemic corticosteroids is also warranted, because these medications can result in suppression of growth and adrenal function and altered skin and bone metabolism. In children who achieve sustained asthma control over 3 or more months, corticosteroid doses should be gradually tapered to the lowest possible dose that maintains control.

Other recommended secondary controller medications for children with severe asthma include LABAs, LTRAs, and/or theophylline. LABAs are the preferred secondary treatment and are superior to LTRA for the prevention of exacerbations and for the improvement of lung function and symptoms in adults inadequately controlled on low doses of ICS.[70] In children, the addition of LABAs to ICS does not significantly reduce exacerbations or healthcare utilization for asthma but does significantly improve lung function compared with doubling of the ICS dose.[71] LABA add-on therapy is also associated with better asthma symptom control and lung function than LTRA add-on therapy in children,[72] although treatment responses can vary. Although questions have been raised regarding the safety profile of LABA, namely the risk of severe asthma exacerbations in patients of African ancestry,[73] a large Phase 4 study found that LABA in a fixed-dose combination inhaler did not result in a higher rate of serious asthma-related events in adults[74] or children.[75] Nonetheless, providers and parents may remain hesitant about the use of LABA medications in children.[76] In those cases, the addition of an LTRA to high-dose ICS may be warranted. LTRA therapy (i.e., montelukast) improves asthma symptoms as compared with ICS monotherapy in adults[77] and may result in similar control of eosinophilic airway inflammation.[78] LTRAs also have good safety profiles,[79] although efficacy and safety data for LTRA

add-on therapy in children are somewhat limited.[77] Current guidelines do not recommend the routine use of theophylline in children, given the potential for side effects[13]; however, sustained-release low-dose theophylline may be considered in adolescents and improves lung function measures in a manner similar to high-dose ICS alone.[80] Immunosuppressants such as cyclosporine A, methotrexate, or azathioprine have a limited evidence base and are not recommended for the treatment of severe asthma because of low quality of available evidence and a high risk of side effects.[13]

PHENOTYPE-DIRECTED TREATMENT STRATEGIES

Although the established medication strategies discussed above are intended as first-line therapy for children with severe asthma, there is growing recognition that these children may not have an adequate clinical response to a "one-size-fits-all" treatment approach. Thus, phenotypic-directed treatment strategies may be warranted. However, there is no universal consensus on what constitutes an asthma "phenotype" in children. In many cases, a "phenotype" for the purpose of pharmacotherapy refers to either a cellular pattern of inflammation (i.e., eosinophilic vs. neutrophilic) or a specific molecular marker of inflammation (i.e., interleukin-13 "high" vs. "low"). For the purpose of this review, two broad phenotypes, the eosinophil-predominant type 2 inflammatory phenotype and the neutrophil-predominant inflammatory phenotype, are discussed below. These broad phenotypes do not necessarily have common endotypic/mechanistic underpinnings (in fact each broad phenotype may be composed of subphenotypes) but are useful conceptually in the consideration of alternative therapies (Fig. 4.4).

Eosinophil-Predominant Type 2 Inflammatory Phenotype

Unlike adults with severe asthma, the majority of children with severe asthma have an eosinophilic pattern of airway inflammation associated with multiple aeroallergen sensitization and elevated immunoglobulin E (IgE) concentrations.[39,40,48] A number of these children have persistent airway eosinophils despite treatment with systemic corticosteroids[69] and may therefore benefit from strategies that target eosinophils and related type 2 inflammatory cytokines, or aeroallergen responses (i.e., specific allergen immunotherapy or anti-IgE therapy). Specific allergen immunotherapy has been extensively studied in children with asthma and has documented efficacy with

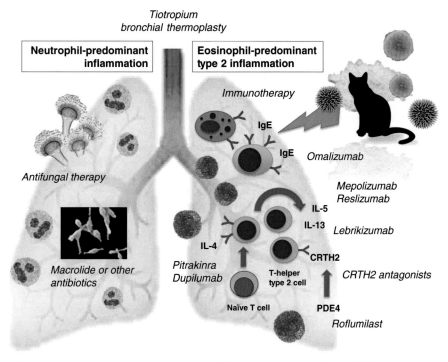

FIG. 4.4 Phenotypic-based treatment strategies for children with severe asthma. *CRTH2*, chemoattractant receptor-homologous molecule expressed on T-helper type 2 cells; *IgE*, immunoglobulin E; *IL*, interleukin; *PDE4*, phosphodiesterase 4.

regard to asthma symptom control, controller medication requirements, and airway hyperresponsiveness.[81] However, current guidelines recommend against the initiation of allergen immunotherapy in unstable children with poor asthma control, and therefore immunotherapy may be difficult to initiate in children with severe asthma.[82] Children with severe asthma also tend to have sensitization to multiple versus single aeroallergens,[23] which may complicate the delivery of therapy.[83] An alternative strategy is treatment with omalizumab, an injectable recombinant humanized IgG1 monoclonal anti-IgE antibody, that is administered to children with severe allergic asthma who have elevated IgE and sensitization to at least one aeroallergen. In a metaanalysis of 25 trials of adults and children, omalizumab reduced asthma exacerbations and hospitalizations when administered as an adjunct to ICS.[84] However, responses to omalizumab are variable and cannot be easily predicted. Given the high cost of the omalizumab, it is recommended that treatment response be globally assessed, with discontinuation of omalizumab if there is no response within 4 months of therapy administration.[13]

Other treatment strategies for eosinophil-predominant type 2 inflammation have shown favorable effects in adults with severe asthma but to date have not been specifically studied in children. These strategies include inhibition of specific cytokines, namely interleukin-5 and interleukin-13, and inhibition of the interleukin-4 receptor. Like omalizumab, mepolizumab, the humanized anti-interleukin-5 monoclonal antibody, reduces annual exacerbation rates and improves quality of life as compared with placebo in adults with eosinophilic asthma.[85] In two large Phase 3 clinical studies, reslizumab, a similar humanized anti-interleukin-5 monoclonal antibody, also improved lung function, asthma control and asthma symptoms in adults with elevated blood eosinophils who were inadequately controlled with ICS.[86,87] Lebrikizumab, a monoclonal antibody to interleukin-13, likewise improved lung function in adults with poor asthma control despite ICS treatment, with the greatest treatment effects in participants with high serum pretreatment levels of the type 2 marker, periostin.[88] Other studies with pitrikinra, an interleukin-4 variant that inhibits binding of interleukin-4 and interleukin-13 to the interleukin-4 receptor alpha complexes, and dupilumab, a human monoclonal antibody to the alpha subunit of the interleukin-4 receptor, have also demonstrated improvements in FEV_1 after allergen challenge[89] and a reduction in airflow obstruction, exacerbations, and biomarkers of type 2 inflammation[90] among patients with elevated eosinophils after treatment.

Antagonism of the chemoattractant receptor-homologous molecule expressed on T-helper type 2 cells (CRTH2) receptor, which is activated by prostaglandin D2, and phosphodiesterase 4 (PDE₄) inhibition are other emerging therapies for eosinophil-predominant type 2 inflammation that have undergone preliminary testing in adults. Although Phase 2 studies of oral CRTH2 antagonists in ICS-treated patients have not had clear efficacy in improving lung function or asthma control, subgroup analyses demonstrated some improvement in these parameters in patients with more severe airflow obstruction.[91] A separate study also found a significant reduction in airway eosinophils in patients with moderate to severe asthma with an elevated sputum eosinophil count despite ICS therapy.[92] Preliminary studies with the anti-PDE₄ agent, roflumilast, have also revealed improvements in FEV1 as compared with placebo in patients treated with ICS.[93] Similar improvements in FEV_1 were also noted when roflumilast was administered with montelukast to patients with uncontrolled moderate to severe asthma despite medium-dose ICS and LABA combination therapy.[94] Further investigations of these agents are ongoing.

Neutrophil-Predominant Inflammatory Phenotype

Although the majority of children with severe asthma have predominant eosinophils and sensitization to aeroallergens, there are children with severe asthma who do not have these features.[95] Although one study of molecular phenotypes in children with asthma found that airway classical type 2 inflammatory cytokines predominated in the airways of children with asthma as compared with controls, other cytokines and chemokines such as C-X-C Motif Chemokine Ligand 1 (CXCL1), C-C Motif Chemokine Ligand 5 (CCL5), interleukin-12, interferon gamma, and interleukin-10 differentiated moderate from severe asthma.[96] A separate study also found undetectable levels of interleukin-4, interleukin-5, and interleukin-13 in the airways of children with asthma as a group,[97] suggesting that the inflammation in these patients may not solely be attributed to type 2 inflammatory cells. Indeed, a recent retrospective review noted that approximately

one-third of children with severe asthma had a neutrophilic pattern of inflammation, which was not consistently associated with pathogenic bacteria or fungi.[95] A separate study also identified a subpopulation of children with severe asthma and increased intraepithelial airway neutrophilia that, unlike in adults, was associated with better lung function and increased expression of interleukin-17 receptor A, which promotes neutrophil maturation.[98] To date, there are no clear therapies for neutrophilic-predominant asthma, as the majority of drug development has focused on type 2 inflammatory phenotypes. Although current ERS/ATS guidelines on severe asthma recommend against routine use of macrolide therapy or antifungals for severe asthma, these may be considered in cases of persistent airway neutrophilia with bacterial infection or when allergic bronchopulmonary aspergillosis is suspected.[13]

OTHER EMERGING TREATMENTS

Tiotropium is an inhaled long-acting muscarinic antagonist that is commonly used for the treatment of chronic obstructive pulmonary disease in adults. Although the precise role of tiotropium in phenotype-directed asthma therapy is not clear, it does have efficacy in chronic obstructive pulmonary disease, which is characterized by predominant airway neutrophils. Tiotropium may therefore be useful in the treatment of severe asthma in children with neutrophilic patterns of airway inflammation, but it could be of benefit to other phenotypes as well. Tiotropium was recently approved for use in patients with asthma and has been shown to improve lung function in adults with poorly controlled asthma despite ICS/LABA combination therapy.[99] Tiotropium also reduces the likelihood of exacerbations requiring systemic corticosteroids in adults treated with ICS monotherapy.[100] Studies in children have yielded similar results. In two recent Phase 3 studies of children aged 6–11 years with severe asthma and adolescents 12–17 years with moderate persistent asthma, tiotropium also improved lung function as an add-on therapy to ICS.[101,102]

Bronchial thermoplasty, which involves direct application of radiofrequency heat to an airway segment to reduce smooth muscle mass, is also available for adults but has not been studied in children. A recent review concluded that bronchial thermoplasty in adults with moderate to severe asthma resulted in lower rates of asthma exacerbations and improved quality of life, but no clear benefit in day-to-day asthma control.[103] Although bronchial thermoplasty is thought to be safe,[104] the ERS/ATS severe asthma guidelines recommended that

---

TABLE 4.4
Priority Research Questions for Children With Severe Asthma

SEVERE ASTHMA ONSET AND DEFINITION

- What is the onset and natural history of severe asthma in children during childhood?
- Can severe asthma be identified in younger preschool children or infants?
- Are there factors associated with progressive versus remitting severe asthma in younger children?
- Are there other proxies or measures in lieu of intensive medication requirements that can be used for the definition of severe asthma in children?

SEVERE ASTHMA PHENOTYPES IN CHILDREN

- What phenotypes are present in children and what are their associated endotypes?
- What is the stability of phenotypes of severe asthma in children and how do they relate to key outcomes such as exacerbations, airway remodeling, and asthma disease burden?
- Do children with severe asthma become adults with severe asthma, and if so, how does the phenotype change?

SEVERE ASTHMA TREATMENT IN CHILDREN

- Are there biomarkers that can be used to guide treatment selection or treatment response in children?
- Can emerging therapies for severe asthma be used safely and effectively in children?
- At which step in the asthma treatment guidelines should phenotype-directed therapy be considered?
- If phenotypic-directed therapy is desired, which treatment should be selected first?
- How should asthma symptom control, treatment feasibility, and treatment costs be weighed and balanced in children with severe asthma?

---

the procedure be performed only in adults with severe asthma in the context of an Institutional Review Board–approved study, given limited available evidence at the time of that report.[13] The role of bronchial thermoplasty in phenotype-directed asthma therapy is also not clear, as there are no current predictors of treatment response.

FUTURE DIRECTIONS AND NEEDS

Severe asthma in children is highly complex and difficult to treat. Although understanding of severe asthma in children has advanced considerably over the past decade, research in this field remains limited and there are still a number of existing knowledge gaps. One major challenge is related to the availability of biomarkers for diagnosis and assessment of treatment response. Pulmonary function testing, although critical for the management of adults with severe asthma, can be challenging in younger children. Furthermore, unlike adults, children with severe asthma can have normal lung function (or lung function values that reverse to normal after bronchodilator administration),[42] with a high degree of discordance between lung function measures, symptoms, and airway inflammation.[15] Moreover, airway biomarkers, such as those obtained from bronchoalveolar lavage or endobronchial brushes or biopsies, are invasive and not always feasible in children. Although blood and urine biomarkers are potentially emerging, these markers may not adequately

reflect the disease processes in the lung. Questionnaire development in children for the purpose of symptom or asthma control standardization can also be challenging because these tools require developmentally appropriate language and concepts that may not be cross-culturally relevant.[61]

These issues, as well as the limited number of children with severe asthma and the heterogeneity within the affected population, make drug therapy challenging. As such, many emerging medications for the treatment of severe asthma do not have pediatric indications and are instead reserved for older adolescents and adults. Thus while phenotype-directed therapy is likely needed for children with severe asthma, there are practical limitations including not only treatment availability but also treatment-related safety, feasibility of administration, and cost. As more treatments become available for children, other challenges include which medication to administer first after first-line therapy with high-dose ICS plus a second controller medication has failed (for example, anti-IgE–directed treatment with omalizumab vs. anti-interleukin-5 inhibition with mepolizumab). The role of other emerging treatments such as tiotropium in phenotype-directed care is also unclear. These questions, as well as other priority research questions for children with severe asthma, are listed in Table 4.4 and highlight the need for continued work in this area before the vision of personalized medicine can become a reality for all children with severe asthma.

REFERENCES

1. Ward BW, Clarke TC, Freeman G, Schiller JS. *Early Release of Selected Estimates Based on Data from the January-June 2016 National Health Interview Survey.* Center for Disease Control and Prevention, National Center for Health Statistics; 2016.
2. National Health Interview Survey (NHIS) Data. *Table 6-1: Asthma Attack Prevalence Percents Among Those with Current Asthma by Age.* Centers for Disease Control and Prevention. United States: National Health Interview Survey; 2014.
3. Barnett SB, Nurmagambetov TA. Costs of asthma in the United States: 2002-2007. *J Allergy Clin Immunol.* 2011;127:145–152.
4. Szefler SJ, Zeiger RS, Haselkorn T, et al. Economic burden of impairment in children with severe or difficult-to-treat asthma. *Ann Allergy Asthma Immunol.* 2011;107:110–119.e1.
5. Nurmagambetov T, Khavjou O, Murphy L, Orenstein D. State-level medical and absenteeism cost of asthma in the United States. *J Asthma.* 2016:1–14.
6. *The Global Asthma Report 2014.* Auckland, New Zealand: Global Asthma Network; 2014.
7. Linneberg A, Dam Petersen K, Hahn-Pedersen J, Hammerby E, Serup-Hansen N, Boxall N. Burden of allergic respiratory disease: a systematic review. *Clin Mol Allergy.* 2016;14:12.
8. Slejko JF, Ghushchyan VH, Sucher B, et al. Asthma control in the United States, 2008-2010: indicators of poor asthma control. *J Allergy Clin Immunol.* 2014;133:1579–1587.
9. Anto JM, Bousquet J, Akdis M, et al. Mechanisms of the development of allergy (MeDALL): introducing novel concepts in allergy phenotypes. *J Allergy Clin Immunol.* 2017;139:388–399.
10. Sheehan WJ, Permaul P, Petty CR, et al. Association between allergen exposure in inner-city schools and asthma morbidity among students. *JAMA Pediatr.* 2017;171:31–38.
11. Puranik S, Forno E, Bush A, Celedon JC. Predicting severe asthma exacerbations in children. *Am J Respir Crit Care Med.* 2016;195(7):854–859.
12. Ahmadizar F, Vijverberg SJ, Arets HG, et al. Childhood obesity in relation to poor asthma control and exacerbation: a meta-analysis. *Eur Respir J.* 2016;48:1063–1073.
13. Chung KF, Wenzel SE, Brozek JL, et al. International ERS/ATS guidelines on definition, evaluation and treatment of severe asthma. *Eur Respir J.* 2014;43:343–373.
14. Phipatanakul W, Mauger DT, Sorkness RL, et al. Effects of age and disease severity on systemic corticosteroid responses in asthma. *Am J Respir Crit Care Med.* 2016;195(11):1439–1448.
15. Fitzpatrick AM, Stephenson ST, Brown MR, Nguyen K, Douglas S, Brown LA. Systemic corticosteroid responses in children with severe asthma: phenotypic and endotypic features. *J Allergy Clin Immunol Pract.* 2016;5(2).
16. Stephenson ST, Brown LA, Helms MN, et al. Cysteine oxidation impairs systemic glucocorticoid responsiveness in children with difficult-to-treat asthma. *J Allergy Clin Immunol.* 2015;136:454–461.e9.
17. Nordlund B, Melen E, Schultz ES, Gronlund H, Hedlin G, Kull I. Prevalence of severe childhood asthma according to the WHO. *Respir Med.* 2014;108:1234–1237.
18. Sullivan PW, Campbell JD, Ghushchyan VH, Globe G. Outcomes before and after treatment escalation to global initiative for asthma steps 4 and 5 in severe asthma. *Ann Allergy Asthma Immunol.* 2015;114:462–469.
19. Sullivan PW, Campbell JD, Ghushchyan VH, Globe G, Lange J, Woolley JM. Characterizing the severe asthma population in the United States: claims-based analysis of three treatment cohorts in the year prior to treatment escalation. *J Asthma.* 2015;52:669–680.
20. Sullivan PW, Slejko JF, Ghushchyan VH, et al. The relationship between asthma, asthma control and economic outcomes in the United States. *J Asthma.* 2014;51:769–778.
21. Wysocki K, Park SY, Bleecker E, et al. Characterization of factors associated with systemic corticosteroid use in severe asthma: data from the Severe Asthma Research Program. *J Allergy Clin Immunol.* 2014;133:915–918.
22. Walter H, Sadeque-Iqbal F, Ulysse R, Castillo D, Fitzpatrick A, Singleton J. Effectiveness of school-based family asthma educational programs in quality of life and asthma exacerbations in asthmatic children aged five to 18: a systematic review. *JBI Database Syst Rev Implement Rep.* 2016;14:113–138.
23. Fitzpatrick AM. Severe asthma in children: lessons learned and future directions. *J Allergy Clin Immunol Pract.* 2016;4:11–19. quiz 20–21.
24. Taylor DR, Bateman ED, Boulet LP, et al. A new perspective on concepts of asthma severity and control. *Eur Respir J.* 2008;32:545–554.
25. Bousquet J, Mantzouranis E, Cruz AA, et al. Uniform definition of asthma severity, control, and exacerbations: document presented for the World Health Organization Consultation on Severe Asthma. *J Allergy Clin Immunol.* 2010;126:926–938.
26. Bush A, Zar HJ. WHO universal definition of severe asthma. *Curr Opin Allergy Clin Immunol.* 2011;11:115–121.
27. Global Initiative for Asthma. *Global Strategy for Asthma Management and Prevention*; 2017. Available from: http://www.ginasthma.org.
28. Krishnan JA, Bender BG, Wamboldt FS, et al. Adherence to inhaled corticosteroids: an ancillary study of the Childhood Asthma Management Program clinical trial. *J Allergy Clin Immunol.* 2012;129:112–118.
29. Melani AS, Bonavia M, Cilenti V, et al. Inhaler mishandling remains common in real life and is associated with reduced disease control. *Respir Med.* 2011;105:930–938.
30. Sleath B, Ayala GX, Gillette C, et al. Provider demonstration and assessment of child device technique during pediatric asthma visits. *Pediatrics.* 2011;127:642–648.

31. Reznik M, Silver EJ, Cao Y. Evaluation of MDI-spacer utilization and technique in caregivers of urban minority children with persistent asthma. *J Asthma*. 2014;51:149–154.

32. Juniper EF, Gruffydd-Jones K, Ward S, Svensson K. Asthma Control Questionnaire in children: validation, measurement properties, interpretation. *Eur Respir J*. 2010;36:1410–1416.

33. Juniper EF, O'Byrne PM, Guyatt GH, Ferrie PJ, King DR. Development and validation of a questionnaire to measure asthma control. *Eur Respir J*. 1999;14:902–907.

34. Schatz M, Sorkness CA, Li JT, et al. Asthma Control Test: reliability, validity, and responsiveness in patients not previously followed by asthma specialists. *J Allergy Clin Immunol*. 2006;117:549–556.

35. Liu AH, Zeiger R, Sorkness C, et al. Development and cross-sectional validation of the childhood asthma control test. *J Allergy Clin Immunol*. 2007;119:817–825.

36. National Asthma Education, Prevention Panel. Expert Panel report 3 (EPR-3): guidelines for the diagnosis and management of asthma-summary report 2007. *J Allergy Clin Immunol*. 2007;120:S94–S138.

37. Quanjer PH, Stanojevic S, Cole TJ, et al. Multi-ethnic reference values for spirometry for the 3-95-yr age range: the global lung function 2012 equations. *Eur Respir J*. 2012;40:1324–1343.

38. Denlinger LC, Phillips BR, Ramratnam S, et al. Inflammatory and comorbid features of patients with severe asthma and frequent exacerbations. *Am J Respir Crit Care Med*. 2017;195:302–313.

39. Fitzpatrick AM, Gaston BM, Erzurum SC, Teague WG. National institutes of health/national heart lung and blood Institute severe asthma research program. Features of severe asthma in school-age children: atopy and increased exhaled nitric oxide. *J Allergy Clin Immunol*. 2006;118:1218–1225.

40. Fleming L, Murray C, Bansal AT, et al. The burden of severe asthma in childhood and adolescence: results from the paediatric U-BIOPRED cohorts. *Eur Respir J*. 2015;46:1322–1333.

41. Jarjour NN, Erzurum SC, Bleecker ER, et al. Severe asthma: lessons learned from the national Heart, lung, and blood Institute severe asthma research program. *Am J Respir Crit Care Med*. 2012;185:356–362.

42. Moore WC, Fitzpatrick AM, Li X, et al. Clinical heterogeneity in the severe asthma research program. *Ann Am Thorac Soc*. 2013;(suppl 10):S118–S124.

43. Fitzpatrick AM, Teague WG, National Institutes of Health/National Heart L, Blood Institute's Severe Asthma Research P. Progressive airflow limitation is a feature of children with severe asthma. *J Allergy Clin Immunol*. 2011;127:282–284.

44. Sorkness RL, Teague WG, Penugonda M, Fitzpatrick AM. National institutes of health national heart, lung and blood Institute's severe asthma research P. Sex dependence of airflow limitation and air trapping in children with severe asthma. *J Allergy Clin Immunol*. 2011;127:1073–1074.

45. Tai A, Tran H, Roberts M, et al. Outcomes of childhood asthma to the age of 50 years. *J Allergy Clin Immunol*. 2014;133:1572–1578.e3.

46. Tai A, Tran H, Roberts M, Clarke N, Wilson J, Robertson CF. The association between childhood asthma and adult chronic obstructive pulmonary disease. *Thorax*. 2014;69:805–810.

47. Schatz M, Hsu JW, Zeiger RS, et al. Phenotypes determined by cluster analysis in severe or difficult-to-treat asthma. *J Allergy Clin Immunol*. 2014;133:1549–1556.

48. Fitzpatrick AM, Teague WG, Meyers DA, et al. Heterogeneity of severe asthma in childhood: confirmation by cluster analysis of children in the national institutes of health/national Heart, lung, and blood Institute severe asthma research program. *J Allergy Clin Immunol*. 2011;127:382–389.e1–e13.

49. Just J, Saint-Pierre P, Gouvis-Echraghi R, et al. Childhood allergic asthma is not a single phenotype. *J Pediatr*. 2014;164:815–820.

50. Just J, Gouvis-Echraghi R, Rouve S, Wanin S, Moreau D, Annesi-Maesano I. Two novel, severe asthma phenotypes identified during childhood using a clustering approach. *Eur Respir J*. 2012;40:55–60.

51. Chang TS, Lemanske Jr RF, Mauger DT, et al. Childhood asthma clusters and response to therapy in clinical trials. *J Allergy Clin Immunol*. 2014;133:363–369.

52. Haland G, Carlsen KC, Sandvik L, et al. Reduced lung function at birth and the risk of asthma at 10 years of age. *N Engl J Med*. 2006;355:1682–1689.

53. Stern DA, Morgan WJ, Wright AL, Guerra S, Martinez FD. Poor airway function in early infancy and lung function by age 22 years: a non-selective longitudinal cohort study. *Lancet*. 2007;370:758–764.

54. Altes TA, Mugler 3rd JP, Ruppert K, et al. Clinical correlates of lung ventilation defects in asthmatic children. *J Allergy Clin Immunol*. 2016;137:789–796.e7.

55. Saglani S, Malmstrom K, Pelkonen AS, et al. Airway remodeling and inflammation in symptomatic infants with reversible airflow obstruction. *Am J Respir Crit Care Med*. 2005;171:722–727.

56. Saglani S, Payne DN, Zhu J, et al. Early detection of airway wall remodeling and eosinophilic inflammation in preschool wheezers. *Am J Respir Crit Care Med*. 2007;176:858–864.

57. Lezmi G, Gosset P, Deschildre A, et al. Airway remodeling in preschool children with severe recurrent wheeze. *Am J Respir Crit Care Med*. 2015;192:164–171.

58. Hauk PJ, Krawiec M, Murphy J, et al. Neutrophilic airway inflammation and association with bacterial lipopolysaccharide in children with asthma and wheezing. *Pediatr Pulmonol*. 2008;43:916–923.

59. Marguet C, Bocquel N, Benichou J, et al. Neutrophil but not eosinophil inflammation is related to the severity of a first acute epidemic bronchiolitis in young infants. *Pediatr Allergy Immunol*. 2008;19:157–165.

60. Marguet C, Jouen-Boedes F, Dean TP, Warner JO. Bronchoalveolar cell profiles in children with asthma, infantile wheeze, chronic cough, or cystic fibrosis. *Am J Respir Crit Care Med*. 1999;159:1533–1540.

61. Szefler SJ, Chmiel JF, Fitzpatrick AM, et al. Asthma across the ages: knowledge gaps in childhood asthma. *J Allergy Clin Immunol.* 2014;133:3–13. quiz 4.

62. Murphy KR, Zeiger RS, Kosinski M, et al. Test for respiratory and asthma control in kids (TRACK): a caregiver-completed questionnaire for preschool-aged children. *J Allergy Clin Immunol.* 2009;123: 833–839.e9.

63. Chipps B, Zeiger RS, Murphy K, et al. Longitudinal validation of the test for respiratory and asthma control in kids in pediatric practices. *Pediatrics.* 2011;127: e737–e747.

64. Zeiger RS, Mellon M, Chipps B, et al. Test for respiratory and asthma control in kids (TRACK): clinically meaningful changes in score. *J Allergy Clin Immunol.* 2011;128:983–988.

65. Guilbert TW, Mauger DT, Allen DB, et al. Growth of preschool children at high risk for asthma 2 years after discontinuation of fluticasone. *J Allergy Clin Immunol.* 2011;128:956–963.e1–e7.

66. Ducharme FM, Lemire C, Noya FJ, et al. Preemptive use of high-dose fluticasone for virus-induced wheezing in young children. *N Engl J Med.* 2009;360:339–353.

67. Barnes PJ. Corticosteroid resistance in patients with asthma and chronic obstructive pulmonary disease. *J Allergy Clin Immunol.* 2013;131:636–645.

68. Bossley CJ, Saglani S, Kavanagh C, et al. Corticosteroid responsiveness and clinical characteristics in childhood difficult asthma. *Eur Respir J.* 2009;34:1052–1059.

69. Bossley CJ, Fleming L, Ullmann N, et al. Assessment of corticosteroid response in pediatric patients with severe asthma by using a multidomain approach. *J Allergy Clin Immunol.* 2016;138:413–420.e6.

70. Ducharme FM, Lasserson TJ, Cates CJ. Long-acting beta2-agonists versus anti-leukotrienes as add-on therapy to inhaled corticosteroids for chronic asthma. *Cochrane Database Syst Rev.* 2006. http://dx.doi.org/10.1002/14651858. CD003137.pub2.

71. Chauhan BF, Chartrand C, Ni Chroinin M, Milan SJ, Ducharme FM. Addition of long-acting beta2-agonists to inhaled corticosteroids for chronic asthma in children. *Cochrane Database Syst Rev.* 2015. http://dx.doi.org/10.1002/14651858. CD007949.pub2.

72. Lemanske Jr RF, Mauger DT, Sorkness CA, et al. Step-up therapy for children with uncontrolled asthma receiving inhaled corticosteroids. *N Engl J Med.* 2010;362: 975–985.

73. Wechsler ME, Castro M, Lehman E, et al. Impact of race on asthma treatment failures in the asthma clinical research network. *Am J Respir Crit Care Med.* 2011;184:1247–1253.

74. Stempel DA, Raphiou IH, Kral KM, et al. Serious asthma events with fluticasone plus Salmeterol versus fluticasone alone. *N Engl J Med.* 2016;374:1822–1830.

75. Stempel DA, Szefler SJ, Pedersen S, et al. Safety of adding Salmeterol to fluticasone propionate in children with asthma. *N Engl J Med.* 2016;375:840–849.

76. Butler MG, Zhou EH, Zhang F, et al. Changing patterns of asthma medication use related to US Food and Drug Administration long-acting beta2-agonist regulation from 2005-2011. *J Allergy Clin Immunol.* 2016;137:710–717.

77. Chauhan BF, Ben Salah R, Ducharme FM. Addition of anti-leukotriene agents to inhaled corticosteroids in children with persistent asthma. *Cochrane Database Syst Rev.* 2013. http://dx.doi.org/10.1002/14651858.CD009585. pub2.

78. Pavord I, Woodcock A, Parker D, Rice L, group Ss. Salmeterol plus fluticasone propionate versus fluticasone propionate plus montelukast: a randomised controlled trial investigating the effects on airway inflammation in asthma. *Respir Res.* 2007;8:67.

79. Joos S, Miksch A, Szecsenyi J, et al. Montelukast as add-on therapy to inhaled corticosteroids in the treatment of mild to moderate asthma: a systematic review. *Thorax.* 2008;63:453–462.

80. Evans DJ, Taylor DA, Zetterstrom O, Chung KF, O'Connor BJ, Barnes PJ. A comparison of low-dose inhaled budesonide plus theophylline and high-dose inhaled budesonide for moderate asthma. *N Engl J Med.* 1997;337:1412–1418.

81. Kim JM, Lin SY, Suarez-Cuervo C, et al. Allergen-specific immunotherapy for pediatric asthma and rhinoconjunctivitis: a systematic review. *Pediatrics.* 2013;131:1155–1167.

82. Cox L, Nelson H, Lockey R, et al. Allergen immunotherapy: a practice parameter third update. *J Allergy Clin Immunol.* 2011;127:S1–S55.

83. Ciprandi G, Incorvaia C, Frati F, Italian Study Group on P. Management of polysensitized patient: from molecular diagnostics to biomolecular immunotherapy. *Expert Rev Clin Immunol.* 2015;11:973–976.

84. Normansell R, Walker S, Milan SJ, Walters EH, Nair P. Omalizumab for asthma in adults and children. *Cochrane Database Syst Rev.* 2014. http://dx.doi.org/10.1002/14651858. CD003559.pub4.

85. Powell C, Milan SJ, Dwan K, Bax L, Walters N. Mepolizumab versus placebo for asthma. *Cochrane Database Syst Rev.* 2015. http://dx.doi.org/10.1002/14651858.CD010834. pub2.

86. Bjermer L, Lemiere C, Maspero J, Weiss S, Zangrilli J, Germinaro M. Reslizumab for inadequately controlled asthma with elevated blood eosinophil levels: a randomized phase 3 study. *Chest.* 2016;150:789–798.

87. Corren J, Weinstein S, Janka L, Zangrilli J, Garin M. Phase 3 study of reslizumab in patients with poorly controlled asthma: effects across a broad range of eosinophil counts. *Chest.* 2016;150:799–810.

88. Corren J, Lemanske RF, Hanania NA, et al. Lebrikizumab treatment in adults with asthma. *N Engl J Med.* 2011;365:1088–1098.

89. Wenzel S, Wilbraham D, Fuller R, Getz EB, Longphre M. Effect of an interleukin-4 variant on late phase asthmatic response to allergen challenge in asthmatic patients: results of two phase 2a studies. *Lancet.* 2007;370:1422–1431.

90. Wenzel S, Ford L, Pearlman D, et al. Dupilumab in persistent asthma with elevated eosinophil levels. *N Engl J Med.* 2013;368:2455–2466.

91. Erpenbeck VJ, Popov TA, Miller D, et al. The oral CRTh2 antagonist QAW039 (fevipiprant): a phase II study in uncontrolled allergic asthma. *Pulm Pharmacol Ther.* 2016;39:54–63.

92. Gonem S, Berair R, Singapuri A, et al. Fevipiprant, a prostaglandin D2 receptor 2 antagonist, in patients with persistent eosinophilic asthma: a single-centre, randomised, double-blind, parallel-group, placebo-controlled trial. *Lancet Respir Med.* 2016;4:699–707.

93. Meltzer EO, Chervinsky P, Busse W, et al. Roflumilast for asthma: efficacy findings in placebo-controlled studies. *Pulm Pharmacol Ther.* 2015;(suppl 35):S20–S27.

94. Bateman ED, Goehring UM, Richard F, Watz H. Roflumilast combined with montelukast versus montelukast alone as add-on treatment in patients with moderate-to-severe asthma. *J Allergy Clin Immunol.* 2016;138:142–149.e8.

95. O'Brien CE, Tsirilakis K, Santiago MT, Goldman DL, Vicencio AG. Heterogeneity of lower airway inflammation in children with severe-persistent asthma. *Pediatr Pulmonol.* 2015;50:1200–1204.

96. Fitzpatrick AM, Higgins M, Holguin F, Brown LA, Teague WG. National institutes of health/national Heart lung and blood Institute severe asthma research program. The molecular phenotype of severe asthma in children. *J Allergy Clin Immunol.* 2010;125:851–857.e18.

97. Bossley CJ, Fleming L, Gupta A, et al. Pediatric severe asthma is characterized by eosinophilia and remodeling without T(H)2 cytokines. *J Allergy Clin Immunol.* 2012;129:974–982.e13.

98. Andersson CK, Adams A, Nagakumar P, et al. Intraepithelial neutrophils in pediatric severe asthma are associated with better lung function. *J Allergy Clin Immunol.* 2016;139(6).

99. Kew KM, Dahri K. Long-acting muscarinic antagonists (LAMA) added to combination long-acting beta2-agonists and inhaled corticosteroids (LABA/ICS) versus LABA/ICS for adults with asthma. *Cochrane Database Syst Rev.* 2016. http://dx.doi.org/10.1002/14651858.CD011721.pub2.

100. Anderson DE, Kew KM, Boyter AC. Long-acting muscarinic antagonists (LAMA) added to inhaled corticosteroids (ICS) versus the same dose of ICS alone for adults with asthma. *Cochrane Database Syst Rev.* 2015. http://dx.doi.org/10.1002/14651858.CD011437.pub2.

101. Szefler SJ, Murphy K, Harper 3rd T, et al. A phase III randomized controlled trial of tiotropium add-on therapy in children with severe symptomatic asthma. *J Allergy Clin Immunol.* 2017. http://dx.doi.org/10.1016/j.jaci.2017.01.014.

102. Hamelmann E, Bateman ED, Vogelberg C, et al. Tiotropium add-on therapy in adolescents with moderate asthma: a 1-year randomized controlled trial. *J Allergy Clin Immunol.* 2016;138:441–450.e8.

103. Torrego A, Sola I, Munoz AM, et al. Bronchial thermoplasty for moderate or severe persistent asthma in adults. *Cochrane Database Syst Rev.* 2014;3. http://dx.doi.org/10.1002/14651858.CD009910.pub2.

104. Zhou JP, Feng Y, Wang Q, Zhou LN, Wan HY, Li QY. Long-term efficacy and safety of bronchial thermoplasty in patients with moderate-to-severe persistent asthma: a systemic review and meta-analysis. *J Asthma.* 2016;53:94–100.

CHAPTER 5

Exhaled Nitric Oxide as a Biomarker for Asthma Management

JOSEPH D. SPAHN, MD • JONATHAN MALKA, MD

ABBREVIATIONS

ACT   Asthma Control Test
ATS   American Thoracic Society
BHR   Bronchial hyperresponsiveness
BDR   Bronchodilator response
cACT   Childhood Asthma Control Test
EG2+   Activated eosinophils
FeNO   Fraction of exhaled nitric oxide
FEV1   Forced expiratory volume in 1 s
GATA   DNA sequence characterized by "GATA"
GERD   Gastroesophageal reflux disease
GC   Glucocorticoid
ICU   Intensive care unit
IFNγ   Interferon gamma
IL   Interleukin
IL-4Rα   Interleukin-4 receptor-α
LABA   Long-acting β-agonist
NO   Nitric oxide
NOS   Nitric oxide synthase
PEF   Peak expiratory flow
RBM   Reticular basement membrane
RR   Relative risk
RTI   Respiratory tract infection
TARC   Thymus and activation-regulated chemokine
Th2   T-helper cell type 2
TLC   Total lung capacity

INTRODUCTION

Although exhaled nitric oxide (termed fraction of exhaled nitric oxide, or FeNO) testing has been available for nearly 15 years, its use as a tool in the management asthma has been limited because of issues with insurance reimbursement, delay in the publication of an American Thoracic Society (ATS) practice guideline for the clinical use of FeNO (2011),[1] and controversy whether FeNO measurement provides added information to that achieved by following guidelines-based management (as reviewed in Ref. 2). As will be

discussed in this chapter, numerous studies evaluating FeNO's use in clinical practice have shown it aids in determination of asthma severity and control and in making the diagnosis of asthma. FeNO can also provide information that lung function or symptoms cannot provide, such as predicting response to glucocorticoid (GC) therapy, and more recently biologic agents such as omalizumab, lebrikizumab, and dupilumab. In addition, FeNO provides information regarding the presence and degree of airway inflammation; it can be used as an objective measure of adherence with inhaled GC therapy in many asthmatics, although a subgroup of severe asthmatics will continue to display elevated FeNO levels despite adequate adherence. FeNO can also be used to predict asthma exacerbations, and it can identify asthmatics with a more reactive phenotype independent of asthma severity.

HOW IS NITRIC OXIDE MEASURED AND HOW IS IT PRODUCED?

FeNO is measured by inhaling to total lung capacity (TLC), followed by exhalation at a steady flow rate (50 mL/s) for 6–10 s. It takes minutes to perform and only one successful effort is required. Children as young as 5 years can perform this test if the exhalation time is reduced to 6 s. FeNO levels are elevated in allergic/eosinophilic-driven lung diseases, while levels are low/normal in neutrophil-mediated diseases. The ATS uses cut-points, rather than reference ranges, when interpreting FeNO levels. Levels of <25 in adults (<20 children) are considered low, intermediate levels are 25–50 in adults (20–35 children), while high levels are >50 ppb in adults (>35 children). FeNO is not correlated with baseline FEV1, while being positively correlated with the change in FEV1 following the administration of a bronchodilator. FeNO can be influenced by a number of factors including age and height (levels rise in childhood because of increases in both lung and airway size as children grow), cigarette smoking (associated with reductions in FeNO), ingestion of nitrate-rich foods (increases FeNO), allergic rhinitis (slight elevations in FeNO), and lastly, measurement should come before spirometry and/or bronchodilator administration as both may slightly increase FeNO levels.

NO is synthesized by inducible NOS (iNOS) that is constitutively expressed in respiratory epithelium, but it can also be upregulated by inflammatory cytokines.[3] In nonasthmatics, IFNγ appears to be involved in the continuous expression of iNOS, while in asthmatics, interleukin (IL)-4 and IL-13 induce iNOS expression. IL-4 and IL-13 expression is regulated by the transcription factor GATA-3, which is expressed predominantly by T-helper type 2 (Th2) cells.[3] Inducible NOS is markedly upregulated in the bronchial epithelium of asthmatics and its expression correlates with FeNO levels.[4]

FRACTION OF EXHALED NITRIC OXIDE IS A MARKER INTERLEUKIN-4 AND INTERLEUKIN-13-MEDIATED INFLAMMATION

FeNO levels are elevated in atopic or "Th2-mediated" asthma, while often being normal in nonatopic or "non-Th2" asthma.[5] Over 80% of children and 50%–60% of adults have the Th2-mediated phenotype of asthma. FeNO correlates positively with total and specific IgE levels and increases during environmental allergen exposure.[6] Although associated with atopy, FeNO is more than just a marker of atopy. Rather, it is a noninvasive measure of Th2-mediated airway inflammation.[7] As FeNO is positively correlated with sputum eosinophils,[8-10] it has long been considered a surrogate of eosinophilic inflammation that has been the "gold standard" noninvasive measure of asthmatic inflammation. With the realization that FeNO is produced as a consequence of IL-4 and IL-13 expression, while eosinophilia is the result of IL-5 expression, FeNO is not a surrogate of eosinophilic inflammation at all, but rather a marker of allergic (IL-4 and IL-13-mediated) inflammation (see Fig. 5.1). The association between FeNO and sputum eosinophilia likely exists because IL-5 is often produced in parallel with IL-4 and IL-13 by activated Th2 cells. Evidence for this "paradigm shift" comes from the finding that FeNO is not influenced by mepolizumab, an anti-IL-5 monoclonal antibody that abolishes circulating and airway eosinophils,[11,12] while dupilumab, an IL-4 receptor α (IL-4Rα) antagonist, which inhibits the function of both IL-4 and IL-13, has no effect on eosinophils, while significantly reducing in FeNO levels.[13,14]

Thus, both biomarkers likely measure distinct aspects of Th2-mediated airway inflammation and should be viewed as equally important in the assessment of this phenotype of asthma. IL-4 and IL-13, acting alone or in concert, are required for IgE synthesis and the expansion of Th2 cells. They are also involved in goblet cell hyperplasia and mucus production, smooth muscle hyperplasia, and subepithelial fibrosis.[15-17] IL-5-mediated eosinophil activation is associated with airway epithelial damage and in the pathogenesis of asthma exacerbations.[18,19] Studies to date have demonstrated anti-IL-5 therapy to significantly reduce exacerbations in severe eosinophilic asthmatics,[11,12,20] while having little effect on lung function, symptoms, bronchial hyperresponsiveness (BHR), and no effect on the allergen-induced late-phase response, despite inhibiting the influx of eosinophils into the airway postchallenge.[21] Anti-IL-4Rα therapy reduces asthma exacerbations, improves lung function, and reduces symptoms, while significantly inhibiting FeNO, even after inhaled GC therapy is withdrawn[13,14] (see Fig. 5.1).

A study comparing the clinical utility of both FeNO and sputum eosinophils was the goal of a study by Covar et al,[10] where over 100 children with mild to moderate asthma performed both measures on completion of long-term inhaled GC therapy and after a 4-month washout period. Both measures provided similar information with respect to asthma severity and control, but from a practical standpoint, FeNO was felt to be superior to sputum induction. Sputum induction was time-consuming (2.5 h for collection and processing), required technical expertise, and could only be performed serially in 66% of children, whereas FeNO took minutes to perform, over 90% of were able to successfully perform serial FeNO measures, and technical expertise was not required. The authors concluded that sputum induction was not a practical method of assessing airway inflammation, while FeNO, which provided similar information, could be easily and quickly performed.

FRACTION OF EXHALED NITRIC OXIDE IS A DIAGNOSTIC TEST FOR ASTHMA

Once it was established that FeNO was elevated in patients with asthma, a number of studies were performed to determine if FeNO could be used to diagnose asthma. The first study evaluated the ability of FeNO to diagnose asthma in 250 adults with respiratory symptoms consistent with asthma.[22] Patients diagnosed with asthma (≥12% improvement in FEV1 following bronchodilator administration or positive

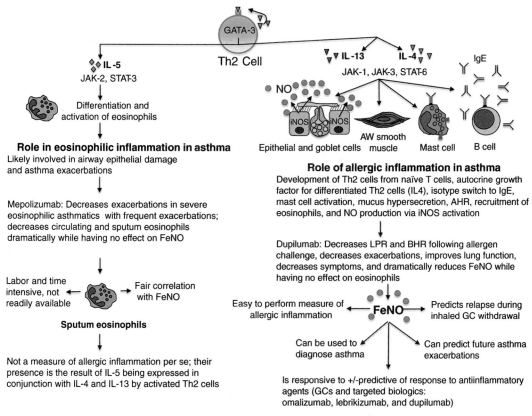

FIG. 5.1 FeNO is produced as a consequence of interleukin (IL)-13 and IL-4-mediated allergic inflammation. Allergic inflammation is involved in both the initiation and maintenance of airway inflammation seen in asthma, while eosinophilic inflammation is likely involved in epithelial damage and in the pathogenesis of asthma exacerbations. Because FeNO is a direct measure of local airway inflammation, it is an ideal noninvasive measure of Th2-mediated inflammation. FeNO levels fall with dupilumab therapy (an inhibitor of both IL-4 and IL-13), while mepolizumab therapy (an inhibitor of IL-5) has no effect on FeNO, suggesting that these are two distinct aspects of airway inflammation. *AW*, airway; *BHR*, bronchial hyperresponsiveness; *FeNO*, fraction of exhaled nitric oxide; *GC*, glucocorticoid; *iNOS*, inducible nitric oxide synthase; *JAK*, Janus kinase; *LPR*, late-phase asthmatic response; *mAB*, monoclonal antibody; *NO*, nitric oxide; *STAT*, signal transducer and activator of transcription; *Th2*, T-helper type 2 cell. (From Spahn JD, et al. Current application of exhaled nitric oxide in clinical practice. *J Allergy Clin Immunol.* 2016;138:1296–1298 with permission.)

methacholine challenge) had elevated FeNO levels compared with those who did not have asthma. At a cutoff of 16 ppb, there was 90% specificity and >90% positive predictive value (PPV) for asthma, while the best specificity (80%) and sensitivity (85%) for asthma occurred at a cut-point of 13 ppb. Asthma could be excluded in 95% of patients whose values were <8 ppb, while asthma could be diagnosed 95% if the FeNO was >18 ppb. A similarly designed study compared the predictive values of FeNO and sputum eosinophils with those of spirometry.[23] Sputum eosinophilia (>3%) and a FeNO level of >20 ppb had similar specificities (~79%) and sensitivities (~88%) and both were superior to a baseline FEV1 <80% predicted or an FEV1/FVC <70% in diagnosing asthma. FeNO was deemed superior to sputum induction in diagnosing asthma because of its ease of use.

Similar findings were noted in studies using FeNO in children with suspected asthma. Children diagnosed with asthma had elevated FeNO levels and sputum eosinophilia compared with those without asthma, with the area under the receiver operating curve for FeNO 0.906, for sputum eosinophils 0.921, and for FEV1 0.606.[24] The best FeNO cut-point for asthma diagnosis was 19 ppb and for sputum eosinophils 2.7%. Both biomarkers were far superior to FEV1. Based on the above studies, patients with suspected asthma with low eNO levels are unlikely to have asthma, whereas patients with elevated FeNO levels have a high probability of having asthma. Although not specifically addressed in the above studies, FeNO's utility in diagnosing asthma is likely limited to patients who have a Th2-mediated phenotype of asthma.

FRACTION OF EXHALED NITRIC OXIDE AND WHEEZING PHENOTYPES

Only one-third of infants/young children with recurrent wheeze will develop childhood asthma, with early-onset aeroallergen sensitization the most strongly associated risk factor for subsequent asthma.[25] As FeNO is a marker of allergic inflammation, it may serve to identify wheezing phenotypes that are likely to result in asthma. A number of studies have found FeNO to be a measure/predictor of asthma in infants who have persistent wheeze. FeNO seems to be elevated early in this group of wheezing infants as described by Debley et al.,[26] who compared lung function with FeNO in wheezing toddlers followed over time. Toddlers with elevated FeNO had a bronchodilator response (BDR) and were likely to experience lung function decline over time. In addition, FeNO best predicted exacerbations, with the risk of an exacerbation increasing 3.3-fold for every 10 ppb increase in FeNO. FeNO has also been compared with interrupter resistance (Rint) in preschool-aged wheezers to predict asthma in grade school.[27] After adjustment for maternal atopy, eczema, and symptom frequency, FeNO was identified as an independent predictor of asthma at 8 years. Two large birth cohort studies using cluster analyses identified either four or six clusters, half being associated with transient, nonatopic wheeze phenotypes, while the other half is associated with persistent wheeze phenotypes and early-onset aeroallergen sensitization. The transient wheezers, when assessed in midchildhood were less likely to have asthma, did not have BHR, and had normal FeNO levels. Children with histories of persistent wheezing phenotypes were more likely to have asthma, have BHR, and have associated elevated FeNO levels.[27,28] Lastly, the functional outcome of early life airway inflammation and airway wall remodeling was assessed in a cohort of children with severe early-onset

wheezing.[29] Lung function impairment was already evident by age 5 years, yet there was no correlation between reticular basement membrane (RBM) thickening and any lung function measurement. In contrast, FeNO correlated with the number of EG2+ cells (activated eosinophils) and RBM, suggesting that allergic airway inflammation as measured by FeNO persisted from 2 to 5 years of life.

FRACTION OF EXHALED NITRIC OXIDE IS A MEASURE OF ASTHMA SEVERITY AND CONTROL

FeNO can be used to provide complementary information to that achieved by symptom frequency and lung function as demonstrated by a number of studies. A large study of adult asthmatics tested the ability of FeNO to both reflect and predict improving or worsening asthma control.[30] Approximately 75% of newly diagnosed asthmatics were poorly controlled as measured by symptoms and lung function. Poorly controlled asthmatics had elevated FeNO levels at baseline, but following institution of inhaled GC therapy, over two-thirds of these subjects were considered well controlled. A baseline FeNO >35 ppb or a fall in FeNO of >40% was predictor of a positive response to inhaled GC therapy. In contrast, an improvement in FEV1 of ≥5% was not predictive of a favorable response. During the study, 20% of the well-controlled asthmatics lost control. A ≥30% increase in FeNO was associated with loss of asthma control in these subjects, while patients with normal FeNO levels at baseline were likely to remain well controlled.

In a private practice setting, FeNO was found to correlate with recent asthma symptoms, need for daily rescue bronchodilator therapy, dyspnea, and BDR, while having no relationship to asthma severity.[31] In a childhood asthma study, FeNO was compared with lung function and the childhood Asthma Control Test (cACT).[32] Suboptimal control (cACT ≤19) was identified in 43% of the newly diagnosed asthmatics versus only 14% of the established patients, while elevated FeNO levels were noted in 66% versus 44% of newly diagnosed and established asthmatics, respectively. FeNO correlated with cACT only in newly diagnosed asthmatics. Even though most established asthmatics had cACT scores of >19, FeNO was elevated in many, suggesting that despite good symptom control, ongoing allergic inflammation persisted. A small group of asthmatics with poor control also had low FeNO levels, suggesting that poor asthma control may have been due to comorbid conditions such as gastroesophageal reflux or sinusitis, as opposed to inadequately treated airway inflammation.

FRACTION OF EXHALED NITRIC OXIDE IS A PREDICTOR OF ASTHMA RELAPSE DURING INHALED GLUCOCORTICOID REDUCTION

As FeNO levels fall rapidly when inhaled GC therapy is initiated and rise as rapidly when they are withdrawn,[33] studies were designed to determine if FeNO could be used to predict worsening asthma control during inhaled GC reduction or withdrawal. Studies in children with varying levels of disease severity addressed this hypothesis with all reaching the same conclusion[34–36] that elevated FeNO levels at baseline or increasing FeNO levels during the inhaled GC taper predicted children who would fail inhaled GC reduction or withdrawal.

Studies in adult asthmatics have yielded conflicting results. One study where inhaled GC therapy was discontinued found highly significant correlations between the change in FeNO after withdrawal and increased symptoms, sputum eosinophils, and BHR in the subjects who exacerbated.[37] A similarly designed study evaluating adult asthmatics failed to identify FeNO as a predictor for loss of asthma control.[38] Hyperresponsiveness to histamine and mannitol at baseline and elevated sputum eosinophils before the last successful iGC reduction predicted a failed inhaled GC reduction, while FeNO, spirometry, and symptoms did not.

Thus, children with elevated FeNO levels at baseline or children whose FeNO levels rise during an inhaled GC taper are not good candidates for inhaled GC reduction, while children with normal baseline FeNO levels and those whose FeNO levels do not rise during the inhaled GC reduction are likely to be successfully tapered. This is an important use for FeNO, because all who care for children with asthma want to use the lowest inhaled GC as possible to maintain good asthma control. Of note, many of the children studied were able to safely tolerate some degree of reduction in their inhaled GC dose.

FRACTION OF EXHALED NITRIC OXIDE IS A PREDICTOR OF ASTHMA EXACERBATIONS

The above studies demonstrated that FeNO could predict "induced-exacerbations" in patients who had their inhaled GC dose tapered or withdrawn. Whether FeNO could predict asthma exacerbations in a "real-world" setting was then evaluated. Adults with moderate persistent

asthma on a fixed dose of inhaled GC/LABA therapy were prospectively studied over 1-year.[39] Diminished FEV1 and elevated FeNO at baseline were independent predictors of an exacerbation in the 50% of subjects who exacerbated during the 1-year study. A baseline FeNO ≥28 ppb increased the relative risk (RR) for an exacerbation by 3.4-fold, while an FEV1 ≤76%, increased the RR by 1.7-fold. Patients with low lung function and elevated FeNO were at greatest risk, while none of the patients with normal FeNO and FEV1 levels suffered an exacerbation.

FeNO, FEV1, and quality of life (QOL) scores at the time of a routine clinic visit were evaluated to predict subsequent exacerbations in adults with severe asthma.[40] At the initial clinic visit, there were no differences in FEV1 or QOL scores, while FeNO levels were twice as high in subjects who exacerbated compared with those who did not exacerbate. A large retrospective study of atopic asthmatics assessed of the utility of FeNO, independent of ACT or FEV1, to predict an asthma exacerbation in the preceding year.[41] Higher FeNO levels correlated with a greater number of asthma exacerbations and were associated with overuse of short-acting β-agonists. A prospective study using the same cohort of asthmatics was then performed that replicated the above findings.[42]

Whether FeNO or a BDR, individually or in combination, could predict subsequent loss of asthma control was studied in inhaled GC naïve asthmatic children.[43] During the monitoring period, 77% of the children had at least one elevated FeNO (≥35 ppb). Children with ≥1 elevated FeNO level were 4.6 times more likely to lose asthma control during the observation period, while children with a BDR had a 3.3-fold increased risk. Children with an elevated FeNO level and a positive BDR were 6.9 times as likely to exacerbate. Lastly, whether FeNO was related to respiratory tract illnesses (RTIs) in preschool children with recurrent wheezing found FeNO to be associated with increased risk of developing an RTI (OR 3.0), and after controlling for confounding factors, the risk increased further to 3.8.[44]

FRACTION OF EXHALED NITRIC OXIDE IS A PREDICTOR OF NONADHERENCE TO INHALED GLUCOCORTICOID THERAPY

Although suboptimal adherence to inhaled GC therapy is an important reason for poor asthma control, it has been difficult to assess. Delgado-Corcoran et al. found FeNO to be inversely related to inhaled GC adherence (r = −0.76; P = .001).[45] Children with good adherence had significantly lower FeNO levels (35 ppb) compared with those with moderate (96 ppb) or poor adherence (130 ppb). FEV1, on the other hand, was unable to distinguish children with good compared with poor adherence. Another study found FeNO to be more responsive to changes in inhaled GC dosing than spirometry. FeNO was also found to be inversely related to adherence.[46] A third study found that the magnitude of change in FeNO after directly observed inhaled GC therapy predicted good versus poor adherence among adults with severe persistent asthma.[47] A fall in FeNO of 42% between day 1 and 5 of observed therapy identified patients who were poorly adherent, with a sensitivity 0.67, a specificity 0.95, a negative predictive value (NPV) 78%, and a PPV of 92%.

FRACTION OF EXHALED NITRIC OXIDE AS A MARKER OF SEVERE ASTHMA

There was initial concern that FeNO monitoring in severe asthma would not be useful, given that GC, when administered in high doses, could directly suppress iNOS expression independent of its ability to inhibit airway inflammation. This concern ended up being unfounded, when Silkoff et al.[48] reported that 50% of adults with severe asthma had elevated FeNO levels and airway eosinophilia. Those with elevated FeNO levels were younger, more symptomatic, and had greater RBM thickening compared with the severe asthmatics with normal FeNO values. FeNO also identified a phenotype of reactive and at-risk asthmatics independent of asthma severity based on asthma guidelines.[49] Subjects with elevated FeNO (≥35 ppb) had greater BHR, BDR, air-trapping, higher circulating and sputum eosinophils, and greater atopy, and were more likely to had a past intensive care unit (ICU) admission or intubation compared with subjects with low FeNO levels. FeNO has also been used as a biomarker to better investigate the molecular basis of asthma phenotypes. By linking FeNO to bronchial airway epithelial cell gene expression, over 500 genes were identified that either positively or negatively correlated with FeNO.[50] Three of the five subject clusters (SCs) identified were associated with elevated FeNO levels, with majority of severe asthmatics found within these clusters.

Elevated FeNO levels are also seen in children with severe asthma.[51] All of the children with severe asthma were atopic and had FeNO levels twice that of children with moderate asthma. Children with severe asthma also had greater airflow limitation and BHR and had required more prednisone, ED visits, and hospitalizations. Lastly, during a 5-year observation period, adults with severe asthma who displayed an accelerated decline in FEV1 (40 mL/year) had elevated FeNO levels at baseline compared with those without a rapid decline.[52] Of interest, those at greatest risk of accelerated lung function decline had normal lung function while having elevated FeNO levels.

FRACTION OF EXHALED NITRIC OXIDE IS A PREDICTOR OF RESPONSE TO GLUCOCORTICOID THERAPY

Soon after it was discovered that sputum eosinophilia predicted response to inhaled GC therapy,[53] studies were performed to determine if FeNO could also predict response to GCs. The first study compared FeNO and sputum eosinophilia to predict a ≥15% improvement in FEV1 following a short course of prednisone.[54] Both biomarkers predicted a favorable response, but FeNO had a higher PPV compared with sputum eosinophilia (83 vs. 68%). A dose escalating study of fluticasone propionate (FP) and beclomethasone dipropionate (BDP) found significant variability in response to both FEV1 and methacholine responsiveness.[55] Elevated FeNO levels predicted an FEV1 response, while sputum eosinophilia predicted a favorable methacholine response. Studies in children with mild to moderate asthma have also found FeNO to be both a short- and long-term predictor of inhaled GC response.[56,57] Smith et al.,[58] compared FeNO with several conventional predictors of inhaled GC response and evaluated several measures of response (improvement in FEV1, AM PEF, symptoms, and reduction in BHR). Response to inhaled GC therapy was greatest in patients with the highest FeNO levels for all response measures. FeNO was also found to be superior to the conventional predictors of response. Response (change in FEV1 ≥10%) to intramuscular triamcinolone in adults with stable yet severe asthma found 20% to have favorable response. Although a number of response predictors were studied, only elevated FeNO and a BDR at baseline predicted response to triamcinolone therapy. Patients with a baseline FeNO ≥20 ppb were three times more likely to respond to triamcinolone compared with those with FeNO <20 ppb.

In contrast to the above positive studies, FeNO did not predict response to low-dose BDP in adults with moderate asthma not already receiving inhaled GC therapy.[59] A positive response, defined as ≥5% improvement in baseline FEV1, was noted in only half of the patients studied. Predictors of response included baseline FEV1, FEV1/FVC ratio, and BDR. These subjects may have been non-Th2 asthmatics, as their median FeNO at entry was normal at 13 ppb. FeNO cannot be used to predict inhaled GC response in non-Th2 asthmatics, and this asthma phenotype is also less responsive to inhaled GC therapy. With the above caveat in mind, FeNO seems to be the best predictor of response to inhaled GC therapy. This is an important use of FeNO because it has become clear that not all asthmatics will respond favorably to inhaled GC therapy. In these subjects, the potential adverse effects of inhaled GC therapy can be avoided.

FRACTION OF EXHALED NITRIC OXIDE IS A PREDICTOR OF RESPONSE TO BIOLOGIC AGENTS

Mepolizumab has been shown to be effective in reducing exacerbations in severe eosinophilic asthmatics with frequent exacerbations[11,12,20] (see Fig. 5.1). Although a FeNO level of ≥50 ppb served as a surrogate for eosinophilic inflammation and as such was an inclusion criterion, mepolizumab had no effect on FeNO levels.[12] Neither atopy nor FeNO predicted response to mepolizumab, while baseline circulating eosinophils and exacerbations in the previous year were the only predictors of response. Lebrikizumab, an anti-IL-13 monoclonal antibody, was studied in atopic asthmatics with enrollment criteria elevated FeNO or serum periostin levels.[50] Although lebrikizumab resulted in a modest improvement in FEV1 over placebo, subjects with high periostin or FeNO levels had the largest FEV1 response, while subjects with low periostin and/or FeNO levels had no FEV1 response. As IL-13 induces both epithelial periostin and NO production, both biomarkers were suppressed by and predicted response to lebrikizumab.

Dupilumab, an anti-IL-4 receptor α (IL-4Rα) monoclonal antibody that blocks the effects of both IL-4 and IL-13, reduced asthma exacerbations and symptoms while improving lung function in adults with moderate to severe eosinophilic asthma suboptimally controlled on combination inhaled GC/LABA therapy[13] (see Fig. 5.1). Although, eosinophilia was an entry requirement, dupilumab therapy had no effect on eosinophils, while it significantly decreased FeNO, IgE, eotaxin-3, and thymus and activation-regulated chemokine (TARC) levels. A subsequent dose-ranging study of dupilumub replicated the previous study's findings. Of interest, dupilumab was found to be effective in patients with (≥300/μL) or without eosinophilia (<300/μL), although its effect was greatest in the eosinophilic group.[14] FeNO not only predicted response but was also a response indicator. Eosinophils, on the other hand, were neither predictive of response, nor were they a response measure.

Although omalizumab has been used to treat patients with allergic asthma since 2003, only recently have biomarkers been identified that can predict response to omalizumab therapy. Predictors of response were evaluated in a post hoc analysis of a large study of omalizumab therapy in patients with severe asthma. In that study, there was a 25% reduction in exacerbations in patients treated with omalizumab compared with placebo.[60] FeNO, circulating eosinophils, and serum periostin obtained at baseline were then assessed to determine if they could predict a favorable response to omalizumab therapy.[61] Subjects were divided into "biomarker high" or "biomarker low" groups based on whether the biomarkers were above or below the median. Patients in the "high biomarker" group had the greatest reductions in exacerbations during omalizumab therapy. Specifically, the "high FeNO" group had a 53% reduction, the "high eosinophil" group had a 32% reduction, while the "high periostin" group had a 30% reduction in exacerbations. In contrast, omalizumab did not significantly reduce exacerbations in the "low biomarker" asthmatics compared with placebo. Although FeNO was a predictor of effect, it was not a response marker.

SUMMARY

FeNO is an important tool in the management of asthma. It is an easily and quickly performed maneuver that provides information regarding the type of airway inflammation (elevated in Th2-mediated asthma, low or normal in non-Th2 asthma) in addition to the degree of allergic inflammation. In patients with Th2-mediated phenotypes of asthma, FeNO is superior to symptoms and baseline FEV1, when used to diagnose asthma, to predict response to antiinflammatory therapy, to assess adherence to inhaled GC therapy, to predict exacerbations induced by inhaled GC reduction/withdrawal, and to independently predict future asthma exacerbations. FeNO can also serve as a marker of disease severity and control, providing supplementary information when used in combination with lung function and symptom frequency.

No other single test has been as extensively studied or scrutinized as FeNO, yet its use has been underutilized. Even though FeNO was shown to predict response to inhaled GC therapy a decade ago and could have been an early example of personalized medicine, it was never embraced by the manufacturers of inhaled GCs. Now that expensive biologic agents are available, markers that predict response to these agents will serve an important role in determining the appropriate patients for these drugs. FeNO appears to be among the best markers of response to omalizumab, lebrikizumab, and dupilumab, because it is a point-of-care test and it is quickly, easily, and cheaply measured.

As asthma is a complex disease/syndrome, there is not a single objective measure or tool that has been shown to address every aspect of this disease with respect to its underlying pathophysiology, its many clinical manifestations, or the many aspects of therapy. FeNO, while being a useful tool in patients with Th2-mediated inflammation, has limited its utility in the large number of asthmatics with non-Th2-mediated inflammation[61] where no acceptable markers have been identified. An unresolved question pertains to what constitutes an abnormal FeNO level, and whether validated FeNO cut-points for good, poor, or very poorly controlled asthma will ever be established.

Another important, yet unresolved issue pertains to whether FeNO provides additional information that cannot be obtained by the assessment of symptom control and lung function alone in the day-to-day management of asthma. Although the available data on this important topic are mixed, FeNO is not generally recommended for asthma management, but a systematic assessment of published randomized trials of asthma therapy guided by FeNO concluded that the mixed results of these studies were due to specific design and methodological issues that may have led to incorrect conclusions.[2]

DISCLOSURE
Spahn, JD—has no conflict of interest. Malka, J—has no conflict of interest.

REFERENCES

1. Dweik RA, Boggs PB, Erzurum SC, et al. An official ATS clinical practice guideline: interpretation of exhaled nitric oxide levels (FeNO) for clinical application. *Am J Respir Crit Care Med.* 2011;184:602–615.
2. Gibson PG. Using fractional exhaled nitric oxide to guide asthma therapy: design and methodological issues for ASthma TREatment ALgorithm studies. *Clin Exp Allergy.* 2009;39:478–490.
3. Alving K, Malinvschi A. Basic aspects of exhaled nitric oxide. *Eur Respir Mon.* 2010;49:1–31.
4. Lane C, Knight D, Burgess S, et al. Epithelial inducible nitric oxide synthase activity is the major determinant of nitric oxide concentration in exhaled breath. *Thorax.* 2004;59:757–760.
5. Miraglia del Giudice M, Capasso M, Maiello N, Capristo C, Piacentini GL, Brunese FP. Exhaled nitric oxide and atopy in children. *J Allergy Clin Immunol.* 2003;111:193.
6. Sacco O, Sale R, Silvestri M, et al. Total and allergen-specific IgE levels in serum reflect blood eosinophilia fractional exhaled nitric oxide concentrations but not pulmonary functions in allergic asthmatic children sensitized to house dust mites. *Pediatr Allergy Immunol.* 2003;14:475–481.
7. Lopuhaa CE, Koopmans JG, Jansen HM, et al. Similar levels of nitric oxide in exhaled air in non-asthmatic rhinitis and asthma after bronchial allergen challenge. *Allergy.* 2003;58:300–305.
8. Berlyne GS, Parameswaran K, Kamada D, et al. A comparison of exhaled nitric oxide and induced sputum as markers of airway inflammation. *J Allergy Clin Immunol.* 2000;106:638–644.
9. Warke TJ, Fitch PS, Brown V, et al. Exhaled nitric oxide correlates with airway eosinophils in childhood asthma. *Thorax.* 2002;57:383–387.
10. Covar RA, Spahn JD, Martin RJ, et al. Safety and application of induced sputum analysis in childhood asthma. *J Allergy Clin Immunol.* 2004;114:575–582.
11. Haldar P, Brightling CE, Hargadon B, et al. Mepolizumab and exacerbations of refractory asthma. *N Engl J Med.* 2009;360:973–984.
12. Pavord ID, Korn S, Howarth, et al. Mepolizumab for severe eosinophilic asthma (DREAM): a multicenter, double blind, placebo-controlled trial. *Lancet.* 2012;380:651–659.
13. Wenzel S, Ford L, Pearlman D, et al. Dupilumab in persistent asthma with elevated eosinophil levels. *N Engl J Med.* 2013;368:2455–2466.
14. Wenzel S, Castro M, Corren J, et al. Dupilumab efficacy and safety in adults with uncontrolled persistent asthma despite use of medium-to-high dose inhaled corticosteroids plus a long-acting ß2 agonist: a randomized double-blind placebo-controlled pivotal phase 2b dose ranging trial. *Lancet.* 2016;388:31–34.
15. Izuhara K, Arima K, Kanaji S, et al. IL-13: a promising therapeutic target for bronchial asthma. *Curr Med Chem.* 2006;13:2291–2298.
16. Kuperman DA, Schleimer RP. Interleukin-4, interleukin-13, signal transducer and activator of transcription factor 6, and allergic asthma. *Curr Mol Med.* 2008;8:384–392.
17. Brightling CE, Symon FA, Birring SS, et al. TH2 cytokine expression in bronchoalveolar lavage fluid T lymphocytes and bronchial submucosa is a feature of asthma and eosinophilic bronchitis. *J Allergy Clin Immunol.* 2002;110:899–905.
18. Green RH, Brightling CE, McKenna S, et al. Asthma exacerbations and sputum eosinophil counts: a randomized controlled trial. *Lancet.* 2002;360:1715–1721.
19. Jayaram L, Pizzichini MM, Cook RJ, et al. Determining asthma treatment by monitoring sputum cell counts: effect on exacerbations. *Eur Respir J.* 2006;27:483–494.
20. Nair P, Pizzichini MMM, Kjarsgaard M, et al. Mepolizumab for prednisone-dependent asthma with sputum eosinophilia. *N Engl J Med.* 2009;360:985–993.
21. Leckie MJ, tenBrinke A, Khan J, et al. Effects of an interleukin-5 blocking monoclonal antibody on eosinophils, airway hyperresponsiveness, and the late asthmatic response. *Lancet.* 2000;356:2144–2148.

22. Dupont LJ, Demedts MG, Verleden GM. Prospective evaluation of the validity of exhaled nitric oxide for the diagnosis of asthma. *Chest.* 2003;123:751–756.
23. Smith AD, Cowan JO, Filsell S, et al. Diagnosing Asthma: comparison between exhaled nitric oxide measurements and conventional tests. *Am J Respir Crit Care Med.* 2004;169:473–478.
24. Sivan Y, Gadish T, Fireman E, et al. The use of exhaled nitric oxide in the diagnosis of asthma in school children. *J Pediatr.* 2009;155:211–216.
25. Illi S, von Mutius E, Lau S, et al. Perennial allergen sensitization early in life and chronic asthma: a birth cohort study. *Lancet.* 2006;368:763–770.
26. Debley JS, Stamey DC, Cochrane ES, et al. Exhaled nitric oxide, lung function and, exacerbations in wheezy infants and toddlers. *J Allergy Clin Immunol.* 2010;125: 1228–1234.
27. Caudri D, wijga AH, Hoekstra MO, et al. Prediction of asthma in symptomatic preschool children using exhaled nitric oxide, Rint and specific IgE. *Thorax.* 2010;65: 801–807.
28. Duijts L, Granell R, Sterne JAC, et al. Childhood wheezing phenotypes influence asthma, lung function and exhaled nitric oxide in adolescence. *Eur Respir J.* 2016;47:510–519.
29. Sonnappa S, Bastardo CM, Bush A, et al. Relationship between past airway pathology and current lung function in preschool wheezers. *Eur Respir J.* 2011;38:1431–1436.
30. Michils A, Baldassarre S, Van Muylem A. Exhaled nitric oxide and asthma control: a longitudinal study in unselected patients. *Eur Respir J.* 2008;31:539–546.
31. Sipple JM, Holden WE, Tilles SA, et al. Exhaled nitric oxide levels correlate with measures of disease control in asthma. *J Allergy Clin Immunol.* 2000;106:645–650.
32. Piacentini GL, Peoni DG, Bonafiglia E, et al. Childhood Asthma Control Test and airway inflammation evaluation in asthmatic children. *Allergy.* 2009;64:1753–1757.
33. Kharitonov SA, Donnelly LE, Montuschi P, et al. Dose dependent onset and cessation of action of inhaled budesonide on exhaled nitric oxide and symptoms in mild asthma. *Thorax.* 2002;57:889–896.
34. Zacharasiewicz A, Wilson N, Lex C, et al. Clinical use of noninvasive measurements of airway inflammation in steroid reduction in children. *Am J Respir Crit Care Med.* 2005;171:1077–1082.
35. Pijnenburg MW, Hofhuis W, Hop WC, De Jongste JC. Exhaled nitric oxide predicts asthma relapse in children with clinical asthma remission. *Thorax.* 2005;60:215–218.
36. Jatakkanon A, Lim S, Barnes PJ, et al. Changes in sputum eosinophils predict loss of asthma control. *Am J Respir Crit Care Med.* 2000;161:64–72.
37. Jones SL, McLachlan CR, Kittelson J. The predictive value of exhaled nitric oxide measurements in assessing changes in asthma control. *Am J Respir Crit Care Med.* 2001;164:738–743.
38. Leuppi JD, Salome CM, Jenkins CR, et al. Predictive markers of asthma exacerbation during stepwise dose reduction of inhaled corticosteroids. *Am J Respir Crit Care Med.* 2001;163:406–412.

39. Gelb AF, Taylor CF, Shinar CM, Gutierrez C, Zamel N. Role of spirometry and exhaled nitric oxide to predict exacerbations in treated asthmatics. *Chest.* 2006;129:1492–1499.
40. Harkins MS, Fiato K-L, Iwamoto GK. Exhaled nitric oxide predicts asthma exacerbations. *J Asthma.* 2004;41: 471–476.
41. Zeiger RS, Schatz M, Zhang F, et al. Association of exhaled nitric oxide to asthma burden in asthmatics on inhaled corticosteroids. *J Asthma.* 2011;48:8–17.
42. Zeiger RS, Schatz M, Zhang F, et al. Exhaled nitric oxide is a clinical indicator of future uncontrolled asthma in asthmatic patients on inhaled corticosteroids. *J Allergy Clin Immunol.* 2011;128:412–414.
43. Kim J-K, Jung J-Y, Eom S-Y, et al. Combined use of fractional exhaled nitric oxide and bronchodilator response in predicting future loss of asthma control among children with atopic asthma. *Respirology.* 2016. http://dx.doi.org/10.1111/resp.12934.
44. Beigelman A, Mauger DT, Phillips BR, et al. Effect of elevated exhaled nitric oxide levels on the risk of respiratory tract illness in preschool-aged children with moderate-to-severe intermittent wheezing. *Ann Allergy Asthma Immunol.* 2009;103:108–113.
45. Delgado-Corcoran C, Kissoon N, Murphy SP, et al. Exhaled nitric oxide reflects asthma severity and control. *Pediatr Crit Care Med.* 2004;5:1–10.
46. Beck-Ripp J, Griese M, Arenz S, et al. Changes of exhaled nitric oxide during steroid treatment of childhood asthma. *Eur Respir J.* 2002;19:1015–1019.
47. McNicholl DM, Stevenson M, McGarvey LP, Heaney LG. The utility of fractional exhaled nitric oxide suppression in the identification of nonadherence in difficult asthma. *Am J Respir Crit Care Med.* 2012;186:1102e8.
48. Silkoff PE, Lent AM, Busacker AA, et al. Exhaled nitric oxide identifies the persistent eosinophilic phenotype in severe refractory asthma. *J Allergy Clin Immunol.* 2005;116:1249–1255.
49. Dweik RA, Sorkness RL, Wenzel S, et al. Use of nitric oxide measurement to identify a reactive, at-risk phenotype among patients with asthma. *Am J Respir Crit Care Med.* 2010;181:1033–1041.
50. Modena BD, Tedrow JR, Milosevic J, et al. Gene expression in relation to exhaled nitric oxide identifies novel asthma phenotypes with unique biomolecular pathways. *Am J Respir Crit Care Med.* 2014;190:1363–1372.
51. Fitzpatrick AM, Gaston BM, Erzurum SC, et al. Features of severe asthma in school-age children: atopy and increased nitric oxide. *J Allergy Clin Immunol.* 2006;118:1218–1225.
52. Van Veen IH, Ten Brinke A, Sterk PJ, et al. Exhaled nitric oxide predicts lung function decline in difficult-to-treat asthma. *Eur Respir J.* 2008;32:344–349.
53. Pavord ID, Brightling CE, Woltmann G, et al. Non-eosinophilic corticosteroid unresponsive asthma. *Lancet.* 1999;353:2213–2214.
54. Little SA, Chalmers GW, MacLeod KJ, McSharry C, Thomson NC. Non-invasive markers of airway inflammation as predictors of oral steroid responsiveness in asthma. *Thorax.* 2000;55:232–234.

55. Szefler SJ, Martin RJ, Sharp King T, et al. Significant variability in response to inhaled corticosteroids for persistent asthma. *J Allergy Clin Immunol.* 2002;109:410–418.

56. Szefler SJ, Phillips BR, Martinez, et al. Characterization of within-subject responses to fluticasone and montelukast in childhood asthma. *J Allergy Clin Immunol.* 2005;115:233–242.

57. Knuffman JE, Sorkness CA, Lemanske RF, et al. Phenotypic predictors of long-term response to inhaled corticosteroid and leukotriene modifier therapies in pediatric asthma. *J Allergy Clin Immunol.* 2009;123:411–416.

58. Smith AD, Cowan JO, Brassett KP, et al. Exhaled nitric oxide: a predictor of response. *Am J Respir Crit Care Med.* 2005;172:453–459.

59. Martin RJ, Szefler SJ, King TS, et al. The predicting response to inhaled corticosteroid efficacy (PRICE) trial. *J Allergy Clin Immunol.* 2007;119:73–80.

60. Hanania NA, Alpan O, Hamilos DL, et al. Omalizumab in severe allergic asthma inadequately controlled with standard therapy. *Ann Intern Med.* 2011;154:573–582.

61. Wenzel SE. Asthma phenotypes: the evolution from clinical to molecular approaches. *Nat Med.* 2012;18:716–725.

FURTHER READING

1. Garden FL, Simpson JM, Mellis CM, et al. Change in the manifestations of asthma and asthma-related traits in childhood: a latent transition analysis. *Eur Respir J.* 2016;47:362–365.

2. Phipatanakul W, Mauger DT, Sorkness RL, et al. Effects of age and disease severity on systemic corticosteroid responses in asthma. *Am J Respir Crit Care Med.* 2017;195:1439–1448.

3. Corren JC, Lemanske RF, Hanania NA, et al. Lebrikizumab treatment in adults with asthma. *N Engl J Med.* 2011;365:1088–1098.

4. Hanania NA, Wenzel S, Rosen K, et al. Exploring the effects of omalizumab in allergic asthma: an analysis of biomarkers in the EXTRA study. *Am J Respir Crit Care Med.* 2013;187:804–811.

CHAPTER 6

Blood and Sputum Eosinophils as a Biomarker for Selecting and Adjusting Asthma Medication

CLAUDIA L. GAEFKE, MD • TARA F. CARR, MD

INTRODUCTION

Asthma is a common disorder characterized by chronic inflammation of the airways, bronchial hyperrespon- siveness, and reversible airflow obstruction. Asthma is also a heterogeneous disorder, causing a spectrum of clinical symptoms among patients with varying demo- graphic characteristics. Inherent to the development of personalized medicine approaches to clinical care of asthma is the assumption that underlying the clini- cal heterogeneity is pathobiologic heterogeneity in the processes causing asthma. Determining the inflamma- tory processes relevant to each patient may therefore drive an improved approach to initiating or adjust- ing therapy. Asthma can be dichotomously defined as eosinophilic or noneosinophilic based on the inflam- matory cellular patterns seen in sputum, blood, and tissue compartments, with approximately half of asth- matics falling into each category.[1] Although this distinc- tion does not necessarily elucidate the molecular basis of each individual's asthmatic condition, eosinophilia as a biomarker can be useful toward determining treat- ment options and assessing each patient's response to therapy.

EOSINOPHIL BIOACTIVITY

Eosinophils actively contribute to innate and adaptive immune system responses and inflammatory cascades, through the production and release of diverse chemo- kines, cytokines, lipid mediators, and other growth fac- tors. Eosinophilic granules contain highly charged and active proteins, including major basic protein (MBP)-1 and MBP-2, eosinophil peroxidase (EPX), eosinophil cationic protein, and eosinophil-derived neurotoxin (EDN), that mediate toxicity toward pathogens and tissues and thereby produce a variety of inflammatory

processes that contribute to tissue pathology. MBP-1 and MBP-2 have a markedly basic pH and are directly toxic to host and parasite cells.[2] EDN exerts antiviral effects through RNase activity.[3] EPX catalyzes develop- ment of reactive oxygen species in the presence of hydro- gen peroxide and can induce mast cell degranulation.[4] Eosinophils produce arachidonic acid metabolites such as the cysteinyl leukotrienes and prostaglandins.[5] Eosinophils also store and produce small molecules such as interleukin (IL)-4, IL-5, IL-13, and IL-25, which are pathognomonic of the type-2/type-2-helper (T2/Th2) inflammatory pathway.[6] In turn, IL-5 stimulates bone marrow production and release of eosinophils, which are then recruited to tissues via ICAM-1, P-selectin, and VCAM-1. Following priming with eosinophil hematopoietins, such as IL-5 and GM-CSF, eosinophils exhibit an increased capacity to respond to inflamma- tory mediators. Chemokines, such as CCL5/RANTES, CCL11/eotaxin, and CCL3, are secreted by eosinophils and can recruit leukocytes to the site of eosinophilic inflammation. The recruited Th2 CD4+ lymphocytes chronically contribute to the release of the T2 inflam- matory mediators, which potentiate this cycle. The role of the complex and fascinating cascade of eosinophil bioactivity in the development and potentiation of asthma is an area of active study.

Terms such as "type-2" and "eosinophilic" are not interchangeable, but there is significant overlap in the processes causing each phenotype. Characteristic of atopic disease, the emergent concept of type-2 inflam- mation is initiated by barrier epithelial cells releasing cytokines IL-25, IL-33, and thymic stromal lymphopoi- etin in response to allergen or pathogen stimulation. These cytokines induce dendritic cells toward Th2 cyto- kine production and direct naïve CD4+ cells to develop into Th2 cells. Subsequent secretion of IL-4, IL-5, and

IL-13 results in production of immunoglobulin (Ig)E, IgE-mediated mast cell and basophil degranulation, and eosinophilia.[7] However, while eosinophils are evidence of T2 inflammation, subsets of eosinophilic asthma have divergent cellular pathways, with differences in the degree of atopy and initiating factors.[8] Nonallergic eosinophilic airway inflammation in asthma can be induced by the innate immune pathways via pollutants and microbes inducing epithelial damage, which in turn causes type-2 innate lymphoid cells to release IL-5, stimulating eosinophilia, as well as IL-13, thereby inducing bronchial hyperreactivity and other asthma phenotypic characteristics. Eosinophils are therefore both markers of and contributors to asthma inflammation, through a variety of mechanisms.

CHARACTERISTICS OF EOSINOPHILIC ASTHMA

The identification of asthmatics with significant eosinophilic inflammation is an important step toward understanding the inflammatory processes underlying the disease phenotype. Eosinophilic asthma can be defined as the clinical inflammatory phenotype wherein a significant number of sputum, airway, and/or blood eosinophils are present. Eosinophils may be detected in one or multiple system compartments, including the peripheral blood, the airway submucosa, and the airway lumen. In general, sputum eosinophil levels of >2%–3% and blood eosinophil counts of >240–300 per microliter (µL) may be used to define eosinophilic disease.[9,10]

The phenomenon of airway eosinophilia occurs in ~50% of asthma patients.[1] Eosinophilia in asthma has been linked to a variety of clinical characteristics and outcomes of asthma. Eosinophilia can be detected across the entire spectrum of asthma severity.[11,12] Eosinophilia is a characteristic of both childhood-onset asthma and later-onset asthma.[13] However, eosinophilic inflammation is especially prominent in severe asthmatics with type 2–like late-onset disease.[14] The number of eosinophils in sputum can be used as a marker of asthma severity, with strong associations in some cohorts between airway eosinophilia and severity of symptoms, worsening lung function, and incidence of fatal asthma.[15,16] Eosinophil accumulation in the airways in severe asthma correlates with markers of local tissue and extracellular matrix remodeling, identifying those at risk for more frequent exacerbations.[17,18] Furthermore, an analysis using the National Health and Nutrition Examination Survey, a large cross-sectional survey of the US general population, revealed that individuals with asthma and blood eosinophil count greater than 300 cells per microliter were more likely to report asthma attacks.[19] Finally, patients with severe asthma and blood eosinophils >400/µL are more likely to have an exacerbation than those with lower blood eosinophil counts.[20] The accurate detection of eosinophils in asthma may therefore give clues to disease characteristics, may identify patients at risk for exacerbations, and will help guide targeted treatment for those with severe disease.

MEASURING EOSINOPHILIA

Defining the presence of eosinophilic asthma requires identification of eosinophils in a clinically relevant compartment, that is, the peripheral blood, sputum/lumen, or bronchial wall. Accurate measurement of eosinophils in asthma can be technically and logistically challenging, due to variability in eosinophil presence and collection methods. Measurement of bronchial wall eosinophils requires bronchoscopy with biopsy, which may neither be readily available nor appropriate for routine clinical use. Recommendations from a National Institutes of Health (NIH) expert panel for the standardization of biomarkers for asthma clinical research, including sputum and blood eosinophil determination, can help guide clinical use of these tests.[21] Interestingly, the presence of eosinophilia is not always consistent among these compartments.[22,23] Eosinophils are primarily tissue-dwelling leukocytes, and therefore blood counts do not necessarily indicate the entire extent of eosinophil involvement in the affected tissues.[21,22] The clinical relevance of this finding is not fully understood. However, the extremes of blood eosinophil levels may be more sensitive and specific for identifying sputum eosinophils.[9,24,25] For example, patients with blood eosinophil counts less than 0.09 eosinophils per microliter are highly unlikely to have airway eosinophilia; alternately, almost all patients with more than 0.4 eosinophils per microliter can be expected to have significant sputum eosinophils.[26]

Sputum may be collected through sputum induction or by spontaneous production. Sputum induction is considered safe and reproducible even among patients with moderate to severe asthma.[27] The most commonly used method for sputum induction in the United States used by NIH-funded studies is the whole expectorant method.[28,29] Sputum eosinophils should be reported as a percentage of all nonsquamous cells, rather than total eosinophil count, because the percentage transformation controls for the effects of saliva in the sample, which can dilute the concentration of eosinophils.

Squamous cells are counted independently to determine sample quality; a squamous cell percentage of greater than 80% is taken to indicate a sputum sample of inadequate quality.[21] Through this method, analysis of the cell differential of induced sputum has been a useful noninvasive method for evaluating airway inflammation in asthma in the research setting.[28,30,31] Reference values for sputum eosinophil percentages have been determined through epidemiologic studies. In one study with 118 healthy nonsmoking subjects, the upper range of normal sputum eosinophilia calculated percent was 2.2%.[32] In a second study of 114 healthy subjects, the mean eosinophil percentage was 0.6 with a standard deviation of 0.8 and a normal upper limit of 2.2%.[33] These data provide the rationale for the commonly used cutoff of 2%–3% sputum eosinophils to determine sputum eosinophilia. Sputum processing for eosinophil counts requires laboratory materials not readily available at all clinical centers; determination of the cell differential should be done by an experienced individual trained in cell identification.[34]

Bronchial wash and bronchoalveolar lavage fluid eosinophil counts are also increased in eosinophilic asthma as compared with noneosinophilic asthma.[35] However, when eosinophil counts in induced sputum, bronchial washing, and bronchoalveolar lavage fluid were compared, induced sputum had higher concentrations of eosinophils, as well as eosinophil products, than bronchoalveolar lavage, with similar levels to bronchial wash. This supports using induced sputum for assessment of eosinophilic asthma as a more feasible alternative to bronchial wash or lavage.[36]

Although induced sputum is a less invasive and therefore more feasible approach than bronchoalveolar lavage for obtaining eosinophil counts, blood eosinophilia remains the least invasive and more widely use marker outside the research setting. Peripheral blood eosinophil counts of >240–300 per microliter may be used to define eosinophilic disease in asthma, particularly as it relates to improvement with targeted antieosinophil biologic therapies.[9] However, the correlation between sputum and blood eosinophilia is more accurate at higher blood eosinophil levels, as a cutoff of 0.45×10^9 cells/μL for blood eosinophilia can better predict airway eosinophilia in patients with severe asthma than lower values.[37] To measure blood eosinophils, the total number of white blood cells is multiplied by the percentage of eosinophils to provide the absolute eosinophil count. The percentage should not be reported unless specific reasons exist for knowing the proportions of eosinophils compared with other cells.[21] In addition to the feasibility, accessibility, and low risk of blood eosinophil testing, with an average cost of approximately $10–$13 and low volume of blood needed, comparisons of blood eosinophil counts are consistent among ethnic groups.[38] Blood eosinophil counts therefore continue to be an important and practical tool for implementation in the clinical setting.

FACTORS THAT DRIVE VARIABILITY IN EOSINOPHIL MEASUREMENT

A variety of innate and external factors can influence eosinophil counts over time, impacting the percentages or absolute numbers of eosinophils in each blood or sputum sample. Diurnal variation of eosinophils is well described, with a nadir in the late morning related to morning cortisol release (Fig. 6.1).[39,40] Time of day should therefore be taken into account when monitoring serial eosinophil levels. Eosinophil counts can fluctuate over weeks[27] to months in sputum,[41,42] with estimates of test repeatability to be 0.82. Thus, to definitively determine whether an individual has eosinophilic disease may require repeated sputum evaluations over time.

Inhaled corticosteroids (ICSs) or systemic corticosteroids can decrease eosinophil counts,[43] as can leukotriene receptor antagonists and omalizumab, an anti-IgE antibody. Sputum cell counts can change within hours after an intervention, as has been shown in studies of airway allergen challenge or exposure to ozone.[28,30,36] Exercise and smoking can increase the blood eosinophil count.[44,45] Infection with viruses and bacteria may decrease peripheral blood eosinophilia and suppress bone marrow eosinophil production, possibly through systemic acute inflammation.[46] Systemic diseases, such as parasitic infection, drug allergy, vasculitis, or malignancy can present with markedly elevated blood or organ-specific eosinophilia. Similarly, eosinophilia can be seen in many diseases of the airway other than asthma, such as chronic sinusitis, chronic obstructive pulmonary disease, hypersensitivity pneumonitis, and eosinophilic pneumonia. The detected levels of blood, sputum, and airway eosinophils should be interpreted with the knowledge of these factors, which induce variability in eosinophil counts.

EOSINOPHILS AS PREDICTORS OF RESPONSE TO THERAPY AND THERAPEUTIC RESPONSE

As previously discussed, asthmatics with significant eosinophilia may be at higher risk for more severe disease.

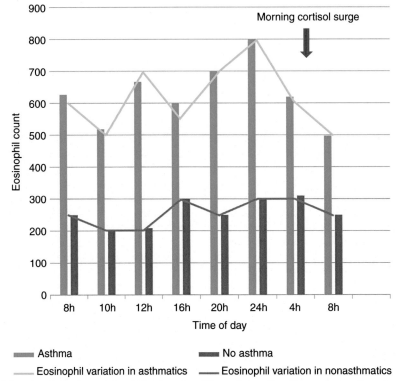

FIG. 6.1 Diurnal variation in peripheral blood eosinophil count, in asthmatics and nonasthmatics. (Adapted from Dahl R. Diurnal variation in the number of circulating eosinophil leucocytes in normal controls and asthmatics. *Acta Allergol.* 1977;32(5):301–303 and Winkel P, Statland BE, Saunders AM, Osborn H, Kupperman H. Within-day physiologic variation of leukocyte types in healthy subjects as assayed by two automated leukocyte differential analyzers. *Am J Clin Pathol.* 1981;75(5):693–700; with permission.)

Therapies that target eosinophils may therefore help control diseases associated with eosinophil-mediated tissue damage and inflammation.[2,47] Irrespective of the pathobiologic pathway contributing to eosinophilia in asthma, the depletion of eosinophils can benefit patients with asthma, such as reducing exacerbations and healthcare utilization for asthma.[48,49] Sputum and blood eosinophils can therefore be used as biomarkers relevant to treatment responses for a spectrum of interventions and should be considered to guide therapy particularly for those with more severe disease (Fig. 6.2).

Response to Steroids

Corticosteroids induce rapid eosinophil apoptosis and inhibit T2 inflammation through multiple other mechanisms including inhibition of cytokine expression and induction of antiinflammatory pathways. Given the many targets of corticosteroids, it is clear why their systemic or topical use has long been the mainstay of pharmacologic asthma control. However, ICSs have

been observed to significantly benefit only approximately half of patients with asthma for symptom control and risk reduction.[1] The presence of eosinophilia may indeed help identify those steroid responders.

Increased blood eosinophil counts have been shown to be a good predictor of treatment response to corticosteroids in asthma.[35,50] In the pediatric population requiring controller therapy for asthma, phenotyping with aeroallergen sensitization and blood eosinophils >300/μL was found to be useful for guiding treatment selection and identifying children with a high exacerbation probability for whom treatment with daily ICSs is beneficial.[51] Furthermore, blood eosinophils have been found to decrease significantly in asthmatics treated with inhaled and systemic steroids, supporting the importance of eosinophil reduction for asthma control.[52,53]

Similarly, there have been many studies reporting sputum eosinophilia as a predictor of response to corticosteroid therapy in eosinophilic asthma. Sputum

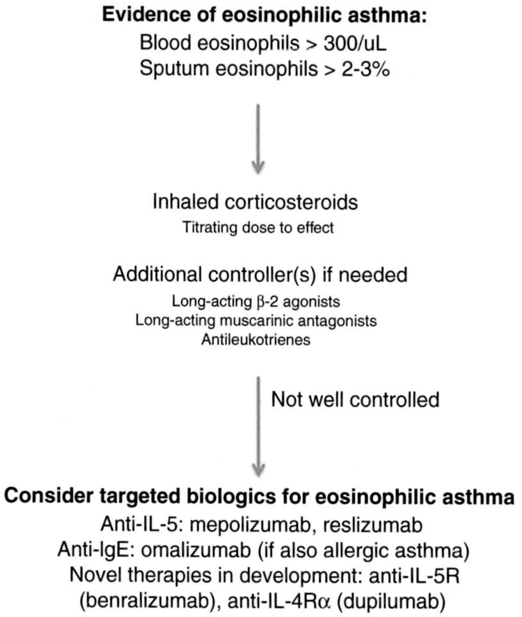

Evidence of eosinophilic asthma:
Blood eosinophils > 300/uL
Sputum eosinophils > 2-3%

↓

Inhaled corticosteroids
Titrating dose to effect

Additional controller(s) if needed
Long-acting β-2 agonists
Long-acting muscarinic antagonists
Antileukotrienes

Not well controlled

↓

Consider targeted biologics for eosinophilic asthma
Anti-IL-5: mepolizumab, reslizumab
Anti-IgE: omalizumab (if also allergic asthma)
Novel therapies in development: anti-IL-5R
(benralizumab), anti-IL-4Rα (dupilumab)

FIG. 6.2 Possible treatment algorithm for eosinophilic asthma.

eosinophilia can identify patients with clinical response to systemic corticosteroids.[54] Pavord et al.[55] and Berry et al.[35] separately demonstrated that treatment with ICSs was also of greater benefit to subjects with sputum eosinophilia than those without. Additionally, Cowan et al. noted a more significant treatment effect of ICSs in patients with sputum eosinophilia, those patients experiencing a loss of control after being weaned off corticosteroids.[43] Similarly, Deykin et al. showed that significant increases in sputum eosinophil counts after patients are weaned off ICSs could identify patients at risk for exacerbations of asthma, in whom ICSs would be protective.[56]

Reassessing and adjusting ICS based on sputum eosinophilia may lead to better clinical outcomes than using empiric clinical guidelines alone.[9] For example, Green et al. compared treatment using guidelines-based or sputum eosinophil–based medication management for individuals with moderate to severe asthma. In this study, treating patients with ICSs or oral corticosteroids with a goal of sputum eosinophil count normalization reduced asthma exacerbations and admissions in the eosinophilic patients.[49] Jayaram et al. found similar benefits in a multicenter intervention.[57] A systematic review and metaanalysis of the literature concluded that tailoring of asthma treatment through titration of corticosteroids based on sputum eosinophilia is effective in decreasing asthma exacerbation risk.[58]

Cell counts and gene expression patterns relevant to eosinophil markers can be detected in the sputum and used to accurately identify steroid responders. For example, expression of the type-2 inflammatory cytokines IL-4, IL-5, and IL-13 correlate with sputum and blood eosinophils[59] and can identify those with benefit from ICSs.[60,61] Increased expression of the gene encoding for the eosinophil's Charcot-Leyden crystal protein can identify the eosinophilic inflammatory phenotype and is observed to predict ICS response.[62] In addition to the presence of eosinophils, markers of eosinophils and their activity, such as the fraction of exhaled nitric oxide, urinary bromotyrosine, and eosinophil peroxidase, in body fluid or tissues can help identify individuals more likely to respond to corticosteroid therapy.[9,50,63]

Biologic Therapies

Despite the benefit of corticosteroids in eosinophilic asthma, there is the observation that half of asthmatics fail to derive significant benefit from ICSs for symptom control and risk reduction, and in some severe asthmatics, high eosinophil levels can persist despite the use of high-dose controller medications, such as corticosteroids.[9] Identification of asthmatics with significant eosinophilic inflammation is an important step toward practicing personalized, precision medicine, which will target relevant pathways (Fig. 6.2, Table 6.1).

Evidence from multicenter, randomized, placebo-controlled clinical trials suggests that targeting the main stimulant of eosinophil recruitment and differentiation, IL-5, can improve outcomes in severe eosinophilic asthma. Currently, in the United States, two anti-IL-5 monoclonal antibodies are available for the treatment of severe eosinophilic asthma. Mepolizumab is administered subcutaneously; reslizumab is administered as an intravenous infusion. Phase 3 studies supported the use of these medications for both reduction of exacerbation frequency and steroid sparing effects in patients with peripheral blood eosinophil counts of >300–400/μL.[64–66] Benralizumab, an IL-5-receptor antagonist that induces rapid eosinophil depletion through antibody-dependent cell-mediated toxicity, is in development for treatment of severe eosinophilic asthma.[67,68] Benralizumab has shown efficacy toward decreasing exacerbations, improving symptoms, and improving lung function in patients with severe eosinophilic asthma. However, not all patients with eosinophilic disease will show clinical improvement with these drugs, underscoring the immunologic complexity of eosinophilic asthma.

TABLE 6.1
Therapies With Evidence for Use in Treatment of Eosinophilic Asthma

Therapeutic Class	Representative Drugs	Effect on Eosinophils	Patient Population	Clinical Outcomes
Corticosteroids	Prednisone (systemic)	Significant reduction	Patients with severe persistent asthma, or in exacerbation	Reduced asthma exacerbations and admissions, improves control
	Fluticasone, mometasone, beclomethasone, ciclesonide, budesonide (inhaled)	No significant effect	Patients requiring controller therapy, evidence of eosinophilic disease	Improves symptoms, lung function, reduces exacerbations
IL-5 inhibition	Mepolizumab, reslizumab (anti-IL-5 antibody)	Significant reduction	Severe asthma, peripheral blood eosinophilia >300–400 cells/µL in the preceding year	Reduced requirements for systemic steroids, reduced exacerbations, improved control
	Benralizumab[a] (anti-IL-5-receptor antibody)	Significant reduction		
IgE	Omalizumab (anti-IgE antibody)	Reduction	Moderate to severe allergic asthma, IgE 30–700 IU/mL, peripheral blood eosinophils >300/µL	Improved asthma symptom control, reduce eosinophil counts, and reduction in exacerbation. Particularly useful in allergic asthma not controlled with increased-dose inhaled steroids
IL-4	Dupilumab[a] (anti-IL-4 receptor-α chain antibody)	No significant effect	Uncontrolled moderate to severe asthma (phase IIb)	Improved lung function, reduced exacerbations

[a]Not FDA approved for treatment of asthma, as of July 27, 2017.

Additional biologic treatments in development for severe eosinophilic asthma directly target other pathways of type-2 inflammation, such as IL-4/IL-13 signaling and IgE function. IgE is an important marker of airway inflammation, in particular playing a key role in allergic asthma. The presence of allergen-specific IgE is required to define atopic asthma, with panels of clinically relevant aeroallergen skin testing or specific IgE-serology functioning as essential biomarkers of allergic asthma. Total serum IgE is considered an outcome for intervention and observation studies.[21]

Binding of IgE to high- and low-affinity receptors and subsequent exposure to allergens initiate the inflammatory cascade inducing mast cell activation and release of inflammatory mediators contributing to acute and chronic symptoms of allergic asthma.[69] Omalizumab is a monoclonal anti-IgE antibody developed for the treatment of severe allergic asthma, which can blunt the allergen-induced early asthmatic responses, producing significant inhibition of allergen-induced bronchoconstriction and suppressing the effect of allergen-induced immediate hypersensitivity responses in the airway.[70] Treatment with omalizumab also decreases the levels of both sputum and blood eosinophils in eosinophilic asthma, as well as depletes IgE from airway tissue.[71] Additionally, in patients with a blood eosinophil count of 300/µL or more, omalizumab treatment can provide a significant reduction in exacerbations.[72] Furthermore, this benefit was shown to be directly related to the decrease in blood eosinophilia,[73] suggesting that the impact of omalizumab on blood eosinophils could be a biomarker of response to therapy. Therefore, omalizumab can be a useful tool in the management of eosinophilic asthma, particularly in allergic asthma not controlled with high-dose inhaled steroids. Finally, while asthma driven by the IL-4/IL-13 inflammatory pathways may present with peripheral blood or airway eosinophils, the presence of eosinophils is not absolutely required to demonstrate efficacy of an IL-4/IL-13 inhibitor, such as in the case of treatment with dupilumab.[74]

CONCLUSIONS

Eosinophils can affect airway biology as both a source of epithelial damage and airway remodeling in asthma. As such, eosinophils contribute to the severity of asthma and may persist despite guideline-based treatment. However, eosinophils can be used as biomarkers to direct therapeutic decision-making and to follow the response to treatment. Most importantly in the clinical setting, eosinophils as biomarkers may allow us to identify populations, particularly among our severe asthmatics, that could respond well to targeted eosinophil-directed or type-2 inflammation–directed biologics.

DISCLOSURE

TFC reports receiving consulting fees from AstraZeneca and the institution has received support from the National Institutes of Health.

REFERENCES

1. McGrath KW, Icitovic N, Boushey HA, et al. A large subgroup of mild-to-moderate asthma is persistently noneosinophilic. *Am J Respir Crit Care Med.* 2012;185(6):612–619.
2. Fulkerson PC, Rothenberg ME. Targeting eosinophils in allergy, inflammation and beyond. *Nat Rev Drug Discov.* 2013;12(2):117–129.
3. Domachowske JB, Dyer KD, Bonville CA, Rosenberg HF. Recombinant human eosinophil-derived neurotoxin/RNase 2 functions as an effective antiviral agent against respiratory syncytial virus. *J Infect Dis.* 1998;177(6):1458–1464.
4. Henderson WR, Chi EY, Klebanoff SJ. Eosinophil peroxidase-induced mast cell secretion. *J Exp Med.* 1980; 152(2):265–279.
5. Carr TF, Berdnikovs S, Simon HU, Bochner BS, Rosenwasser LJ. Eosinophilic bioactivities in severe asthma. *World Allergy Organ J.* 2016;9:21.
6. Ying S, Humbert M, Barkans J, et al. Expression of IL-4 and IL-5 mRNA and protein product by CD4+ and CD8+ T cells, eosinophils, and mast cells in bronchial biopsies obtained from atopic and nonatopic (intrinsic) asthmatics. *J Immunol.* 1997;158(7):3539–3544.
7. Hammad H, Lambrecht BN. Barrier epithelial cells and the control of type 2 immunity. *Immunity.* 2015;43(1):29–40.
8. Lambrecht BN, Hammad H. The immunology of asthma. *Nat Immunol.* 2015;16(1):45–56.
9. Arron JR, Choy DF, Scheerens H, Matthews JG. Noninvasive biomarkers that predict treatment benefit from biologic therapies in asthma. *Ann Am Thorac Soc.* 2013;(10 suppl): S206–S213.
10. Coumou H, Bel EH. Improving the diagnosis of eosinophilic asthma. *Expert Rev Respir Med.* 2016;10(10):1093–1103.
11. Moore WC, Bleecker ER, Curran-Everett D, et al. Characterization of the severe asthma phenotype by the national heart, lung, and blood Institute's severe asthma research program. *J Allergy Clin Immunol.* 2007;119(2): 405–413.
12. Moore WC, Meyers DA, Wenzel SE, et al. Identification of asthma phenotypes using cluster analysis in the Severe Asthma Research Program. *Am J Respir Crit Care Med.* 2010; 181(4):315–323.
13. Fitzpatrick AM, Teague WG, Meyers DA, et al. Heterogeneity of severe asthma in childhood: confirmation by cluster analysis of children in the national Institutes of health/ national heart, lung, and blood institute severe asthma research program. *J Allergy Clin Immunol.* 2011;127(2): 382–389. e381–e313.
14. Denlinger LC, Phillips BR, Ramratnam S, et al. Inflammatory and Co-Morbid features of patients with severe asthma and frequent exacerbations. *Am J Respir Crit Care Med.* 2016;195(3).
15. Trejo Bittar HE, Yousem SA, Wenzel SE. Pathobiology of severe asthma. *Annu Rev Pathol.* 2015;10:511–545.
16. Miranda C, Busacker A, Balzar S, Trudeau J, Wenzel SE. Distinguishing severe asthma phenotypes: role of age at onset and eosinophilic inflammation. *J Allergy Clin Immunol.* 2004;113(1):101–108.
17. Flood-Page PT, Menzies-Gow AN, Kay AB, Robinson DS. Eosinophil's role remains uncertain as anti-interleukin-5 only partially depletes numbers in asthmatic airway. *Am J Respir Crit Care Med.* 2003;167(2):199–204.
18. Lee JJ, Jacobsen EA, McGarry MP, Schleimer RP, Lee NA. Eosinophils in health and disease: the LIAR hypothesis. *Clin Exp Allergy.* 2010;40(4):563–575.
19. Tran TN, Khatry DB, Ke X, Ward CK, Gossage D. High blood eosinophil count is associated with more frequent asthma attacks in asthma patients. *Ann Allergy Asthma Immunol.* 2014;113(1):19–24.
20. Zeiger RS, Schatz M, Li Q, et al. High blood eosinophil count is a risk factor for future asthma exacerbations in adult persistent asthma. *J Allergy Clin Immunol Pract.* 2014;2(6):741–750.
21. Szefler SJ, Wenzel S, Brown R, et al. Asthma outcomes: biomarkers. *J Allergy Clin Immunol.* 2012;129(suppl 3): S9–S23.
22. Desai D, Newby C, Symon FA, et al. Elevated sputum interleukin-5 and submucosal eosinophilia in obese individuals with severe asthma. *Am J Respir Crit Care Med.* 2013;188(6):657–663.
23. Hastie AT, Moore WC, Li H, et al. Biomarker surrogates do not accurately predict sputum eosinophil and neutrophil percentages in asthmatic subjects. *J Allergy Clin Immunol.* 2013;132(1):72–80.
24. Wagener AH, de Nijs SB, Lutter R, et al. External validation of blood eosinophils, FE(NO) and serum periostin as surrogates for sputum eosinophils in asthma. *Thorax.* 2015;70(2):115–120.

25. Zhang XY, Simpson JL, Powell H, et al. Full blood count parameters for the detection of asthma inflammatory phenotypes. *Clin Exp Allergy*. 2014;44(9):1137–1145.

26. Westerhof GA, Korevaar DA, Amelink M, et al. Biomarkers to identify sputum eosinophilia in different adult asthma phenotypes. *Eur Respir J*. 2015;46(3):688–696.

27. Fahy JV, Boushey HA, Lazarus SC, et al. Safety and reproducibility of sputum induction in asthmatic subjects in a multicenter study. *Am J Respir Crit Care Med*. 2001;163(6):1470–1475.

28. Fahy JV, Liu J, Wong H, Boushey HA. Cellular and biochemical analysis of induced sputum from asthmatic and from healthy subjects. *Am Rev Respir Dis*. 1993;147(5):1126–1131.

29. Gershman NH, Wong HH, Liu JT, Mahlmeister MJ, Fahy JV. Comparison of two methods of collecting induced sputum in asthmatic subjects. *Eur Respir J*. 1996;9(12):2448–2453.

30. Pin I, Gibson PG, Kolendowicz R, et al. Use of induced sputum cell counts to investigate airway inflammation in asthma. *Thorax*. 1992;47(1):25–29.

31. Kips JC, Fahy JV, Hargreave FE, Ind PW, in't Veen JC. Methods for sputum induction and analysis of induced sputum: a method for assessing airway inflammation in asthma. *Eur Respir J Suppl*. 1998;26:9S–12S.

32. Belda J, Leigh R, Parameswaran K, O'Byrne PM, Sears MR, Hargreave FE. Induced sputum cell counts in healthy adults. *Am J Respir Crit Care Med*. 2000;161(2 Pt 1):475–478.

33. Spanevello A, Confalonieri M, Sulotto F, et al. Induced sputum cellularity. Reference values and distribution in normal volunteers. *Am J Respir Crit Care Med*. 2000;162 (3 Pt 1):1172–1174.

34. Peters SP. Counterpoint: is measuring sputum eosinophils useful in the management of severe asthma? No, not for the vast majority of patients. *Chest*. 2011;139(6):1273–1275. Discussion 1275–1278.

35. Berry M, Morgan A, Shaw DE, et al. Pathological features and inhaled corticosteroid response of eosinophilic and non-eosinophilic asthma. *Thorax*. 2007;62(12):1043–1049.

36. Fahy JV, Wong H, Liu J, Boushey HA. Comparison of samples collected by sputum induction and bronchoscopy from asthmatic and healthy subjects. *Am J Respir Crit Care Med*. 1995;152(1):53–58.

37. Fowler SJ, Tavernier G, Niven R. High blood eosinophil counts predict sputum eosinophilia in patients with severe asthma. *J Allergy Clin Immunol*. 2014;135(3).

38. Bain B, Seed M, Godsland I. Normal values for peripheral blood white cell counts in women of four different ethnic origins. *J Clin Pathol*. 1984;37(2):188–193.

39. Dahl R. Diurnal variation in the number of circulating eosinophil leucocytes in normal controls and asthmatics. *Acta Allergol*. 1977;32(5):301–303.

40. Winkel P, Statland BE, Saunders AM, Osborn H, Kupperman H. Within-day physiologic variation of leukocyte types in healthy subjects as assayed by two automated leukocyte differential analyzers. *Am J Clin Pathol*. 1981;75(5):693–700.

41. Bacci E, Latorre M, Cianchetti S, et al. Transient sputum eosinophilia may occur over time in non-eosinophilic asthma and this is not prevented by salmeterol. *Respirology*. 2012;17(8):1199–1206.

42. Simpson JL, McElduff P, Gibson PG. Assessment and reproducibility of non-eosinophilic asthma using induced sputum. *Respiration*. 2010;79(2):147–151.

43. Cowan DC, Cowan JO, Palmay R, Williamson A, Taylor DR. Effects of steroid therapy on inflammatory cell subtypes in asthma. *Thorax*. 2010;65(5):384–390.

44. Christensen RD, Hill HR. Exercise-induced changes in the blood concentration of leukocyte populations in teenage athletes. *Am J Pediatr Hematol Oncol*. 1987;9(2):140–142.

45. Mensinga TT, Schouten JP, Weiss ST, Van der Lende R. Relationship of skin test reactivity and eosinophilia to level of pulmonary function in a community-based population study. *Am Rev Respir Dis*. 1992;146(3):638–643.

46. Bass DA. Behavior of eosinophil leukocytes in acute inflammation. II. Eosinophil dynamics during acute inflammation. *J Clin Invest*. 1975;56(4):870–879.

47. Radonjic-Hoesli S, Valent P, Klion AD, Wechsler ME, Simon HU. Novel targeted therapies for eosinophil-associated diseases and allergy. *Annu Rev Pharmacol Toxicol*. 2015;55:633–656.

48. Pavord ID, Korn S, Howarth P, et al. Mepolizumab for severe eosinophilic asthma (DREAM): a multicentre, double-blind, placebo-controlled trial. *Lancet*. 2012;380(9842):651–659.

49. Green RH, Brightling CE, McKenna S, et al. Asthma exacerbations and sputum eosinophil counts: a randomised controlled trial. *Lancet*. 2002;360(9347):1715–1721.

50. Cowan DC, Taylor DR, Peterson LE, et al. Biomarker-based asthma phenotypes of corticosteroid response. *J Allergy Clin Immunol*. 2014;135(4).

51. Fitzpatrick AM, Jackson DJ, Mauger DT, et al. Individualized therapy for persistent asthma in young children. *J Allergy Clin Immunol*. 2016;138(6):1608–1618.e1612.

52. Hodgson D, Anderson J, Reynolds C, et al. A randomised controlled trial of small particle inhaled steroids in refractory eosinophilic asthma (SPIRA). *Thorax*. 2015;70(6):559–565.

53. ten Brinke A, Zwinderman AH, Sterk PJ, Rabe KF, Bel EH. "Refractory" eosinophilic airway inflammation in severe asthma: effect of parenteral corticosteroids. *Am J Respir Crit Care Med*. 2004;170(6):601–605.

54. Little SA, Chalmers GW, MacLeod KJ, McSharry C, Thomson NC. Non-invasive markers of airway inflammation as predictors of oral steroid responsiveness in asthma. *Thorax*. 2000;55(3):232–234.

55. Pavord ID, Brightling CE, Woltmann G, Wardlaw AJ. Non-eosinophilic corticosteroid unresponsive asthma. *Lancet*. 1999;353(9171):2213–2214.

56. Deykin A, Lazarus SC, Fahy JV, et al. Sputum eosinophil counts predict asthma control after discontinuation of inhaled corticosteroids. *J Allergy Clin Immunol*. 2005;115(4):720–727.

57. Jayaram L, Pizzichini MM, Cook RJ, et al. Determining asthma treatment by monitoring sputum cell counts: effect on exacerbations. *Eur Respir J.* 2006;27(3):483–494.

58. Petsky HL, Cates CJ, Lasserson TJ, et al. A systematic review and meta-analysis: tailoring asthma treatment on eosinophilic markers (exhaled nitric oxide or sputum eosinophils). *Thorax.* 2012;67(3):199–208.

59. Peters MC, Mekonnen ZK, Yuan S, Bhakta NR, Woodruff PG, Fahy JV. Measures of gene expression in sputum cells can identify TH2-high and TH2-low subtypes of asthma. *J Allergy Clin Immunol.* 2014;133(2):388–394.

60. Woodruff PG, Boushey HA, Dolganov GM, et al. Genome-wide profiling identifies epithelial cell genes associated with asthma and with treatment response to corticosteroids. *Proc Natl Acad Sci USA.* 2007;104(40):15858–15863.

61. Woodruff PG, Modrek B, Choy DF, et al. T-helper type 2-driven inflammation defines major subphenotypes of asthma. *Am J Respir Crit Care Med.* 2009;180(5):388–395.

62. Baines KJ, Simpson JL, Wood LG, et al. Sputum gene expression signature of 6 biomarkers discriminates asthma inflammatory phenotypes. *J Allergy Clin Immunol.* 2014; 133(4):997–1007.

63. Rao R, Frederick JM, Enander I, Gregson RK, Warner JA, Warner JO. Airway function correlates with circulating eosinophil, but not mast cell, markers of inflammation in childhood asthma. *Clin Exp Allergy.* 1996;26(7):789–793.

64. Bel EH, Wenzel SE, Thompson PJ, et al. Oral glucocorticoid-sparing effect of mepolizumab in eosinophilic asthma. *N Engl J Med.* 2014;371(13):1189–1197.

65. Ortega HG, Liu MC, Pavord ID, et al. Mepolizumab treatment in patients with severe eosinophilic asthma. *N Engl J Med.* 2014;371(13):1198–1207.

66. Castro M, Zangrilli J, Wechsler ME, et al. Reslizumab for inadequately controlled asthma with elevated blood eosinophil counts: results from two multicentre, parallel, double-blind, randomised, placebo-controlled, phase 3 trials. *Lancet Respir Med.* 2015;3(5):355–366.

67. Bleecker ER, FitzGerald JM, Chanez P, et al. Efficacy and safety of benralizumab for patients with severe asthma uncontrolled with high-dosage inhaled corticosteroids and long-acting beta2-agonists (SIROCCO): a randomised, multicentre, placebo-controlled phase 3 trial. *Lancet.* 2016. http://dx.doi.org/10.1016/S0140-6736(16)31324-1.

68. FitzGerald JM, Bleecker ER, Nair P, et al. Benralizumab, an anti-interleukin-5 receptor α monoclonal antibody, as add-on treatment for patients with severe, uncontrolled, eosinophilic asthma (CALIMA): a randomised, double-blind, placebo-controlled phase 3 trial. *Lancet.* 2016;388(10056):2128–2141.

69. Hanf G, Brachmann I, Kleine-Tebbe J, et al. Omalizumab decreased IgE-release and induced changes in cellular immunity in patients with allergic asthma. *Allergy.* 2006; 61(9):1141–1144.

70. Boulet LP, Chapman KR, Côté J, et al. Inhibitory effects of an anti-IgE antibody E25 on allergen-induced early asthmatic response. *Am J Respir Crit Care Med.* 1997;155(6):1835–1840.

71. Djukanović R, Wilson SJ, Kraft M, et al. Effects of treatment with anti-immunoglobulin E antibody omalizumab on airway inflammation in allergic asthma. *Am J Respir Crit Care Med.* 2004;170(6):583–593.

72. Busse W, Spector S, Rosén K, Wang Y, Alpan O. High eosinophil count: a potential biomarker for assessing successful omalizumab treatment effects. *J Allergy Clin Immunol.* 2013;132(2):485–486. e411.

73. Skiepko R, Ziętkowski Z, Lukaszyk M, et al. Changes in blood eosinophilia during omalizumab therapy as a predictor of asthma exacerbation. *Postepy Dermatol Alergol.* 2014;31(5):305–309.

74. Wenzel S, Castro M, Corren J, et al. Dupilumab efficacy and safety in adults with uncontrolled persistent asthma despite use of medium-to-high-dose inhaled corticosteroids plus a long-acting beta2 agonist: a randomised double-blind placebo-controlled pivotal phase 2b dose-ranging trial. *Lancet.* 2016;388(10039):31–44.

Regulatory Aspects of Pediatric Biomarkers for Assessing Medication Response

GILBERT J. BURCKART, PHARMD • DIONNA J. GREEN, MD

INTRODUCTION

Biomarkers are one of the most active areas for discussion in the clinical research and the drug development community. Literally, thousands of publications are being written on this topic every year. The value of understanding biomarkers of disease and drug response to public health is reflected in the work of the Food and Drug Administration (FDA) National Institutes of Health (NIH) Biomarker Working Group and their extensive BEST (Biomarkers, EndpointS, and other Tools) Resource.[1]

However, the machinery of drug evaluation and approval within the regulatory framework, a critical part of the drug development process, cannot stop and wait for biomarker validation and qualification. Decisions by regulators have to be made based on the facts as they exist presently. Unfortunately, any book chapter written about the regulatory aspects of a rapidly moving science has a chance of very quickly becoming outdated.

Our hope is that this chapter will be outdated rapidly, but the history of the development of biomarkers within a therapeutic area says otherwise. The process of scientifically developing, validating, and qualifying a biomarker, whether or not through a formal regulatory process, is very challenging. Often these studies do not attract the types of funding that keep academic researchers interested beyond the publication of a couple of manuscripts. Pharmaceutical companies are hesitant to spend the funds required to study new endpoints when they can fall back on endpoints previously used in drug development programs.

Biomarkers can drive the development of new therapies in a therapeutic area. An increased understanding of the pathophysiology of a disease process can identify new targets, which then may present opportunities to develop, validate, and qualify biomarkers that can be used in a drug development program. Unfortunately, the opposite effect can also be seen in areas of therapeutics that failed to develop new biomarkers and qualified endpoints. Endpoints that are costly, difficult to measure, or take an excessive amount of time to accomplish will not attract new therapies that may be useful in several areas of therapeutics. For example, a warning of the need for validation and qualification of biomarkers was published for the organ transplant community in 2007.[2] No new qualified biomarkers in the organ transplant area have been produced, and few new therapies in organ transplantation have emerged since 1998.

Children do require special consideration for biomarker development, because most research is directed toward adults and adult disease. Because of the challenges of conducting biomarker research in pediatric patients, children have even been referred to as "biomarker orphans."[3] As will be discussed in this chapter, biomarkers and endpoints are frequently different in children than they are in adults for similar indications.

The objective of this chapter is to review the regulatory aspects of biomarkers and endpoints as it relates to pediatric drug development. The types of endpoints that have been used in pediatric drug development will be discussed, and pediatric asthma will be used as the example to describe previous endpoints that have been used for drug approval.

Biomarker Categories and Definitions

The categories of biomarkers are represented in Fig. 7.1 and are defined in the BEST document.[1] A biomarker is defined as a specific characteristic that is measured as an indicator of normal biologic processes, pathogenic processes, or responses to an exposure or intervention, including therapeutic interventions. Molecular, histologic, radiographic, or physiologic characteristics are

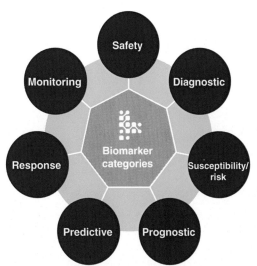

FIG. 7.1 Biomarker categories. (From McCune S. *Outcome Measures, Biomarkers and Endpoints*. 2016. Available at: https://www.fda.gov/downloads/NewsEvents/Meetings ConferencesWorkshops/UCM519805.pdf; with permission.)

types of biomarkers. A biomarker is not a direct assessment of how an individual feels, functions, or survives. Categories of biomarkers include the following:

- susceptibility/risk biomarker
- diagnostic biomarker
- monitoring biomarker
- prognostic biomarker
- predictive biomarker
- pharmacodynamic/response biomarker
- safety biomarker

The BEST document defines each of these types of biomarkers and provides examples. In 2015, the FDA published a survey in the Federal Register entitled, "Identifying Potential Biomarkers for Qualification and Describing Contexts of Use to Address Areas Important to Drug Development." The purpose of the survey was to seek information to inform the development and qualification of biomarkers in areas related to human drug therapeutics. A total of 74 responses were received either online or via submissions to the docket, which closed on May 14, 2015. The primary disease areas and organ toxicities covered by the survey included neurodegenerative, neuromuscular, neurologic and neuropsychiatric, autoimmune and inflammatory, hepatic, musculoskeletal, pulmonary, renal, cardiovascular, metabolic, and infectious diseases and oncology. The pulmonary diseases do not include asthma. The survey designated the biomarker name and context of use and

listed why the biomarker is useful in drug development. The context of use does not line up entirely with the BEST document.

For example, monitoring biomarkers in the BEST document do not entirely align with the FDA survey document. A monitoring biomarker is a biomarker measured serially for assessing status of a disease or a medical condition or for evidence of exposure to (or effect of) a medical product or an environmental agent. One of the examples provided in the BEST document for a monitoring biomarker is B-type natriuretic peptide or BNP. BNP may be used as a monitoring biomarker during follow-up to supplement clinical decision-making in pediatric patients with pulmonary hypertension. BNP is mentioned several times in the 2015 FDA survey, but not in relation to pulmonary hypertension in pediatric patients. Therefore the two documents may be complimentary when an investigator is searching for biomarkers that have been included in FDA-related documents.

Pediatric patients are not excluded from the use of the biomarkers mentioned in these documents, but the applicability of the biomarker to the pediatric patient and disease process has to be evaluated on a case-by-case basis. Perhaps the best example is in the use of predictive genomic biomarkers. A predictive biomarker is a biomarker used to identify individuals who are more likely than individuals without the biomarker to experience a favorable or unfavorable effect from exposure to a medical product or an environmental agent. The application of pharmacogenomic information in FDA labels was recently reviewed,[4] and we found that in 86% of the cases, the information was entirely derived from adult studies. Of the 65 drug labels with pharmacogenomic information, we determined that in 40 (71%) cases the information was suitable for use in pediatric patients. Primarily because of ontogeny of the enzyme, transporter, or receptor, in the other 16 (29%) cases we determined that the application of the predictive information to pediatric patients was unclear.

The most commonly used biomarkers in drug development are the pharmacodynamic/response biomarkers. These biomarkers are defined as a biomarker used to show that a biologic response has occurred in an individual who has been exposed to a medical product or an environmental agent. In a medical product development setting, pharmacodynamic/response biomarkers may be useful to establish proof-of-concept that a drug produces a pharmacologic response in humans thought to be related to clinical benefit and to guide dose-response studies. These biomarkers may also provide useful information for dose adjustment. Although these biomarkers are not always considered surrogate endpoints, some may be accepted as surrogate endpoints in specific contexts.

Surrogate Endpoints

Surrogate endpoints are an important topic in pediatric drug development because the majority of endpoints measured in pediatric drug development efficacy studies are surrogate endpoints. A surrogate endpoint is used in clinical trials as a substitute for a direct measure of how a patient feels, functions, or survives. A surrogate endpoint does not measure the clinical benefit of primary interest in and of itself, but rather is expected to predict the clinical benefit or harm based on epidemiologic, therapeutic, pathophysiologic, or other scientific evidence. From a US regulatory standpoint, surrogate endpoints and potential surrogate endpoints can be characterized by the level of clinical validation:

- validated surrogate endpoint
- reasonably likely surrogate endpoint
- candidate surrogate endpoint

The use of surrogate endpoints in drug development is controversial, because many examples of presumed surrogate endpoints that have turned out to not predict clinical benefit as expected. The reasons for the failure of surrogate endpoints in adult clinical trials have been discussed previously.[5]

Multiple examples of the use of surrogate endpoints in pediatric patients have been noted.[6] Antiviral agents that are used to treat HIV infection in pediatric patients routinely are assessed by reduction in HIV-1 RNA levels <400 copies/mL and increases in CD4 counts. For pediatric asthmatic patients, inhaled corticosteroids are frequently used, but concerns about the effect of these drugs on growth have led to 1-year safety assessments of linear growth in children, which is a surrogate marker for bone health and ultimate adult height. A final statistical approach to surrogate endpoints has not been resolved, but statistical approaches using the proportion of treatment explained have replaced approaches devised three decades earlier.[6]

Regulatory History of Biomarker Qualification

The recognition that biomarkers, or the lack of qualified biomarkers, play a critical role in drug development was highlighted in the 2004 and 2006 US FDA documents referred to as the Critical Path to developing new medical products. As was stated in the forward of the 2004 document,[7] the document "provides FDA's analysis of the *pipeline problem*—the recent slowdown, instead of the expected acceleration, in innovative

medical therapies reaching patients." The 2004 document refers to biomarkers and surrogate endpoints multiple times, and states: "Adopting a new biomarker or surrogate endpoint for effectiveness standards can drive rapid clinical development." This document also establishes the idea of having an expended new drug development toolkit. "A new product development toolkit—containing powerful new scientific and technical methods such as animal or computer-based predictive models, biomarkers for safety and effectiveness, and new clinical evaluation techniques—is urgently needed to improve predictability and efficiency along the critical path from laboratory concept to commercial product." These statements established the need for an FDA Guidance, which will be discussed below, outlining the tools for drug development and how they might function. One of those tools is the biomarker qualification process.

A second FDA Critical Path document was released in 2006, outlining a number of more specific opportunities with the intent of stimulating activity in these areas. The document was titled the Critical Path Opportunities List[8] and contained six topic areas. One of those six areas was "Better Evaluation Tools" including biomarker qualification in disease-specific areas. One of the topic areas that is addressed is biomarker qualification; "The process and criteria for qualifying biomarkers for use in product development should be mapped. Clarity on the conceptual framework and evidentiary standards for qualifying a biomarker for various purposes would establish the path for developing predictive biomarkers."

In addition, the 2006 document[8] discusses disease and disorder-specific biomarkers. Ten years later, some of these biomarkers have worked and some have not. For example, the asthma example provided in the Critical Path Opportunities document lists β-adrenergic receptor polymorphisms and the prediction of long-term asthma outcomes as the opportunity. Many of the asthma biomarkers mentioned in this book were not being considered in 2006, but asthma was obviously identified as one of the more impactful diseases that require qualified biomarkers to expedite drug development.

The following section discusses how biomarkers are validated and qualified.

USING ENDPOINTS AND BIOMARKERS IN DRUG DEVELOPMENT

To obtain marketing approval, drug manufacturers must demonstrate the effectiveness (and safety) of their products, usually through the conduct of adequate and well-controlled investigations.[9,10] Efficacy endpoints are used to assess the effects of a therapeutic intervention being evaluated in a clinical trial and are typically results, conditions, or events. Efficacy endpoints are often categorized as clinical outcomes or biomarkers. A clinical outcome is a direct measure of how a patient feels, functions, and survives. Clinical endpoints are most relevant to the study subject and are considered clinically meaningful. As stated previously, a surrogate measure is a biomarker intended to substitute for a clinically meaningful endpoint and is expected to predict the clinical benefit. In other words, changes in the surrogate endpoint in response to the therapeutic intervention should be reflective of changes in the clinically meaningful endpoint. In the context of drug development, the use of a validated or "reasonably likely" surrogate endpoint in a clinical trial offers several potential advantages including reducing the cost and duration of the trial. These decisions about surrogate endpoints are based on a case-by-case basis.

Endpoints can also be categorized based on their relative subjectivity or objectivity. Subjective endpoints are outcome measures that rely heavily on the assessor's or patient's opinion, interpretation, emotion, or judgment (e.g., symptom scores), whereas objective endpoints are not influenced to a large degree by individual interpretation, emotions, opinions, or personal feelings (e.g., mortality or a laboratory measurement). In asthma clinical research, pulmonary function tests (e.g., FEV1) and inflammatory markers (e.g., sputum eosinophils) are considered objective measures, while symptoms scores or the need for rescue medication is considered subjective measures.[13] Although subjective outcome measures can provide valuable insight into the therapeutic effect of a drug, it is important to be mindful that they have the potential to introduce bias into the trial, particularly in the case of an open-label trial.[14-18]

Establishing Primary and Secondary Endpoints in Drug Development

Endpoints are typically grouped into three categories: primary, secondary, and tertiary (also referred to as exploratory).[19,20] In studies designed to assess drug efficacy, the primary endpoint is a measure by which the effectiveness of a therapeutic intervention is evaluated and is intended to support regulatory action. There is generally only one primary endpoint in a trial, and it should be the outcome measure that provides the most clinically relevant evidence and addresses the primary objective of the trial. The primary endpoint is the outcome measure for which subjects in the trial are randomized and is important in determining the sample size required to adequately power the study to demonstrate a statistically significant difference in the primary endpoint between the randomized groups.

Secondary endpoints are measures that can provide supportive evidence concerning the objectives of the study, only after there is first a demonstration of treatment effect on the primary endpoint. Secondary outcome measures may also provide insight into the underlying mechanism of the drug's effect on the primary endpoint or reveal additional effects on the disease or condition under study. Nevertheless, secondary endpoints may or may not be powered for hypothesis testing within the trial. In the study protocol, it is important that the primary endpoint and secondary endpoints be prespecified and their rationale for selection be clearly stated.

All other endpoints measured within a trial are considered exploratory. Exploratory endpoints are usually not prospectively planned and are not typically rigorously evaluated like primary and secondary endpoints. Although exploratory endpoints have limited value for confirmatory purposes, they can have utility in unplanned subgroup analyses and for hypothesis generation.

Relationship Between Adult Endpoints and Pediatric Endpoints

Given that the primary efficacy endpoint is integral to a well-designed study and serves as the basis for a robust evaluation of the clinical impact of the therapeutic intervention, it is critical that endpoints selected for use in clinical trials be well-defined, reliable, interpretable, and directly applicable to the disease or condition being studied. Past experience has shown that the use of inappropriate or unvalidated endpoints in pediatric trials has led to trial failure.[21] It is important to note that endpoints measured in adult trials may not always be suitable for use in pediatrics.[22] This may be due to a variety of reasons including differences in the pathophysiology, natural history (e.g., migraine),[23] or symptomatology (e.g., acute heart failure)[24] of the disease under study. In other cases, there may be differences in the performance capacity of the pediatric age subgroup being studied as opposed to that of the adult population. For example, the 6-min walk test (6MWT), a measure of exercise capacity, has been frequently assessed as a primary endpoint in interventional trials in adults with pulmonary arterial hypertension (PAH).[25-27] In contrast, for infants and younger children are who are not developmentally and physically able to perform exercise testing, the 6MWT would not be a feasible endpoint to measure.[28,29] The same is true for spirometry as measured by FEV1 (forced expiratory volume in 1 s) as an assessment of asthma control in clinical trials. The successful performance of the forced expiratory maneuver recommended for spirometry is highly dependent on patient cooperation and effort and as such is more suitable for children old enough to comprehend and follow instructions.[13] In other instances, it may not be feasible to incorporate the endpoint used in an adult trial into a pediatric trial because of the relatively small pediatric disease population. For example, mortality is a widely accepted outcome measure for interventional trials in adults with sepsis. However, because of the relatively low incidence of mortality events in children with sepsis, the use of mortality or survival endpoints would require a substantially large number of pediatric subjects to demonstrate differences in treatment effects between study arms.[30] Recruitment of sufficient numbers of pediatric subjects into the study may be extremely difficult.

Experience With Pediatric Endpoints in Drug Development

We have surveyed primary endpoints measured in pediatric efficacy trials submitted to the FDA between 2007 and September 2016. A total of 234 trials evaluating 138 unique drug products were identified. The most frequently studied therapeutic areas with full efficacy studies were pulmonary, antiviral, and allergy (Fig. 7.2). Of the 234 trials, 179 (76.5%) successfully met their primary endpoint and demonstrated the effectiveness of the drug, while 55 (23.3%) failed to establish efficacy in the population studied. The majority of endpoints were objective measures (48.7%), while the remaining were considered subjective (43.2%), or both objective and subjective (9.0%). When the endpoint was an objective measure, 20.2% of trials failed, whereas 31.3% of trials failed when the endpoint was subjective. Only 4.8% of trials failed when the endpoint measured was composed of both objective and subjective components ($P<0.05$) (Fig. 7.3).

In 93/234 (39.7)% of the cases, the endpoint assessed in the pediatric trial differed from the endpoint

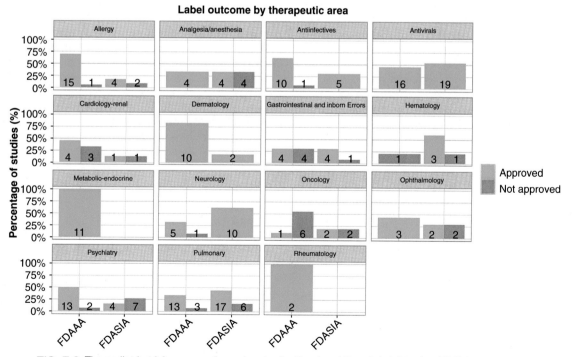

FIG. 7.2 The pediatric trials were performed under the Food and Drug Administration (FDA) Amendments Act (FDAAA; 2007–12) and the FDA Safety and Innovation Act (FDASIA; 2012–16). The *green bars* represent those trials that were approved for pediatric labeling of the indication following the trial. Some of the trials were conducted with pediatric extrapolation of adult efficacy to pediatric patients (e.g., antiinfectives).

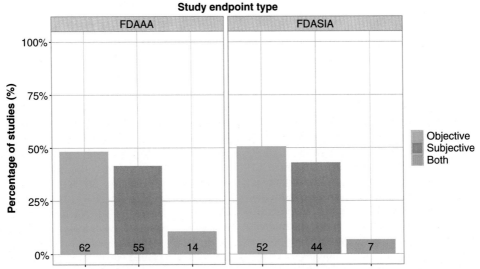

FIG. 7.3 Breakdown of pediatric endpoints used in efficacy trials under the Food and Drug Administration (FDA) Amendments Act (FDAAA; 2007–12) and the FDA Safety and Innovation Act (FDASIA; 2012–16). The comparison is the use of objective endpoints and subjective endpoints, and some trials used both types of endpoints.

measured in the correlate adult trial for the same indication. When the pediatric and adult endpoint differed, these trials failed more often than when the endpoint in the pediatric and adult trials was the same (38.7% vs. 13.3%, $P<0.01$) (Fig. 7.4). In the total cohort of trials, 95 (40.6%) enrolled both adult and pediatric patients into the same trial. The trial success rate was higher when pediatric patients were able to be included in the adult trial as opposed to when the pediatric and adult trials were conducted separately (89.5% vs. 67.6%, $P<0.01$) (Fig. 7.5).

Endpoints Used Previously in Pediatric Asthma Research

Numerous endpoints have been used in asthma.[13,31] More and more often biomarkers beyond FEV1 are being incorporated into clinical research studies of asthma to further define and characterize the population under study and to assess therapeutic effect.[32]

When reviewing drug development studies submitted to the FDA since 2012, there were a total of 28 pediatric efficacy trials for asthma-related indications, including acute and maintenance treatment, prevention, reduction of exacerbations, and prevention of exercise-induced bronchospasm (Table 7.1). Within these trials, 10 drug products were evaluated. The age range across all of the trials spanned from infancy through adolescence and 19 of the 28 (67.9%) asthma

trials enrolled both adults and adolescent patients 12 years of age and older into a single trial. For the majority of treatment and prevention trials (60.7%), the surrogate marker FEV1 served as the primary endpoint. However, for trials enrolling pediatric subjects 4 years of age and younger, the primary endpoint involved an assessment tool such as the Respiratory Status Scale, Pediatric Asthma Caregiver Assessment, and the Pediatric Asthma Questionnaire. Examples of other primary endpoints measured in the remaining trials included exacerbation rates, percent reduction in steroid use, and hospital admission rates and total length of stay.

BIOMARKER QUALIFICATION

Food and Drug Administration Experience With Biomarker Qualification

The critical regulatory question for most investigators and sponsors when using a biomarker is: "Is this biomarker fit-for-purpose for use in a drug development program?" Although the Biomarker Qualification program of the US FDA was developed to assist in answering this question, in fact, most biomarkers are not approved via this program.

There are three general pathways to acceptance of a biomarker for drug development (Fig. 7.6).[33] The most common pathway for acceptance is through the drug

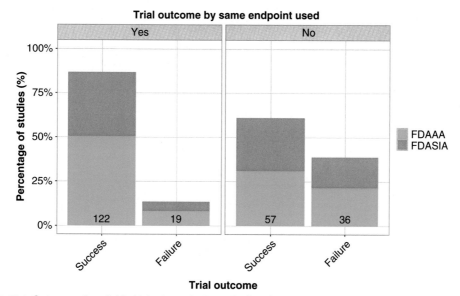

FIG. 7.4 Outcome of pediatric trials dependent on whether they used the same endpoint as in adults. The pediatric trials were performed under the Food and Drug Administration (FDA) Amendments Act (FDAAA; 2007–12) and the FDA Safety and Innovation Act (FDASIA; 2012–16). Failed trials did not receive pediatric labeling for the indication that was being studied. When the pediatric and adult endpoint differed, these trials failed more often than when the endpoint in the pediatric and adult trials was the same (38.7% vs. 13.5%, $P<0.01$).

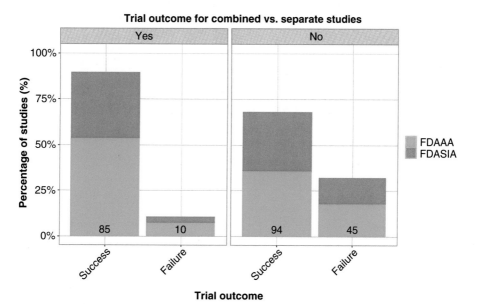

FIG. 7.5 Outcome of pediatric trials dependent on whether pediatric patients were studied in the same trial as adults. The pediatric trials were performed under the Food and Drug Administration (FDA) Amendments Act (FDAAA; 2007–12) and the FDA Safety and Innovation Act (FDASIA; 2012–16). Failed trails did not receive pediatric labeling for the indication that was being studied. The trial success rate was higher when pediatric patients were able to be included in the adult trial as opposed to when the pediatric and adult trials were conducted separately (89.5% vs. 67.6%, $P<0.01$).

TABLE 7.1
Endpoints Measured in Pediatric Asthma Trials Submitted to the Food and Drug Administration (2012–17)

Drug Name	Indication	Age Group Studied	Primary Endpoint(s)	Secondary Endpoints
ProAir Respiclick (albuterol)	Treatment/prevention	12 years and older	Change in FEV_1	Baseline-adjusted area-under-the effect curve for percent-predicted FEV_1 over 6 h ($PPFEV_1$ $AUEC_{0-6}$), measured in percent-predicted FEV_1 hours (%h)
	Treatment/prevention	12 years and older	Change in FEV_1	Baseline-adjusted FEV_1 AUC_{0-6} at day 1; baseline-adjusted FEV_1 AUC_{0-6} at day 8; baseline-adjusted FEV_1 AUC_{0-6} at day 85
	Treatment/prevention	12 years and older	Change in FEV_1	Baseline-adjusted FEV_1 AUC_{0-6} at day 1; baseline-adjusted FEV_1 AUC_{0-6} at day 85
	Prevention of exercise-induced bronchospasm	12 years and older	Change in FEV_1 postexercise challenge	Percentage of patients whose maximum percentage fall from the baseline FEV_1 postexercise challenge was <10%
	Treatment/prevention	4–11 years	Change in FEV_1	FEV_1 AUC_{0-6}; baseline-adjusted maximum FEV_1 (FEV_{1max}) within 6 h after treatment; baseline-adjusted maximum $PPFEV_1$ ($PPFEV_{1max}$) within 6 h after treatment
	Treatment/prevention	4–11 years	Change in FEV_1	Baseline-adjusted area under the curve for peak expiratory flow (PEF) over 6 h postdose (PEF AUC_{0-6}) over the 3-week treatment period
Arnuity Ellipta (fluticasone furoate)	Maintenance treatment	12 years and older	Change in FEV_1	Mean change from baseline in the percentage of rescue-free 24-h periods during the 24-week treatment period; mean change from baseline in daily trough (predose and prerescue bronchodilator); PM PEF averaged over the 24-week treatment period; mean change from baseline in daily AM PEF averaged over the 24-week treatment period; mean change from baseline in the percentage of symptom-free 24-h periods during the 24-week treatment period; change from baseline in total Asthma Quality of Life Questionnaire (AQLQ) (+12) score at the end of week 12 and to the end of the 24-week treatment period; change in Asthma Control Test (ACT) score from baseline (visit 2), at the end of week 12 (visit 6), and at the end of the 24-week treatment period (visit 9); the number of withdrawals due to lack of efficacy during the 24-week treatment period; Global Assessment of Change at the end of week 4 (visit 4), week 12 (visit 6), and 24 weeks' of treatment (visit 9); unscheduled healthcare contacts/resource utilization (for severe asthma exacerbations and other asthma-related healthcare)

| Maintenance treatment | 12 years and older | Change in FEV1 | Mean change from baseline in the percentage of rescue-free 24-h periods during the 12-week treatment period; change from baseline in the percentage of symptom-free 24-h periods during the 12-week treatment period; change from baseline in total AQLQ (+12) score at the end of 12-week treatment period; the number of withdrawals due to lack of efficacy during the 12-week treatment period; clinic visit 12-h FEV1 at the end of the 84-day treatment period and was assessed in the subset of subjects who were performing serial FEV1 assessments; weighted mean serial FEV1 over 0–24 h postdose calculated in a subset of subjects on day 0; weighted mean serial FEV1 over 0–4 h postdose calculated in the subset of subjects who were performing serial FEV1 assessments, on day 0 and day 84; time to onset of bronchodilator effect taken from serial measurements at visit 3; mean change from baseline in daily PM PEF averaged over the 12-week treatment period; mean change from baseline in daily AM PEF averaged over the 12-week treatment period; change from baseline in ACT at the end of the 12-week treatment period; Global Assessment of Change at the end of 4, 8, and 12 weeks of treatment; unscheduled healthcare contacts/resource utilization (for severe asthma exacerbations and other asthma-related healthcare); inhaler-use assessment at randomization, at the end of 2 weeks and 4 weeks of treatment; ease-of-use questions on inhaler at end of 4 weeks of treatment |
| Maintenance treatment | 12 years and older | Change in FEV1 | Change from baseline in the percentage of rescue-free 24-h periods during the 24-week treatment period; change from baseline in daily PM PEF, averaged over the 24-week treatment period; change from baseline in daily AM PEF, averaged over the 24-week treatment period; change from baseline in the percentage of symptom-free 24-h periods during the 24-week treatment period; change from baseline in ACT score at the end of the 24-week treatment period; percentage of subjects controlled, defined as an ACT score ≥20, at the end of the 24-week treatment period or every week; incidence of protocol defined severe exacerbations throughout the 24-week treatment period; unscheduled healthcare contacts/resource utilization for severe asthma exacerbations and other asthma-related healthcare; inhaler-use assessment at the end of 2 and 4 weeks of treatment; ease-of-use questions on the dry powder inhaler (DPI) at the end of 4 weeks of treatment |

Continued

TABLE 7.1
Endpoints Measured in Pediatric Asthma Trials Submitted to the Food and Drug Administration (2012–17)—cont'd

Drug Name	Indication	Age Group Studied	Primary Endpoint(s)	Secondary Endpoints
	Maintenance treatment	12 years and older	Change in FEV1	Mean change from baseline in the percentage of rescue-free 24-h periods during the 24-week treatment period; change from baseline in the percentage of symptom-free 24-h periods during the 24-week treatment period; change from baseline in total AQLQ (+12) score during 12 and 24 weeks of treatment; clinic visit 12 h FEV1 at the end of the 168-day treatment period and was assessed in the subset of subjects who were performing serial FEV1 assessments; weighted mean serial FEV1 over 0–4 h postdose calculated in the subset of subjects performing serial FEV1 on Day 168; mean change from baseline in daily AM PEF averaged over the first 12 weeks and over the 24-week treatment period; mean change from baseline in daily PM PEF averaged over the first 12 weeks and over the 24-week treatment period; the number of withdrawals due to lack of efficacy during the 24-week treatment period; change from baseline in the ACT at the end of 4, 12, and 24 weeks of treatment; Global Assessment of Change at the end of 4, 12, and 24 weeks of treatment; unscheduled healthcare contacts/resource utilization for severe asthma exacerbations and other asthma-related healthcare
Xopenex (levalbuterol)	Treatment	2–5 years	Pediatric asthma questionnaire total score	Pediatric Asthma Caregiver Assessment completed 3 days after each study visit; PEF rate in clinical and at-home measurements obtained predose and 30–45 min postdose; rescue medicines usage; number of uncontrolled asthma days; number of asthma exacerbations; function status II questionnaire and CHQ-PF50 General Health Perceptions Scale Questionnaire; Pediatric Asthma Caregiver's Quality of Life Questionnaire; Global Assessment by physician and parent/legal guardian at end of study
	Treatment	0–48 months	Respiratory status scale (RSS) total score	Individual RSS parameters; time to meet discharge criteria, time to maximum decrease in RSS total score; rate of hospitalization; rate of relapse; rate of respiratory exacerbations; rescue medication use; daytime and nighttime breathing symptoms assessed by the Children Breathing Questionnaire; relief of bronchoconstriction as assessed by physician and caregiver global evaluations
	Treatment	0–48 months	Pediatric asthma caregiver assessment score	Pediatric Asthma Questionnaire (PAQ); Pediatric Asthma Quality of Life Questionnaire (PAQLQ); PEF Maneuvers in subjects 24–47 months of age; investigator and caregiver global evaluations; and rescue medication use
	Treatment	2–17 years	Hospital admissions rate; total length of stay (LOS)	Emergency department (ED) LOS; Asthma Care Path LOS; number of aerosols required before discharge criteria were met; number of subjects with LOS <24 h in each group; number of subjects requiring intensification therapy, requirement of supplemental oxygen, concurrent medication in the ED, and rates of acute visits or readmissions to the hospital for worsening asthma

Xopenex HFA (levalbuterol)	Treatment	0–48 months	Pediatric asthma caregiver assessment score	Daily Pediatric Asthma Caregiver Assessments (PACA), PAQ, Pediatric Asthma Quality of Life Questionnaire (PACQLQ), PEF maneuvers in subjects 24–47 months of age, investigator and caregiver global evaluations, and rescue medication use
Nucala (mepolizumab)	Maintenance treatment	12 years and older	Annualized rate of asthma exacerbations	Time to first clinically significant exacerbation; frequency of exacerbations requiring hospitalization or ED visit; frequency of investigator-defined exacerbations; time to first investigator-defined exacerbation; mean change from baseline in clinical prebronchodilator FEV_1 over the 52-week treatment period; mean change from baseline in clinical postbronchodilator FEV_1 over the 52-week treatment period; time to first exacerbation requiring hospitalization or ED visit; blood eosinophil count; annual rate of exacerbations by blood eosinophil count
	Maintenance treatment	12 years and older	Annualized rate of asthma exacerbations	Rate of asthma exacerbations; frequency of exacerbations requiring hospitalization or ED visit; frequency of exacerbations requiring hospitalization; mean change from baseline in clinic prebronchodilator FEV_1; mean change in St. George Respiratory Questionnaire
	Maintenance treatment	12 years and older	% reduction in oral corticosteroid (OCS) dose	Proportion of subjects who achieve a 50% reduction or greater in their daily OCS dose, compared with baseline dose during 20–24 weeks while maintaining asthma control; the proportion of subjects who achieve a reduction of their daily OCS dose to less than or equal 5 mg during weeks 20–24, while maintaining asthma control; the proportion of subjects who achieve a total reduction of OCS dose during 20–24 weeks, while maintaining asthma control; median percentage reduction from baseline in daily OCS dose during weeks 20–24 while maintaining asthma control
Asmanex HFA (mometasone furoate)	Maintenance treatment	12 years and older	Change in FEV_1	Trough FEV_1; change from baseline in ACQ; change from baseline in AQLQ; change from baseline in AM and PM PEF rates; change from baseline in AM and PM asthma symptom scores; proportion of nights with nocturnal awakenings; rescue medication usage
	Maintenance treatment	12 years and older	Change in FEV_1	Time to first severe asthma exacerbation; trough FEV_1; change from baseline in the AQLQ; change from baseline in the ACQ; change from baseline in AM and PM PEF rates; change from baseline in AM and PM asthma symptom scores; proportion of nights with nocturnal awakenings; rescue medication usage
Dulera (mometasone furoate/formoterol)	Treatment	5–11 years	Change in FEV_1	Change from baseline in AM PEF at week 12 using diary data; change from baseline in PAQLQ; the percent-predicted FEV_1 compared with MF DPI

Continued

TABLE 7.1
Endpoints Measured in Pediatric Asthma Trials Submitted to the Food and Drug Administration (2012–17)—cont'd

Drug Name	Indication	Age Group Studied	Primary Endpoint(s)	Secondary Endpoints
Xolair (omalizumab)	Maintenance treatment	6–11 years	Rate of asthma exacerbations	The rate of clinically significant asthma exacerbations during the 52-week double-blind treatment period; change in nocturnal clinical symptom score from baseline to the end (last 4 weeks) of the 24 week double-blind fixed steroid treatment period (time adjusted); change in β-agonist rescue medication use from baseline to the end (last 4 weeks) of the 24-week double-blind fixed steroid treatment period; change in quality of life (PAQLQ[S]) in overall score from baseline to the end (last visit) of the 24-week double-blind fixed steroid treatment period
Cinqair (reslizumab)	Maintenance treatment	12 years and older	Change in FEV1	ACQ: change from baseline to weeks 4, 8, 12, 16, and endpoint; AQLQ: change from baseline to week 16, and endpoint; forced vital capacity (FVC): change from baseline to weeks 4, 8, 12, 16, and endpoint; forced expiratory flows (FEF25%–75%); change from baseline to weeks 4, 8, 12, 16, and endpoint; Asthma Symptom Utility Index (ASUI): change from baseline to weeks 4, 8, 12, 16, and endpoint; short-acting β-agonist (SABA) use: change from baseline to weeks 4, 8, 12, 16, and endpoint; blood eosinophils (EOS): change from baseline to weeks 4, 8, 12, 16, and endpoint; % predicted FEV1: change from baseline to weeks 4, 8, 12, 16, and endpoint
	Maintenance treatment	12 years and older	Annualized rate of asthma exacerbations	FEV1: change from baseline to week 16; FEV1: change from baseline over 16 weeks; AQLQ: change from baseline to week 16; ACQ: change from baseline to week 16; time to first clinical asthma exacerbation; ASUI: change from baseline over 16 weeks; SABA use: change from baseline over 16 weeks; blood eosinophils: change from baseline over 16 weeks and 52 weeks
	Maintenance treatment	12 years and older	Annualized rate of asthma exacerbations	FEV1: change from baseline to week 16; FEV1: change from baseline over 16 weeks; AQLQ: change from baseline to week 16; ACQ: change from baseline to week 16; time to first clinical asthma exacerbation; ASUI: change from baseline over 16 weeks; SABA use: change from baseline over 16 weeks; blood eosinophils: change from baseline over 16 and 52 weeks

| Spiriva Respimat (tiotropium bromide) | Maintenance treatment | 12 years and older | Peak FEV1 | Predose FEV1 measured just before the last administration of randomized treatment; (trough FEV1 [L]), determined as a response from baseline at the end of the 4-week treatment period; maximum FVC measured within the first 3 h after dosing (FVC Peak0–3 h [L]), determined as a response from baseline at the end of each 4-week treatment period; predose FVC measured just before the last administration of randomized treatment (trough FVC [L]), determined as a response from baseline at the end of each 4-week treatment period; AUCs from 0 to 3 h for FEV1 (FEV1 AUC0–3 h) and FVC (FVC AUC0–3 h [L]); the AUC was calculated by using the trapezoidal rule divided by the observation time (3 h) and was determined as a response from baseline at the end of each 4-week treatment period. The trough values were assigned to 0 time; individual FEV1 [L] and FVC [L] measurements at each time point ("personal best"); mean FEF between 25% and 75% of the FVC (also known as maximum midexpiratory flow; FEF25%–75% [L]), which was determined as a response at the end of each 4-week treatment period; control of asthma as assessed by the ACQ, which was determined at the end of each 4-week treatment period. This endpoint was not analyzed as a response; predose morning and evening peak expiratory flow (PEF am/pm [L/min]), determined as a response from baseline based on the weekly mean of the last week of treatment; for each treatment period. This was measured by patients at home using the Asthma Monitor AM3 (AM3) device; use of PRN (pro re nata, or as necessary) rescue medication, determined as a response from baseline based on the weekly mean of the last week of treatment for each treatment period. This was recorded by patients at home using the AM3 device; nighttime awakenings due to asthma symptoms, determined as a response from baseline based on the weekly mean of the last week of treatment for each treatment period. This was assessed by the patient's electronic diary incorporated in the AM3 device |

Continued

TABLE 7.1
Endpoints Measured in Pediatric Asthma Trials Submitted to the Food and Drug Administration (2012–17)—cont'd

Drug Name	Indication	Age Group Studied	Primary Endpoint(s)	Secondary Endpoints
	Maintenance treatment	12 years and older	Peak and trough FEV1	Trough FEV1 at 24 weeks; peak (within 3 h postdosing) and trough FVD at the end of the 24-week treatment period; FEV(AUC0-3) and FVC (AUC0-3) at the end of the 24-week treatment period; individual FEV1 and FVC measurements at all time points including peak, trough, and AUC0-3 during the 48-week treatment period; PEF am/pm mean predose morning and evening PEF measured by patients at home; number of asthma exacerbations per patient based on severity of the asthma exacerbation; number of patients with at least one asthma exacerbation based on severity during the 48-week treatment period; time to first hospitalization during the 48-week treatment period; number of hospitalizations for asthma exacerbations per patient during the 48-week treatment period; number of patients with at least one hospitalization for asthma exacerbation during the 48-week treatment period; quality of life as assessed by standardized AQLQ at all time points during the 48-week treatment period; control of asthma assessed by the ACQ at all time points during the 48-week treatment period; asthma symptoms as assessed by the patients' electronic diary during the 48-week treatment period; asthma symptom–free days during the 48-week treatment period defined as no days reported symptoms and no use of rescue medication; use of PRN salbutamol rescue medication during the 48-week treatment period: number of puffs used per 24-h period; mean FEF between 25% and 75% of the FVC or maximum expiratory flow
	Maintenance treatment	12 years and older	Peak FEV1	Trough FEV1 at 12 weeks; peak (within 3 h postdosing) and trough FVD at the end of the 12-week treatment period; FEV(AUC0-3) and FVC (AUC0-3) at the end of the 12-week treatment period; individual FEV1 and FVC measurements at all time points including peak, trough, and AUC0-3 during the 12-week treatment period; PEF am/pm mean predose morning and evening PEF measured by patients at home; number of asthma exacerbations per patient based on severity of the asthma exacerbation; number of patients with at least one asthma exacerbation based on severity during the 12-week treatment period; time to first hospitalization during the 12-week treatment period; number of hospitalizations for asthma exacerbations per patient during the 12-week treatment period; number of patients with at least one hospitalization for asthma exacerbation during the 12-week treatment period; quality of life as assessed by standardized AQLQ at all time points during the 12-week treatment period; control of asthma assessed by the ACQ at all time points during the 12-week treatment period; asthma symptoms as assessed by the patients' electronic diary during the 12-week treatment period; asthma symptom–free days during the 12-week treatment period defined as no days reported symptoms and no use of rescue medication; use of PRN salbutamol rescue medication during the 12-week treatment period: number of puffs used per 24-h period; mean FEF between 25% and 75% of the FVC or maximum expiratory flow

FEV1, forced expiratory volume in 1 s.

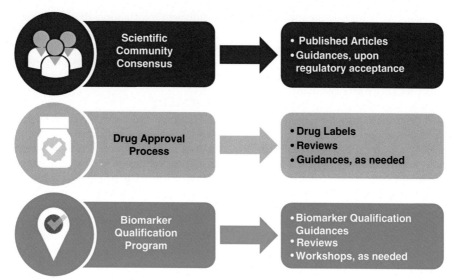

FIG. 7.6 The biomarker acceptance pathways. (From McCune S. *Outcome Measures, Biomarkers and Endpoints*; 2016. Available at: https://www.fda.gov/downloads/NewsEvents/MeetingsConferencesWorksho ps/UCM519805.pdf; with permission.)

approval process. The endpoints that have been used in previous drug development programs have been "qualified" by their use in prior programs. These biomarkers and endpoints can be found in FDA reviews and in the FDA-approved drug labels.

Predictive enrichment biomarkers are frequently used in pediatric patients. A good example of a predictive biomarker in pediatric patients is the use of ivacaftor in cystic fibrosis patients. Ivacaftor was designed for use in cystic fibrosis patients with the *G551D* mutation in the *CFTR* gene, the third most common mutation in cystic fibrosis patients. Ivacaftor was studied in two double-blind, placebo-controlled trials in cystic fibrosis patients. The primary efficacy endpoint in these studies was improvement in lung function as determined by the mean absolute change from baseline in percent-predicted predose FEV1 through 24 weeks of treatment. This is an example of the approval of a biomarker through the drug approval process.

A second mechanism is through a scientific community consensus regarding the use of a biomarker as a valid indirect measure of how a patient feels, functions, or survives. For the biomarker to be used in a drug development program, some discussion with regulators needs to take place, and a guidance would probably be needed to indicate regulatory acceptance of this biomarker. The guidance could then also clarify the context of use for the biomarker, which could be quite specific and may or may not apply to pediatric patients.

An example is the use of total kidney volume in studies of polycystic kidney disease, for which a guidance has been issued.[34]

The third mechanism is the FDA's biomarker qualification program, which has a dedicated website.[35] This process is the most structured program for biomarker qualification for drug development, and a 2014 FDA Guidance explaining the qualification process is available.[36] The US FDA also makes available an educational program about the integration of biomarkers into drug development programs.[37] Therefore the US FDA is actively involved in promoting and assisting with biomarker validation and qualification.

The terms "validation" and "qualification" are often used interchangeably and incorrectly regarding biomarkers. The Guidance on the qualification of drug development tools does mention the validity if analytical methods, but not the validation process. Analytical validation is establishing that the performance characteristics of a test, tool, or instrument are acceptable in terms of its sensitivity, specificity, accuracy, precision, and other relevant performance characteristics using a specified technical protocol (which may include specimen collection, handling and storage procedures). This is validation of the test's, tool's, or instrument's technical performance but is not validation of the item's usefulness.[33] There is also clinical validation that establishes that the test, tool, or instrument acceptably identifies, measures, or predicts the concept of interest.

A concept in a regulatory context is the aspect of an individual's clinical, biologic, physical, or functional state, or experience that the assessment is intended to capture or reflect.

Qualification, on the other hand, is a conclusion, based on a formal regulatory process, that within the stated context of use, a medical product development tool can be relied on to have a specific interpretation and application in medical product development and regulatory review. While the Guidance does provide information about the process, the FDA has a webpage that specifically discusses the three stages (initiation, consultation and advice, and review) of biomarker qualification.[38]

The biomarker qualification process has been active since 2008, but three nonclinical and three clinical biomarkers have now been approved.[39] The clinical biomarkers were approved in 2015–16. For example, galactomannan was approved as a serum/bronchoalveolar lavage fluid biomarker for enrollment of patients into clinical trials for invasive aspergillosis, and a Guidance related to this biomarker is now available.[40] Now that three clinical biomarkers have been approved, the expectation is that the pace of submission to the Biomarker Qualification Program will increase.

Codevelopment of a Companion Diagnostic With a Therapeutic Product

The development of a biomarker with a therapeutic product often involves formalization of the test (device) for the biomarker of interest. Such a program would be codevelopment of the drug and device, and the FDA has a Guidance directed at the process by which the two entities are codeveloped.[41] The Guidance is extensive (48 pages), and the process of codevelopment should start very early in the drug development process.

The process of codevelopment started in 1998 with the approval of trastuzumab (Herceptin) and a test for HER-2 positivity in breast cancer tissue. According to the Guidance, "companion diagnostics are, by definition, essential for the safe and effective use of a corresponding therapeutic product and may be used to: 1) identify patients who are most likely to benefit from the therapeutic product; 2) identify patients likely to be at increased risk for serious adverse reactions as a result of treatment with the therapeutic product; 3) monitor response to treatment with the therapeutic product for the purpose of adjusting treatment (e.g., schedule, dose, discontinuation) to achieve improved safety or effectiveness; or 4) identify patients in the population for whom the therapeutic product has been adequately studied and found to be safe and effective (i.e., there is insufficient information about the safety and effectiveness of the therapeutic product in any other population)." Each of these scenarios could also be referred to as a biomarker used for these purposes.

SUMMARY

Having qualified biomarkers and endpoints for drug development is a critical part of the process. The US FDA established biomarkers as an essential component of improving the drug development process in 2004. Therefore the FDA established a Biomarker Qualification Program to encourage the qualification of both nonclinical and clinical biomarkers.

Most biomarkers are, however, qualified by being part of a successful drug development program. New biomarkers in asthma will have to choose one of the three routes mentioned to be validated and qualified for use in drug development. From our experience with endpoints in pediatric efficacy trials, we know that establishing a qualified biomarker in an adult program is more likely to lead to a successful program in pediatric patients if the same endpoint can be used. Including adolescent pediatric patients in the adult trial will be one additional means of improving the chances for labeling the product for the intended context of use in pediatric patients.

However, the Biomarker Qualification Program still holds considerable promise for qualifying new asthma biomarkers. With the qualification of three clinical biomarkers in 2015–16, the agency now seems poised to assist sponsors and academic investigators with the validation and qualification process. The regulatory pathway for biomarker qualification now seems to be supportive of the submission of new means of applying the multifaceted aspects of biomarkers to improve drug development and public health.

DISCLAIMER

The opinions expressed in this chapter are those of the authors and do not necessarily represent the position of the U.S. Food and Drug Administration.

REFERENCES

1. Group F-N-BW. *BEST (Biomarkers, EndpointS, and Other Tools) Resource*; 2016. Access at: https://www.ncbi.nlm.nih .gov/books/NBK326791/pdf/Bookshelf_NBK326791.pdf.
2. Burckart GJ, Amur S, Goodsaid FM, et al. Qualification of biomarkers for drug development in organ transplantation. *Am J Transpl.* 2007;8(2):267–270.

3. Savage W, Everett A. Biomarkers in pediatrics: children as biomarker orphans. *Proteomics Clin Appl.* 2010;4:915–921.

4. Green DJ, Mummaneni P, Kim IW, Oh JM, Pacanowski M, Burckart GJ. Pharmacogenomic information in FDA-approved drug labels: application to pediatric patients. *Clin Pharmacol Ther.* 2016;99:622–632.

5. Fleming TR, DeMets DL. Surrogate end points in clinical trials: are we being misled? *Ann Intern Med.* 1996;125:605–613.

6. Molenberghs G. Surrogate endpoints: applications in pediatric clinical trials. In: Mulberg AE, Murphy D, Dunne J, Mathis LL, eds. *Pediatric Drug Development: Concepts and Applications.* Hoboken, NJ, USA: Wiley Blackwell; 2013.

7. US Food and Drug Administration. *Challenge and Opportunity on the Critical Path to New Medical Products;* 2004. Available at: https://www.fda.gov/downloads/ScienceResearch/SpecialTopics/CriticalPathInitiative/CriticalPathOpportunitiesReports/ucm113411.pdf.

8. US Food and Drug Administration. *Critical Path Opportunities List;* 2006. Access at: https://www.fda.gov/downloads/ScienceResearch/SpecialTopics/CriticalPathInitiative/CriticalPathOpportunitiesReports/UCM077258.pdf.

9. Guidance for Industry. *Providing Clinical Evidence of Effectivess for Human Drug and Biological Products.* U.S FDA; 1998. Access at: https://www.fda.gov/ohrms/dockets/98p0311/Tab0035.pdf.

10. Downing NS, Aminawung JA, Shah ND, Krumholz HM, Ross JS. Clinical trial evidence supporting FDA approval of novel therapeutic agents, 2005–2012. *JAMA.* 2014;311(4): 368–377.

11. Kakkis ED, O'Donovan M, Cox G, et al. Recommendations for the development of rare disease drugs using the accelerated approval pathway and for qualifying biomarkers as primary endpoints. *Orphanet J Rare Dis.* 2015;10:16.

12. Johnson JR, Ning YM, Farrell A, Justice R, Keegan P, Pazdur R. Accelerated approval of oncology products: the food and drug administration experience. *J Natl Cancer Inst.* 2011;103(8):636–644.

13. de Benedictis FM, Guidi R, Carraro S, Baraldi E, Excellence TENo. Endpoints in respiratory diseases. *Eur J Clin Pharmacol.* 2011;67(suppl 1):49–59.

14. Hrobjartsson A, Thomsen AS, Emanuelsson F, et al. Observer bias in randomized clinical trials with measurement scale outcomes: a systematic review of trials with both blinded and nonblinded assessors. *CMAJ.* 2013;185(4):E201–E211.

15. Hrobjartsson A, Thomsen AS, Emanuelsson F, et al. Observer bias in randomised clinical trials with binary outcomes: systematic review of trials with both blinded and non-blinded outcome assessors. *BMJ.* 2012;344:e1119.

16. Moustgaard H, Bello S, Miller FG, Hrobjartsson A. Subjective and objective outcomes in randomized clinical trials: definitions differed in methods publications and were often absent from trial reports. *J Clin Epidemiol.* 2014;67(12):1327–1334.

17. Kahan BC, Cro S, Dore CJ, et al. Reducing bias in open-label trials where blinded outcome assessment is not feasible: strategies from two randomised trials. *Trials.* 2014;15:456.

18. Kahan BC, Dore CJ, Murphy MF, Jairath V. Bias was reduced in an open-label trial through the removal of subjective elements from the outcome definition. *J Clin Epidemiol.* 2016;77:38–43.

19. *Guidance for Industry: Multiple Endpoints in Clinical Trials.* US FDA; 2017. Access at: https://www.fda.gov/downloads/Drugs/GuidanceComplianceRegulatoryInformation/Guidances/UCM536750.pdf.

20. *Guidance for Industry: E9 Statistical Principles for Clinical Trials US.* FDA (ICH); 1998. Access at: https://www.fda.gov/downloads/drugs/guidancecomplianceregulatoryinformation/guidances/ucm073137.pdf.

21. Momper JD, Mulugeta Y, Burckart GJ. Failed pediatric drug development trials. *Clin Pharmacol Ther.* 2015;98(3): 245–251.

22. Wang S, Laitinen-Parkkonen P. Efficacy assessment in paediatric studies. *Handb Exp Pharmacol.* 2011;205:149–168.

23. Sun H, Bastings E, Temeck J, et al. Migraine therapeutics in adolescents: a systematic analysis and historic perspectives of triptan trials in adolescents. *JAMA Pediatr.* 2013;167(3):243–249.

24. Shaddy RE, Olsen SL, Bristow MR, et al. Efficacy and safety of metoprolol in the treatment of doxorubicin-induced cardiomyopathy in pediatric patients. *Am Heart J.* 1995;129(1):197–199.

25. Farber HW, Miller DP, McGoon MD, Frost AE, Benton WW, Benza RL. Predicting outcomes in pulmonary arterial hypertension based on the 6-minute walk distance. *J Heart Lung Transplant.* 2015;34(3):362–368.

26. Fritz JS, Blair C, Oudiz RJ, et al. Baseline and follow-up 6-min walk distance and brain natriuretic peptide predict 2-year mortality in pulmonary arterial hypertension. *Chest.* 2013;143(2):315–323.

27. Demir R, Kucukoglu MS. Six-minute walk test in pulmonary arterial hypertension. *Anatol J Cardiol.* 2015;15(3):249–254.

28. Cappelleri JC, Hwang LJ, Mardekian J, Mychaskiw MA. Assessment of measurement properties of peak VO_2 in children with pulmonary arterial hypertension. *BMC Pulm Med.* 2012;12:54.

29. Zijlstra WM, Ploegstra MJ, Vissia-Kazemier T, et al. Physical activity in pediatric pulmonary arterial hypertension measured by accelerometry: a candidate clinical endpoint. *Am J Respir Crit Care Med.* 2017. http://dx.doi.org/10.1164/rccm.201608-1576OC.

30. Curley MA, Zimmerman JJ. Alternative outcome measures for pediatric clinical sepsis trials. *Pediatr Crit Care Med.* 2005;6(3 suppl):S150–S156.

31. Krishnan JA, Lemanske RF Jr, Canino GJ, et al. Asthma outcomes: symptoms. *J Allergy Clin Immunol.* 2012;129(3 suppl):S124–S135.

32. Szefler SJ, Wenzel S, Brown R, et al. Asthma outcomes: biomarkers. *J Allergy Clin Immunol.* 2012;129(3 suppl): S9–S23.

33. McCune S. *Outcome Measures, Biomarkers and Endpoints;* 2016. https://www.fda.gov/downloads/NewsEvents/MeetingsConferencesWorkshops/UCM519805.pdf.

34. US Food and Drug Administration. *Qualification of Biomarker – Total Kidney Volume in Studies for Treatment of Autosomal Dominant Polycystic Kidney Disease;* 2015. Access at: https://www.fda.gov/downloads/Drugs/Guidances/UCM458483.pdf.

35. US Food and Drug Administration. *Biomarker Qualification Program.* Access at: https://www.fda.gov/Drugs/DevelopmentApprovalProcess/DrugDevelopmentToolsQualificationProgram/BiomarkerQualificationProgram/ucm20086360.htm.

36. US Food and Drug Administration. *Guidance for Industry and FDA Staff: Qualification Process for Drug Development Tools.* Access at: https://www.fda.gov/downloads/drugs/guidances/ucm230597.pdf.

37. US Food and Drug Administration. *Pathways for Biomarker Integration in Drug Developemnt.* Access at: https://www.fda.gov/Drugs/DevelopmentApprovalProcess/DrugDevelopmentToolsQualificationProgram/BiomarkerQualificationProgram/ucm536403.htm.

38. US Food and Drug Administration. *Information for Biomarker Qualification Submitters.* Access at: https://www.fda.gov/Drugs/DevelopmentApprovalProcess/DrugDevelopmentToolsQualificationProgram/BiomarkerQualificationProgram/ucm535115.htm.

39. US Food and Drug Administration. *List of Qualified Biomarkers.* Access at: https://www.fda.gov/Drugs/DevelopmentApprovalProcess/DrugDevelopmentToolsQualificationProgram/BiomarkerQualificationProgram/ucm-535383.htm.

40. US Food and Drug Administration. *Guidance on Qualification of Biomarker—Galactomannan in Studies of Treatments of Invasive Aspergillosis.* Access at: https://www.fda.gov/downloads/Drugs/GuidanceComplianceRegulatoryInformation/Guidances/UCM472606.pdf.

41. US Food and Drug Administration. *Draft Guidance for Industry and FDA Staff: Principles for Codevelopment of an In Vitro Companion Diagnostic Device With a Therapeutic Product.* Access at: https://www.fda.gov/downloads/MedicalDevices/DeviceRegulationandGuidance/GuidanceDocuments/UCM510824.pdf.

CHAPTER 8

Discovery and Validation of New Biomarkers for Personalizing Asthma Therapy

KIAN FAN CHUNG, MD, DSC, FRCP

INTRODUCTION

Despite the recognition that asthma is a disease with many faces, the introduction of biomarkers in the management of asthma has become a matter of interest only in recent years. Phenotypes of asthma have been identified regarding causal or triggering factors such as allergen-induced or aspirin-induced, in relation to the type of airflow obstruction, according to the severity and response to treatments, radiologic findings, and the nature of airway inflammation.[1,2] Clinicians have also long recognized certain types of asthma defined according to the age of onset of symptoms of asthma. The early-onset asthma in childhood associated with allergies usually has a favorable outcome with disappearance of symptoms by adolescence or early adulthood; on the other hand, late-onset asthma is usually associated with nasal polyps and eosinophilia, with a more chronic course often needing maintenance oral corticosteroid therapy. In addition, blood eosinophilia was recognized to be associated with a good response to inhaled and oral corticosteroid therapy and also with the severity of asthma. With the recent development of the concept of personalized medicine and the introduction of drugs that target specific pathways, it is now imperious to consider a more rationalized approach toward the phenotyping of asthma and with it the development of new biomarkers. This has also become a necessity because of the 5% of patients with severe refractory asthma where phenotyping remains incomplete with a lack of understanding of underlying mechanisms with consequent unmet need of novel effective therapies.[3]

PERSONALIZED MEDICINE FOR ASTHMA

Personalized medicine is an emerging approach for disease treatment and prevention that takes into account individual variability in genes, environment, and lifestyle for each person. It is also often described as providing the right patient with the right drug at the right time.[4] Therefore, personalized medicine is the tailoring of medical management to the individual characteristics and preferences of an individual patient. Other terms that are used sometimes interchangeably with personalized medicine include precision medicine, stratified medicine, or targeted medicine. The practice of medicine since the time of Hippocrates has been to treat the individual patient, but only recent developments in technology has enabled the medical practitioner to use tools that will predict how an individual patient may respond to a medical therapy or experience side effects from that treatment. This will ultimately lead to the development of targeted therapeutics. The delivery of personalized medicine will depend on the availability of accurate and reliable diagnostics with the identification of predictive biomarkers that need to be reliable and accurate.

TYPES OF BIOMARKERS IN ASTHMA

The importance of having biomarkers in asthma is to define the phenotypes that constitute the whole range of asthma and to find the patients who will respond to specific therapies. A biomarker is defined as a characteristic that can be measured and evaluated as an indicator of normal or pathologic biologic processes or the biologic response to a therapeutic intervention.[5] Therefore, biomarkers can be used to increase our understanding of the pathways that lead to disease progression or drug toxicity. Thus, under this class, diagnostic biomarkers may be used to distinguish between different phenotypes of asthma to ensure, for example, that the patients selected for a clinical study are of the appropriate phenotype required for the study in question or can be used to stratify patients in clinical trials. On the other hand, prognostic biomarkers provide some information about the course of the disease, if left untreated. Predictive biomarkers allow a prediction of the likelihood of therapeutic response of a particular patient to a specific therapeutic intervention, and a response biomarker would be a biomarker that shows that a biologic response has occurred after receiving an intervention. Biomarkers can also be used as substitute for primary clinical efficacy endpoints or as surrogate markers, i.e., used as predictive or response biomarkers. It is therefore important to note that a biomarker may be useful in more than one category. For the development of new treatments, there are various biomarker qualification processes put forward by regulatory bodies.

CURRENT BIOMARKERS USED IN ASTHMA MANAGEMENT

A handful of biomarkers mostly indicative of T2-high asthma are used in the management of asthma, namely blood eosinophil count, serum IgE and serum periostin levels, levels of nitric oxide in exhaled breath (FeNO), and sputum eosinophil count. The focus has been on the use of these biomarkers in the management of asthma. First, there has been interest in determining whether sputum eosinophil counts or FeNO could help in shaping better outcome measures mainly in terms of exacerbations if they were used as response to treatment with corticosteroid therapy. In a metaanalysis of six (two adults and four children/ adolescents) studies utilizing FeNO[6-10] and three adult studies utilizing sputum eosinophils,[11-13] tailoring of asthma treatment based on sputum eosinophils was effective in decreasing asthma exacerbations, whereas that based on FeNO levels was not effective in improving asthma outcomes in children and adults.[14] However, routine use of sputum analysis to determine eosinophil counts is not advocated for adjusting the levels of corticosteroid therapy because of the technical expertise needed and the costs of the test and neither the use of FeNO proposed for its lack of effectiveness. However, sputum-guided treatment has been recommended with moderate or severe asthma where patients are managed in centers experienced in this technique by the ERS/ATS guidelines.[3] Usefulness of FeNO measurements has been provided for assessing adherence to corticosteroid therapy, but this remains to be validated.[15]

Blood eosinophil counts have also been shown to predict responsiveness to corticosteroid therapy particularly in children, but there is as yet a study on blood eosinophil–guided clinical trial.[16] They appear to be the best surrogate marker for sputum eosinophil in comparison with FeNO and serum periostin levels.[17] Interleukin (IL)-5 is a T2 cytokine that is involved in the terminal differentiation of eosinophils in the bone marrow and in its recruitment, and two anti-IL-5 monoclonal antibodies, mepolizumab[18,19] and reslizumab,[20] and one anti-IL5Rα antibody, benralizumab,[21,22] have been shown to reduce exacerbations and improve FEV_1, in patients with eosinophilic moderate to severe asthma characterized by high blood eosinophil counts. In two clinical trials of mepolizumab,[18,23] a close relationship between baseline blood eosinophil count and clinical efficacy of mepolizumab in patients with severe eosinophilic asthma and a history of exacerbations was shown, with clinically relevant reductions in exacerbation frequency in patients with a count of 150 cells/μL or more at baseline.[24] Interestingly, sputum eosinophil counts did not predict treatment response to mepolizumab.[25]

Total serum IgE level has been used as a response biomarker for the use of anti-IgE antibody, omalizumab, in the treatment of severe allergic asthma. Only recently has predictive biomarkers been assessed in omalizumab response: increased levels of FeNO (>19.5 parts per billion) and blood eosinophil count (>260/μL) significantly predicted those responding with a reduction in exacerbations while serum periostin (>50 ng/mL) did not achieve this at the 5% level.[26]

Periostin is a protein induced by IL-13 and produced by many cells in the airways. Serum levels of periostin were better at detecting airway eosinophilia than blood eosinophil counts or FeNO.[27] Increased serum periostin levels were found in patients who showed a greater increase in FEV_1 when treated with the anti-IL-13 antibody, lebrikizumab.[28] In those with high periostin levels, a larger reduction in FeNO was found. Thus, serum periostin could be a predictive biomarker for identification of responders to anti-IL-13 therapy. However, this was not supported in phase 3 studies where lebrikizumab did not consistently show significant reduction in asthma exacerbations in patients with serum periostin levels.[29] Dupilumab, an anti-IL4Rα monoclonal antibody that inhibits both IL-4 and IL-13 signaling, increased lung function and reduced severe exacerbations in patients with uncontrolled persistent asthma irrespective of whether the baseline eosinophil count was above or below the count of 300/μL.[30] This might suggest that for dupilumab blood eosinophil count is not the best predictive biomarker. It also means that for each of those specific antibody therapies, more specific

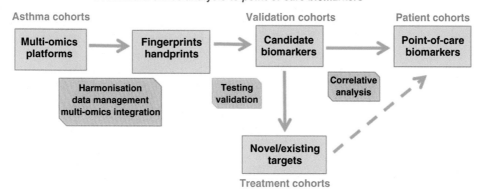

FIG. 8.1 Schematic approach to endotyping and biomarker discovery. Unbiased clustering of omics data leading to the identification of endotypes and candidate biomarkers. This will lead to target identification and potential new therapies. From candidate biomarkers, point-of-care biomarkers need to be derived.

biomarkers are needed for prediction of therapeutic response, rather than using generic ones related to T2 pathways.

CURRENT UNMET NEEDS IN BIOMARKERS IN ASTHMA

The present use of biomarkers in asthma has therefore been limited to the determination of the response of patients to new medications such as anti-IgE therapy or anti-IL-5 therapy.[4] The important reason why the use of biomarkers is currently very restrictive is because knowledge of the phenotypes of asthma is incomplete. A severe eosinophilic asthma phenotype has been characterized by severe refractory asthma with an exacerbation frequency ≥2 per year, dependence on oral corticosteroid therapy for asthma control, and a high circulating blood eosinophil count.[31] Other criteria may include raised FeNO level, late-onset disease, the presence of nasal polyps, fixed airflow obstruction, and air trapping with mucus plugging. On the other hand, a Th2 or T2 molecular phenotype has been characterized by the expression of genes that are upregulated in epithelial cells by the Th2 cytokine, IL-13, and this molecular phenotype was associated with high blood and sputum eosinophils.[32] This indicated that eosinophilic asthma is associated with a Th2 molecular phenotype. However, very little is known of either the noneosinophilic or the low Th2 or T2 asthma.[33]

The following areas must be considered as unmet needs in the field of biomarkers in asthma: (1) delineation of molecular phenotypes of asthma, particularly those in the non-T2/Th2 pathways; (2) lack of more phenotypic and predictive biomarkers to delineate

these molecular phenotypes of asthma; and (3) lack of specific biomarkers to predict therapeutic outcomes to more specific targeted therapies.

An unbiased approach is necessary to define the phenotypes of asthma. Although this can be determined on the basis of clinical parameters, the use of omics data from transcriptomics, proteomics, lipidomics, or metabolonomics holds the best chance of obtaining phenotypes on the basis of mechanisms, named as endotypes[34,35] (Fig. 8.1). This approach will also be best for obtaining composite biomarkers that would differentiate the different endotypes being described.

UNBIASED CLASSIFICATION USING CLINICAL, PHYSIOLOGIC, AND INFLAMMATORY FEATURES

Asthma is a heterogeneous condition that can present with diverse clinical traits, and several different molecular mechanisms may be driving these different phenotypes.[36,37] Biomarker research has been focused on the patient category of severe refractory asthma. Using partition-around-medoids clustering in the U-BIO-PRED severe asthma cohort, the phenotypes obtained were characterized by one well-controlled moderate to severe asthma, with three severe asthma phenotypes with (1) late-onset with past or current smoking and chronic airflow obstruction, predominantly eosinophilic; (2) nonsmoking severe asthma with chronic airflow obstruction and using oral corticosteroid therapy; and (3) obese female patients with frequent exacerbations but with normal lung function.[38] In the SARP cohort, phenotypes of early-onset atopic asthma with mild to moderate severity; obese, late-onset nonatopic asthma female patients with frequent exacerbations; and those with severe airflow obstruction with use of oral corticosteroid therapy were identified.[39] In the Leicester cohorts that also used sputum eosinophilia as a marker of eosinophilic asthma,[40] one cluster was that of an early-onset, symptom-predominant group with minimal eosinophilic disease, with a high prevalence of obesity and female gender, while the other cluster consisted of an eosinophilic inflammation-predominant group with few symptoms, late-onset disease, and a greater proportion of males, with a high prevalence of rhinosinusitis, aspirin sensitivity, and exacerbations. In the SARP unsupervised clustering using eosinophilic variables in blood, sputum, and bronchoalveolar lavage (BAL) fluid, patients with severe asthma were distributed among four clusters: early-onset allergic asthma with low lung function and eosinophil inflammation, late-onset asthma with nasal polyps and eosinophilia, persistent eosinophilia in blood and BAL fluid, and exacerbations despite high systemic corticosteroid use.[41] This clustering based on clinical, physiologic, and inflammatory parameters while yielding distinct phenotypes have not in general led to the elaboration of phenotypic biomarkers. Indeed, use of currently available biomarkers such as blood eosinophil counts or FeNO was not able to distinguish between these phenotypes.

MOLECULAR PHENOTYPING OF SEVERE ASTHMA

The approach of phenotyping on the basis of gene or protein expression seems to be more promising in terms of finding biomarkers and particularly in terms of developing phenotypic biomarkers that may be used to define a particular phenotype/endotype.[42] One mechanism underlying the eosinophilic asthma phenotype has been established, referred to as Th2-high or T2-high characterized by expression of genes stimulated by exposure to the Th2/T2 cytokine, IL-13, in airway epithelial cells.[32] The clinical counterpart of this gene-based phenotype is that these mild to moderate asthma patients have more blood and BAL eosinophils, increased levels of serum IgE, increased expression of mucin MUC5AC, increased expression of IL-5 and IL-13 in biopsies, and increased bronchial hyperresponsiveness, and respond to inhaled corticosteroids by an increase in FEV_1 compared with Th2-low. However, the pathways underling the Th2-low group remained unclear.

Recent studies have now elucidated pathways involved in these non-T2-high groups. In SARP, clustering of genes that were correlated with levels of FeNO

using K-means led to five clusters that were differentiated by 1584 genes. Hierarchic clustering of these genes led to the identification of nine gene clusters that were associated not only with T2-like genes but also with other pathways not usually associated with asthma such as neuronal pathways, WNT/β-catenin signaling pathway, and actin cytoskeleton pathways.[43] Using the technique of Weighted Gene Co-expression Network Analysis (WGCNA) to associate gene networks in epithelial cells with severe asthma traits in SARP, Modena et al. also found gene networks linked to epithelial growth and repair and decreased neuronal function in severe asthma.[44] T2 genes were increased in those treated with corticosteroids, and T1 inflammation in association with T2 gene expression was increased in a subgroup of severe asthma patients.

Using analysis of sputum transcriptomics, a six-gene signature including Charcot-Leyden crystal protein (CLC), carboxypeptidase A3 (CPA3), deoxyribonuclease I-like 3 (DNASE1L3), IL-1β, alkaline phosphatase, tissue-nonspecific isozyme (ALPL), and chemokine (C-X-C motif) receptor 2 (CXCR2), identified from gene expression profiles from induced sputum, could discriminate eosinophilic asthma from other phenotypes of noneosinophilic asthma, paucigranulocytic, and neutrophilic asthma. This six-gene signature also predicted response to inhaled corticosteroid therapy.[45] In neutrophilic asthma, there was significantly elevated gene expression of NLRP3, caspase-1, and IL-1β in sputum macrophages, providing evidence for NLRP3 inflammasome being upregulated in neutrophilic asthma.[46]

U-BIOPRED OMICS ANALYSIS

U-BIOPRED is a unique European research project that has recruited a severe asthma cohort with the aim of determining biomarker profiles from high-dimensional molecular, physiologic, and clinical data integrated by an innovative systems medicine approach into distinct handprints with the hope that these will enable the prediction of clinical course and therapeutic efficacy and identification of potential targets in the treatment of severe asthma.[47]

In the U-BIOPRED analysis of sputum omics data, an unbiased hierarchic clustering of differentially expressed genes between eosinophilic and noneosinophilic inflammatory profiles led to the description of three molecular phenotypes each characterized by 30-gene signatures representing different pathways.[48] Further characterization of these clusters was possible through proteomic analysis and gene expression

TABLE 8.1

Transcriptome-Associated Clusters (TACs) of Moderate to Severe Asthma From Sputum Analysis (U-BIOPRED)

	TAC 1	TAC 2	TAC 3
Mechanisms	T2 associated	Inflammasome	Mitochondrial oxidative stress
Affymetrix microarray	IL33R, TSLPR, CCR3, IL3RA	IFN and TNF superfamily, CASP4	Metabolic genes
Gene set variation analysis	Th2/ILC2	NLPR3/DAMP-associated	Th17; OXPHOS; aging
Protein (somalogic)	IL-16, periostin, serpin peptidase inhibitor 1, adiponectin, PAPPA	TNFAIP6, MIF, Tyrosine kinase src	Cathepsin B, G
Blood eosinophil count (/µL)	430	250	200
Sputum eosinophils (%)	30.9 (15–51)	0.6 (0.2–2.4)	1.0 (0.2–4.5)
Sputum neutrophil (%)	49.0 (26–71)	90.0 (85–94)	48.8 (33–64)
CRP (mg/L)	2.5 (1.0–3.4)	5.4 (3.0–7.2)	1.9 (1.0–5.0)
FeNO (ppb)	29.5	22.0	27.5
Clinical features	Severe asthma Highest nasal polyps Oral OCS-dependent Severe airflow obstruction	Moderate to severe asthma Moderate airflow obstruction High blood CRP levels More eczema	Moderate to severe asthma Mild airflow obstruction Lowest oral prednisolone Less frequent exacerbations

CRP, C-reactive protein; *FeNO*, level of nitric oxide in exhaled breath; *OCS*, oral corticosteroid. Numbers in brackets are 95th centile range of the median. Adapted from Kuo CS, Pavlidis S, Loza M, et al. T-helper cell type 2 (Th2) and non-Th2 molecular phenotypes of asthma using sputum transcriptomics in U-BIOPRED. *Eur Respir J.* 2017;49(2):pii: 1602135; with permission.

by gene set variation analysis. Three transcriptome-associated clusters (TACs) were defined (Table 8.1). TAC1 was characterized by immune receptors IL33R, CCR3, and TSLPR with the highest enrichment of gene signatures for IL-13/T-helper cell type 2 (Th2) and innate lymphoid cell type 2 associated with the highest sputum eosinophilia and exhaled nitric oxide fraction and was restricted to severe asthma with oral corticosteroid dependency, frequent exacerbations, and severe airflow obstruction. TAC2 was characterized by interferon-associated, tumor necrosis factor-α–associated, and inflammasome-associated genes with the highest sputum neutrophilia, serum C-reactive protein levels, and prevalence of eczema. TAC3 was characterized by genes of metabolic pathways, ubiquitination, and mitochondrial function with normal to moderately high sputum eosinophils and better preserved FEV$_1$.[48]

In a second analysis of U-BIOPRED database, the transcriptome derived from bronchial biopsies and epithelial brushings of 107 subjects with moderate to severe asthma were annotated by gene set variation analysis using 42 gene signatures relevant to asthma, inflammation, and immune function.[49] Nine gene set variation analysis signatures expressed in bronchial biopsies and airway epithelial brushings that included Th2-high, Th1-high, corticosteroid insensitivity, and oxidative stress signatures distinguished two distinct asthma subtypes with contrasting high blood and sputum eosinophils associated with high CD4$^+$ and CD8$^+$ T cells in biopsies. The eosinophilic group was subdivided into highest submucosal eosinophils, as well as high fractional exhaled nitric oxide levels, exacerbation rates, and oral corticosteroid use, and into a highest level of sputum eosinophils with a high body mass index. In contrast, the other two groups had a high likelihood of having noneosinophilic inflammation. Using machine-learning tools, an inference scheme was described using the biomarkers, sputum eosinophilia, and fractional exhaled nitric oxide levels, along with oral corticosteroid use, that could predict the subtypes of gene expression within bronchial biopsies and epithelial cells with good sensitivity and specificity. This analysis showed that different pathways are important in different compartments of the lungs and that the Th2 pathway can be associated with other pathways such as Th1 and corticosteroid insensitivity.

WHAT SHOULD CONSTITUTE A USEFUL BIOMARKER(S)?

It should be clear that a useful biomarker is one that represents the underlying pathologic mechanisms of disease; if the biomarker correlates with the mechanism of action of a biologic targeted therapy, then this will allow for targeted therapy through personalized medicine. Another important quality of a biomarker is that it should be assayed in a minimally invasive accessible medium and the measurement should be easily done and reproducible; these are the characteristics of "point-of-care" biomarkers, i.e., the biomarkers that can be used by the clinician in the clinic. It is possible that a combination of composite biomarkers, a reflection of several pathway interactions, might be more useful as diagnostic or predictive biomarkers. In the end, personalized medicine should not be solely based on a biomarker(s) but should be used together with the patient's clinical traits, particularly if these traits are amenable to therapy. Finally, biomarkers should be validated and reproduced in independent cohorts.

The molecular analyses described above provided biomarkers such as mRNA expression in airway samples that are not easily accessible. Therefore, these biomarkers need to be translated into point-of-care biomarkers that can be measured in the most minimally invasive specimens including blood, urine, and exhaled breath in relation to chronic airways disease such as asthma (Fig. 8.1). Thus, samples of blood, urine, or exhaled breath that have been stored can be used to analyze metabolites/analytes that reflect the biomarker expression derived from the omics analysis. This would be of importance particularly for cohorts that are undergoing clinical trials of drug therapy (Fig. 8.1). It is of the opinion of the author that more efforts should be put into obtaining lower airway samples such as sputum from subjects because these are valuable samples from the site of the disease that might provide better information. Unbiased analysis of other omics data, such as metabolonomics in exhaled breath through the use of eNOSE or lipidomics (focused on eicosanoids) in urine through the use of mass spectrometry in U-BIOPRED, has also yielded phenotypes of asthma.

Analysis of noninvasive metabolonomics of the exhaled breath consisting of volatile organic compounds (VOCs) is a promising point-of-care biomarker

approach for chronic obstructive airways disease such as asthma.[50] Analysis of VOC changes in asthmatic patients can be a useful tool for the diagnosis of asthma in conjunction with other tests.[51] The breath of patients with asthma versus those with chronic obstructive pulmonary disease can be distinguished with some degree of accuracy.[52,53] Exhaled breath profiles have been associated with pulmonary eosinophilia in asthma.[54] Breath analysis with an electronic nose could be used to predict oral steroid responsiveness in patients with mild to moderate asthma who had previously stopped steroid therapy.[55]

One approach taken by U-BIOPRED is to combine the analysis of more than one omics platform to produce fingerprints of asthma. It is the hope that this approach will provide more refined and precise endotypes of asthma, and this is currently being investigated.

PEDIATRIC CONSIDERATIONS

I have focused on adult asthma where most of the efforts have been centerd in terms of personalized medicine. However, pediatric asthma also represents a significant burden of disease, where there are still important knowledge gaps and unmet needs.[56] There is a need to define effective ways to prevent exacerbations and the progression of disease, and the focus continues to be on the improvement in asthma control so as to avert any potential adverse disease progression occurring later in life.[57] However, the optimal treatment strategy for pediatric asthma is not yet defined, but it is likely that this will depend on the characteristics of the patient and the disease. As for adult asthma, a better definition of the phenotypes of asthma and targeting of therapy based on phenotypes or, even better, on endotypes are likely to improve the management of pediatric asthma.

Cluster analysis of pediatric patients in the Severe Asthma Research Program (SARP) has identified four phenotype clusters differentiated by level of lung function, of which three clusters are atopic.[58] Another study (CAMP study) using spectral clustering defined five clusters on the basis of atopic status, degree of airflow obstruction, and exacerbation rates.[59] There are reports of asthmatic children with an atopic background having high blood eosinophils or a T2 profile,[60,61] but a study of severe therapy-resistant asthma reported that increased eosinophil counts in BAL fluid was not accompanied by increased levels of the T2 cytokines IL-4, IL-5, or IL-13.[62] One recent molecular phenotyping analysis of blood[63] yielded molecular phenotypes that demonstrated an interplay between innate and adaptive immunity. More molecular phenotyping studies are needed. In the field of biologic treatments for asthma that lags behind adult asthma, anti-IgE therapy is now available for the treatment of moderate to severe persistent asthma for allergic patients 12 years of age or older. With the promise of more biologic therapies becoming available for pediatric asthma, it would be important to do more molecular phenotyping in pediatric asthma, which may be different in many ways from adult asthma and derive useful biomarkers that will characterize phenotypes (endotypes) and those responsive to targeted therapies.

CONCLUSION

The heterogeneity and complexity of the asthma syndrome necessitates a different approach to phenotyping these patients. Use of clinical features and physiologic and inflammatory data are no longer sufficient to segment this condition. Use of omics data and unbiased clustering will provide greater chance of phenotyping asthma according to the mechanisms driving the disease in each phenotype from which a composite set of biomarkers could be used to define and categorize these endotypes. In the immediate future, it is envisaged that these new biomarkers might replace currently available biomarkers for both specific T2 and non-T2 pathways. Personalized medicine will allow for more precise treatment aims and also provide a source of novel targets and hence new treatments for each defined endotype.

ACKNOWLEDGMENT

The author would like to thank members of the U-BIO-PRED Consortium for interactions and discussion of the personalized approach to asthma.

REFERENCES

1. Nair P, Dasgupta A, Brightling CE, Chung KF. How to diagnose and phenotype asthma. *Clin Chest Med.* 2012;33(3):445–457.
2. Chung KF. Inflammatory biomarkers in severe asthma. *Curr Opin Pulm Med.* 2012;18(1):35–41.
3. Chung KF, Wenzel SE, Brozek JL, et al. International ERS/ATS guidelines on definition, evaluation and treatment of severe asthma. *Eur Respir J.* 2014;43(2):343–373.
4. Chung KF. New treatments for severe treatment-resistant asthma: targeting the right patient. *Lancet Respir Med.* 2013;1(8):639–652.
5. Amur S, LaVange L, Zineh I, Buckman-Garner S, Woodcock J. Biomarker qualification: toward a multiple mtakeholder framework for biomarker development, regulatory acceptance, and utilization. *Clin Pharmacol Ther.* 2015; 98(1):34–46.
6. Shaw DE, Berry MA, Thomas M, et al. The use of exhaled nitric oxide to guide asthma management: a randomized controlled trial. *Am J Respir Crit Care Med.* 2007;176(3):231–237.
7. Smith AD, Cowan JO, Brassett KP, Herbison GP, Taylor DR. Use of exhaled nitric oxide measurements to guide treatment in chronic asthma. *N Engl J Med.* 2005;352(21): 2163–2173.
8. de Jongste JC, Carraro S, Hop WC, Baraldi E. Daily telemonitoring of exhaled nitric oxide and symptoms in the treatment of childhood asthma. *Am J Respir Crit Care Med.* 2009;179(2):93–97.
9. Pijnenburg MW, Floor SE, Hop WC, De Jongste JC. Daily ambulatory exhaled nitric oxide measurements in asthma. *Pediatr Allergy Immunol.* 2006;17(3):189–193.
10. Szefler SJ, Mitchell H, Sorkness CA, et al. Management of asthma based on exhaled nitric oxide in addition to guideline-based treatment for inner-city adolescents and young adults: a randomised controlled trial. *Lancet.* 2008;372(9643):1065–1072.
11. Chlumsky J, Striz I, Terl M, Vondracek J. Strategy aimed at reduction of sputum eosinophils decreases exacerbation rate in patients with asthma. *J Int Med Res.* 2006;34(2):129–139.
12. Green RH, Brightling CE, McKenna S, et al. Asthma exacerbations and sputum eosinophil counts: a randomised controlled trial. *Lancet.* 2002;360(9347):1715–1721.
13. Jayaram L, Pizzichini MM, Cook RJ, et al. Determining asthma treatment by monitoring sputum cell counts: effect on exacerbations. *Eur Respir J.* 2006;27(3): 483–494.
14. Petsky HL, Cates CJ, Lasserson TJ, et al. A systematic review and meta-analysis: tailoring asthma treatment on eosinophilic markers (exhaled nitric oxide or sputum eosinophils). *Thorax.* 2012;67(3):199–208.
15. McNicholl DM, Stevenson M, McGarvey LP, Heaney LG. The utility of fractional exhaled nitric oxide suppression in the identification of nonadherence in difficult asthma. *Am J Respir Crit Care Med.* 2012;186(11): 1102–1108.
16. Gaillard EA, McNamara PS, Murray CS, Pavord ID, Shields MD. Blood eosinophils as a marker of likely corticosteroid response in children with preschool wheeze: time for an eosinophil guided clinical trial? *Clin Exp Allergy.* 2015;45(9):1384–1395.
17. Wagener AH, de Nijs SB, Lutter R, et al. External validation of blood eosinophils, FE(NO) and serum periostin as surrogates for sputum eosinophils in asthma. *Thorax.* 2015;70(2):115–120.
18. Ortega HG, Liu MC, Pavord ID, et al. Mepolizumab treatment in patients with severe eosinophilic asthma. *N Engl J Med.* 2014;371(13):1198–1207.

19. Bel EH, Wenzel SE, Thompson PJ, et al. Oral glucocorticoid-sparing effect of mepolizumab in eosinophilic asthma. *N Engl J Med.* 2014;371(13):1189–1197.

20. Corren J, Weinstein S, Janka L, Zangrilli J, Garin M. Phase 3 study of reslizumab in patients with poorly controlled asthma: effects across a broad range of eosinophil counts. *Chest.* 2016;150(4):799–810.

21. FitzGerald JM, Bleecker ER, Nair P, et al. Benralizumab, an anti-interleukin-5 receptor alpha monoclonal antibody, as add-on treatment for patients with severe, uncontrolled, eosinophilic asthma (CALIMA): a randomised, double-blind, placebo-controlled phase 3 trial. *Lancet.* 2016;388:2128–2141. http://dx.doi.org/10.1016/S0140-6736(16)31322-8.

22. Bleecker ER, FitzGerald JM, Chanez P, et al. Efficacy and safety of benralizumab for patients with severe asthma uncontrolled with high-dosage inhaled corticosteroids and long-acting beta2-agonists (SIROCCO): a randomised, multicentre, placebo-controlled phase 3 trial. *Lancet.* 2016;388:2115–2127. http://dx.doi.org/10.1016/S0140-6736(16)31324-1.

23. Pavord ID, Korn S, Howarth P, et al. Mepolizumab for severe eosinophilic asthma (DREAM): a multi-centre, double-blind, placebo-controlled trial. *Lancet.* 2012;380(9842):651–659.

24. Ortega HG, Yancey SW, Mayer B, et al. Severe eosinophilic asthma treated with mepolizumab stratified by baseline eosinophil thresholds: a secondary analysis of the DREAM and MENSA studies. *Lancet Respir Med.* 2016;4(7):549–556.

25. Katz LE, Gleich GJ, Hartley BF, Yancey SW, Ortega HG. Blood eosinophil count is a useful biomarker to identify patients with severe eosinophilic asthma. *Ann Am Thorac Soc.* 2014;11(4):531–536.

26. Hanania NA, Wenzel S, Rosen K, et al. Exploring the effects of omalizumab in allergic asthma: an analysis of biomarkers in the EXTRA study. *Am J Respir Crit Care Med.* 2013;187(8):804–811.

27. Jia G, Erickson RW, Choy DF, et al. Periostin is a systemic biomarker of eosinophilic airway inflammation in asthmatic patients. *J Allergy Clin Immunol.* 2012;130(3):647–654. e10.

28. Corren J, Lemanske RF, Hanania NA, et al. Lebrikizumab treatment in adults with asthma. *N Engl J Med.* 2011;365(12):1088–1098.

29. Hanania NA, Korenblat P, Chapman KR, et al. Efficacy and safety of lebrikizumab in patients with uncontrolled asthma (LAVOLTA I and LAVOLTA II): replicate, phase 3, randomised, double-blind, placebo-controlled trials. *Lancet Respir Med.* 2016;4:781–796. http://dx.doi.org/10.1016/S2213-2600(16)30265-X.

30. Wenzel S, Castro M, Corren J, et al. Dupilumab efficacy and safety in adults with uncontrolled persistent asthma despite use of medium-to-high-dose inhaled corticosteroids plus a long-acting beta2 agonist: a randomised double-blind placebo-controlled pivotal phase 2b dose-ranging trial. *Lancet.* 2016;388(10039):31–44.

31. de Groot JC, Storm H, Amelink M, et al. Clinical profile of patients with adult-onset eosinophilic asthma. *ERJ Open Res.* 2016;2(2).

32. Woodruff PG, Modrek B, Choy DF, et al. T-helper type 2-driven inflammation defines major subphenotypes of asthma. *Am J Respir Crit Care Med.* 2009;180(5):388–395.

33. Chung KF. Defining phenotypes in asthma: a step towards personalized medicine. *Drugs.* 2014;74(7):719–728.

34. Anderson GP. Endotyping asthma: new insights into key pathogenic mechanisms in a complex, heterogeneous disease. *Lancet.* 2008;372(9643):1107–1119.

35. Chung KF, Adcock IM. Clinical phenotypes of asthma should link up with disease mechanisms. *Curr Opin Allergy Clin Immunol.* 2015;15(1):56–62.

36. Wenzel SE. Asthma phenotypes: the evolution from clinical to molecular approaches. *Nat Med.* 2012;18(5):716–725.

37. Chung KF. Asthma phenotyping: a necessity for improved therapeutic precision and new targeted therapies. *J Intern Med.* 2016;279(2):192–204.

38. Lefaudeux D, De Meulder B, Loza MJ, et al. U-BIOPRED clinical adult asthma clusters linked to a subset of sputum omics. *J Allergy Clin Immunol.* 2016;139(6).

39. Moore WC, Meyers DA, Wenzel SE, et al. Identification of asthma phenotypes using cluster analysis in the Severe Asthma Research Program. *Am J Respir Crit Care Med.* 2010;181(4):315–323.

40. Haldar P, Pavord ID, Shaw DE, et al. Cluster analysis and clinical asthma phenotypes. *Am J Respir Crit Care Med.* 2008;178(3):218–224.

41. Wu W, Bleecker E, Moore W, et al. Unsupervised phenotyping of Severe Asthma Research Program participants using expanded lung data. *J Allergy Clin Immunol.* 2014;133(5):1280–1288.

42. Chung KF, Adcock IM. How variability in clinical phenotypes should guide research into disease mechanisms in asthma. *Ann Am Thorac Soc.* 2013;10 (suppl):S109–S117.

43. Modena BD, Tedrow JR, Milosevic J, et al. Gene expression in relation to exhaled nitric oxide identifies novel asthma phenotypes with unique biomolecular pathways. *Am J Respir Crit Care Med.* 2014;190(12):1363–1372.

44. Modena BD, Bleecker ER, Busse WW, et al. Gene expression correlated to severe asthma characteristics reveals heterogeneous mechanisms of severe disease. *Am J Respir Crit Care Med.* 2017;195:1449–1463.

45. Baines KJ, Simpson JL, Wood LG, et al. Sputum gene expression signature of 6 biomarkers discriminates asthma inflammatory phenotypes. *J Allergy Clin Immunol.* 2014; 133(4):997–1007.

46. Simpson JL, Phipps S, Baines KJ, Oreo KM, Gunawardhana L, Gibson PG. Elevated expression of the NLRP3 inflammasome in neutrophilic asthma. *Eur Respir J.* 2014;43(4):1067–1076.

47. Auffray C, Adcock IM, Chung KF, Djukanovic R, Pison C, Sterk PJ. An integrative systems biology approach to understanding pulmonary diseases. *Chest.* 2010;137(6):1410–1416.

48. Kuo CS, Pavlidis S, Loza M, et al. T-helper cell type 2 (Th2) and non-Th2 molecular phenotypes of asthma using sputum transcriptomics in U-BIOPRED. *Eur Respir J.* 2017;49(2):1602135.

49. Kuo CS, Pavlidis S, Loza M, et al. A transcriptome-driven analysis of epithelial brushings and bronchial biopsies to define asthma phenotypes in U-BIOPRED. *Am J Respir Crit Care Med.* 2017;195(4):443–455.

50. Bos LD, Sterk PJ, Fowler SJ. Breathomics in the setting of asthma and chronic obstructive pulmonary disease. *J Allergy Clin Immunol.* 2016;138(4):970–976.

51. Rufo JC, Madureira J, Fernandes EO, Moreira A. Volatile organic compounds in asthma diagnosis: a systematic review and meta-analysis. *Allergy.* 2016;71(2):175–188.

52. de Vries R, Brinkman P, van der Schee MP, et al. Integration of electronic nose technology with spirometry: validation of a new approach for exhaled breath analysis. *J Breath Res.* 2015;9(4):046001. http://dx.doi.org/10.1088/1752-7155/9/4/046001.

53. Fens N, Zwinderman AH, van der Schee MP, et al. Exhaled breath profiling enables discrimination of chronic obstructive pulmonary disease and asthma. *Am J Respir Crit Care Med.* 2009;180(11):1076–1082.

54. Fens N, van der Sluijs KF, van de Pol MA, et al. Electronic nose identifies bronchoalveolar lavage fluid eosinophils in asthma. *Am J Respir Crit Care Med.* 2015;191(9):1086–1088.

55. van der Schee MP, Palmay R, Cowan JO, Taylor DR. Predicting steroid responsiveness in patients with asthma using exhaled breath profiling. *Clin Exp Allergy.* 2013;43(11):1217–1225.

56. Szefler SJ, Chmiel JF, Fitzpatrick AM, et al. Asthma across the ages: knowledge gaps in childhood asthma. *J Allergy Clin Immunol.* 2014;133(1):3–13, quiz 4.

57. Anderson 3rd WC, Szefler SJ. New and future strategies to improve asthma control in children. *J Allergy Clin Immunol.* 2015;136(4):848–859.

58. Fitzpatrick AM, Teague WG, Meyers DA, et al. Heterogeneity of severe asthma in childhood: confirmation by cluster analysis of children in the National Institutes of Health/National Heart, lung, and blood Institute severe asthma research program. *J Allergy Clin Immunol.* 2011;127(2):382–389.e1–e13.

59. Howrylak JA, Fuhlbrigge AL, Strunk RC, Zeiger RS, Weiss ST, Raby BA. Classification of childhood asthma phenotypes and long-term clinical responses to inhaled anti-inflammatory medications. *J Allergy Clin Immunol.* 2014;133(5):1289–1300. 300.e1–300.e12.

60. Fitzpatrick AM, Gaston BM, Erzurum SC, Teague WG. Features of severe asthma in school-age children: atopy and increased exhaled nitric oxide. *J Allergy Clin Immunol.* 2006;118(6):1218–1225.

61. Zoratti E, Havstad S, Wegienka G, et al. Differentiating asthma phenotypes in young adults through polyclonal cytokine profiles. *Ann Allergy Asthma Immunol.* 2014;113(1):25–30.

62. Bossley CJ, Fleming L, Gupta A, et al. Pediatric severe asthma is characterized by eosinophilia and remodeling without T(H)2 cytokines. *J Allergy Clin Immunol.* 2012;129(4):974–982.

63. George BJ, Reif DM, Gallagher JE, et al. Data-driven asthma endotypes defined from blood biomarker and gene expression data. *PloS One.* 2015;10(2):e0117445.

CHAPTER 9

Pharmacogenomics and Applications to Asthma Management

EMILY J. PENNINGTON, MD • MICHAEL E. WECHSLER, MD • VICTOR E. ORTEGA, MD, PHD

INTRODUCTION

Rationale for Pharmacogenetic Studies in Asthma

Asthma is a disease characterized by chronic airway inflammation that results from interactions between genetic factors, host susceptibility, and environmental exposures. There are three main classes of drugs used in the management of asthma: inhaled corticosteroids (ICSs), short-acting β2-adrenergic receptor agonists (β-agonists, SABA) and long-acting β2 agonists (LABA), and leukotriene modifiers (LTMs). However, a subgroup of patients with persistent asthma remains with poorly controlled symptoms and experiences exacerbations despite treatment with a combination of multiple drugs, including high-dose ICSs.[1,2] Both SABA and LABA therapy have been associated with severe, potentially life-threatening events in a small subgroup of individuals with asthma, and adverse responses to LABA have been observed more frequently in African-Americans compared with non-Hispanic whites.[3-10] The observed interindividual and interethnic variability in therapeutic drug responsiveness suggests that there are heritable factors influencing drug response. The heritable basis of pharmacologic responsiveness has been based on the observation that interindividual (between different individuals) variability in response to asthma therapy is significantly higher than intraindividual (within the same individual) variability in therapeutic response.[11,12] Pharmacogenetics is the study of gene-by-environment interactions in which the environment is the exposure to a drug and the outcome is the response to therapy.

A Primer on Human Genetic Variation and Pharmacogenetic Studies

Information from genetic studies has advanced markedly since the initial sequencing of the human genome in 2001, and early family-based linkage studies revealed that multiple genetic loci determine asthma risk.[13-15] Since then, high-throughput genotyping technologies using chip array technologies have facilitated simultaneous testing or "genotyping" of thousands to millions single nucleotide polymorphisms (SNPs or "snips") in large cohorts. SNPs have also been called point mutations and are two or more variants of a single base pair of DNA usually denoted by a reference sequence number (for example, rs1042713) or by the resulting coding change (for example, Gly16Arg) within an exon, the coding region of a gene (β2-adrenergic receptor or *ADRB2*). SNPs are the most abundant form of genetic variation, occurring once in every 300 nucleotides. They occur in both coding (exons) and noncoding regions of chromosomes (introns, 5′ promoter, and 3′ untranslated regions) and provide comprehensive coverage of biologic candidate gene pathways or entire genomes for genome-wide association studies (GWASs) to discover novel genes.

The ability to evaluate entire genes or genomes using a panel of selected SNPs is based on the fact that two or more neighboring SNPs on a chromosomal region are nonrandomly associated or linked because of close physical distance and an increased likelihood of being inherited from one ancestral chromosomal unit, a relationship described as linkage disequilibrium (LD). Genetic studies based on SNPs selected by LD are advantageous by reducing the number of SNPs required for genetic studies; however, more intensive genotyping or fine mapping of gene regions is usually required to identify a causative genetic variant.

Both candidate gene studies and GWAS have been used to identify genetic loci for asthma risk and therapeutic response phenotypes through pharmacogenetic studies. In pharmacogenetic studies, genetic variants or polymorphisms are associated with a measured clinical trial outcome. Similar to what has been described for the genetic basis of asthma risk and progression, the role of genetic variants in influencing drug response in asthma is the result of multiple different genes from distinct biologic pathways that contain genetic variants. Genetic variants identified through pharmacogenetic studies could regulate drug responsiveness through pharmacodynamic effects, such as altered biologic target receptor or pathway activation, disease pathobiology, or through adverse, unintended effects. Pharmacogenetic variants could also alter drug responsiveness or contribute to adverse toxicity through variation that determines drug distribution, metabolism, or excretion (pharmacokinetic effects).

Most asthma pharmacogenetic studies evaluate pharmacodynamic endpoints, such as lung function, asthma exacerbations, and symptom control. Data are usually obtained from clinical trials that have completed enrollment, which are then analyzed for genetic associations with prespecified clinic trial endpoints using DNA sample previously collected during study enrollment. Many asthma pharmacogenetic studies have focused on candidate genes within the biologic pathways associated with glucocorticoid, β-agonist, and LTM therapies, whereas preliminary studies have shown the promise of pharmacogenetics in the development of biologic drugs. A small number of candidate gene studies have used prospective, genotyped-stratified trials in which subjects are genotyped for a particular variant and randomized to drug or placebo based on specific variant genotypes.[16] This trial design ensures sufficient statistical power to analyze variants that are less common in a population and allows for comparisons between specific genotypes (i.e., homozygotes for alternative alleles of a variant). More recently, asthma clinical cohorts with sufficient sample sizes have also allowed for GWAS to identify novel loci for therapeutic response to commonly used therapies.

This chapter will review pharmacogenetic research for the most commonly used asthma drug classes that have identified variation in multiple genes associated with therapeutic response phenotypes in asthma cohorts. This chapter will then discuss how the information from these and future asthma pharmacogenetic studies based on advancements in DNA whole-genome, high-throughput genotyping, and next-generation sequencing will be applied to future precision medicine approaches.

INHALED CORTICOSTEROIDS
Biologic Candidate Gene Studies of Glucocorticoid Response
ICSs are the first-line therapy in the management of asthma and are the most effective therapy for the majority of asthma patients.[17,18] However, there is a

small subset of patients who have a minimal or negative response to ICS therapy and individuals with refractory asthma who exacerbate or are symptomatic despite the use of multiple therapies combined with ICSs.[19] The genetic basis for the observed interindividual variability in ICS therapeutic responsiveness has been examined with candidate gene studies, GWAS, and integrative analyses to identify the genetic basis for ICS therapy (see Table 9.1).[11,20]

Among the first pharmacogenetic studies of ICS response were biologic candidate gene studies that evaluated the genes encoding important determinants of the glucocorticoid signaling and related inflammatory pathways, including the receptor heterocomplex and chaperone proteins. The glucocorticoid pathway is initiated when glucocorticoids bind and activate a cytosolic chaperone-receptor heterocomplex. This heterocomplex is translocated to the nucleus where proinflammatory gene transcription is repressed and antiinflammatory gene transcription is enhanced.

In a candidate gene study of three clinical trial cohorts with adult and pediatric asthma subjects randomized to ICS therapy, two SNPs (rs242941 and rs1876828) from the corticotropin-releasing hormone receptor 1 (CRHR1) gene were associated with lung function response.[21] A second study found that SNP associations in CRHR1 with lung function change in response to ICS therapy could be related to LD with a 900-kilobase inversion encompassing CRHR1.[22] A more recent candidate gene study also identified three additional SNPs in CRHR1 and three SNPs in the gene encoding α-1(type II) chain of type II collagen (COL2A1) associated with change in asthma control questionnaire scores and lung function, respectively, during ICS therapy.[23] A pathway candidate gene study of glucocorticoid receptor heterocomplex identified three SNPs within a heat shock–organizing protein, STIP1, associated with lung function response to ICS therapy.[24]

Additional candidate gene studies have evaluated inflammatory pathway genes that encode transcription factors that regulate naïve T-lymphocyte development (His^{33}Glu in TBX21 encoding T-bet) and histone deacetylases that regulate Th2-inflammatory pathway gene expression (HDAC1) to identify loci for ICS response phenotypes.[25–27] In addition, CYP3A4, a pharmacokinetic pathway gene study of a cytochrome P450 enzyme gene variant, which metabolizes fluticasone propionate, was associated with improved asthma symptom control.[28]

A candidate gene study of known asthma risk loci in atopic and nonatopic asthma subjects based on

TABLE 9.1
Inhaled Corticosteroid Pharmacogenetic Candidate Genes

Gene	Associated Loci	Study Design	Response Phenotype
CRHR1	rs242941, rs1876828, rs739645, rs1876831, rs1876829	Candidate gene study	FEV1 response
STIP1	rs2236647, rs6591838, rs1011219	Candidate gene study	FEV1 response
COL2A1	rs2276458, rs2276455, rs2276454	Candidate gene study	FEV1 response
TBX21	His33Glu (rs2240017)	Candidate gene study	Bronchial hyperresponsiveness, FEV1 response
HDAC1	rs1741981	Candidate gene study	FEV1 response
CYP3A4	CYP3A4*22	Candidate gene study	Symptom control
T gene	rs3099266, rs1134481, rs2305089	GWAS	FEV1 response
GLCCI1	rs37972	GWAS	FEV1 response
FBXL7	rs10044254	GWAS	Symptom control
CA10	rs967676	GWAS	FEV1 response
SGK493			
CTNNA3	rs1786929	GWAS	FEV1 response
Metabolic genes	rs6924808, rs10481450, rs1353649, rs124388740	GWAS	FEV1 response
CRISPLD2		RNA-Seq	Antiinflammatory effects of glucocorticoids
SPATA20	rs6594666 and rs1380657	eQTL	Bronchial hyperresponsiveness
ACOT4	rs12891009	eQTL	Bronchial hyperresponsiveness
BRWD1	rs2037925 and rs 2836987	eQTL	Bronchial hyperresponsiveness
ALG8	rs1144764	eQTL	Bronchial hyperresponsiveness
NAPRTI	rs2793371	eQTL	Bronchial hyperresponsiveness

eQTL, expression quantitative trait loci; FEV1, forced expiratory volume in 1 s; GWAS, genome-wide association study; RNA-Seq, RNA sequencing.
Genes are listed by gene symbol, associated genetic variant (single nucleotide polymorphism rs number and coding change, if applicable), genetic study design, and response phenotype for which a pharmacogenetic association has been described.

immunoglobulin E (IgE) levels and skin prick testing identified SNPs in the gene encoding carbonic anhydrase X (rs967676 in *CA10*) and α-T-catenin (rs1786929 in *CTNNA3)* associated with lung function change in response to ICS therapy.[29] *CTNNA3* variation has also been associated with toluene diisocyanide–induced asthma and exacerbations possibly through binding of glucocorticoid-induced transcription factors known to regulate inflammatory response in lung epithelium (CCAAT/enhancer binding protein-β, CEBP-B).[30,31] The therapeutic response associated with the *CTNNA3* variant was found with all asthma subjects, but the association with the *CA10* variant was only seen in atopic asthma subjects consistent with its role in mast

cell regulation and suggesting that specific asthma subgroups are important to consider in pharmacogenetic studies.

Genome-Wide Association Studies and Integrative Genomics Identify Novel Inhaled Corticosteroid Pharmacogenetic Loci

GWASs are time-consuming and cost-intensive, requiring large clinical trial cohorts and multiple cohorts to independently replicate initial discoveries followed by function validation with in vitro studies; thus, there are only a small number of pharmacogenetic GWAS in asthma. The first GWAS to evaluate ICS treatment response was in the Childhood Asthma Management

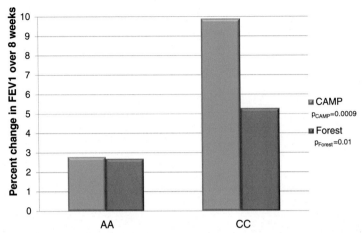

FIG. 9.1 **Genome-Wide Association Studies (GWAS) of the *T* gene and Inhaled Corticosteroid (ICS) Response.** GWAS performed in 418 non-Hispanic white subjects with asthma treated with ICS. The CAMP (Childhood Asthma Management Program) cohort was used for primary analysis. The Forest pharmaceutical study was used for replication. One single nucleotide polymorphism in the *T* gene, rs1134481, showed a two- to three-fold improvement in forced expiratory volume in 1 s (FEV1) in subjects with the minor allele compared with subjects homozygote for the common allele. (Adapted from Tantisira KG, Damask A, Szefler SJ, et al. Genome-wide association identifies the T gene as a novel asthma pharmacogenetic locus. *Am J Respir Crit Care Med*. June 2012;185(12):1286–1291; with permission.)

Program (CAMP) with replication in four clinical trial cohorts.[32] This GWAS identified a promoter SNP in the glucocorticoid-induced transcript-1 gene (*GLCCI1*) associated with decreased forced expiratory volume in 1 s (FEV1) during ICS therapy and demonstrated in vitro to influence *GLCCI1* expression. *GLCCI1* is thought to play an early role in regulating glucocorticoid-induced apoptosis, but this locus is not replicated in a subsequent, independent analysis of an ICS-treated adult trial cohort, suggesting that *GLCCI1* variation could influence ICS response in specific age groups.[33]

Subsequent GWAS identified novel SNPs in the *T* gene (rs3099266, rs1134481, and rs2305089) associated with lung function response (see Fig. 9.1) and the F-box and leucine–rich repeat protein 7 gene (rs10044254 in *FBXL7*) associated with symptomatic response to ICS therapy.[34,35] The *T* gene is coexpressed with three other genes (*NRIP1, FOXA2, and TTPA*) that interact with the glucocorticoid receptor gene (*NR3C1*) while the intronic *FBXL7* variant likely results in either altered IL-33–mediated airway inflammation or dyspnea perception through altered hypoxia-induced factor 1 degradation.[34,35] A pharmacodynamic model GWAS incorporated a therapeutic intervention of increasing doses of ICS therapy, which

identified five novel variants in intergenic, noncoding regions (rs6924808, rs10481450, rs1353649, and rs124388740) associated with dose-dependent changes in lung function. Such an approach demonstrated the importance of considering dose-related drug responsiveness to identify novel loci that could be used to tailor optimal dosing.[36]

Newer genomic analytical methods have integrated GWAS with high-throughput, whole-genome RNA sequencing (RNA-Seq) or RNA expression chip arrays for the identification of expression quantitative trait loci (eQTL) or variants that correlate with gene mRNA expression. eQTL analyses are robust for the discovery of novel gene variation because most variation are in noncoding, regulatory regions making it challenging to map causative variation. RNA-Seq analysis of glucocorticoid-treated human airway smooth muscle led to the identification of *CRISPLD2*, a gene that potentially regulates the antiinflammatory effects of glucocorticoids in airway smooth muscle cells, which was nominally associated with corticosteroid resistance in prior GWAS.[37] Combined eQTL RNA expression analysis with GWAS of lymphoblastoid cell lines from glucocorticoid-treated pediatric asthma trial subjects also identified multiple additional novel loci associated with longitudinal changes in bronchial hyperresponsiveness during ICS therapy including SNPs in *SPATA20*, *BRWD1*, *ACOT4*, *ALG8*, and *NAPRT1*.[38]

These data from biologic candidate gene studies, GWAS, and eQTL analyses of ICS response have identified multiple novel gene loci directly and indirectly related to the glucocorticoid receptor pathway that could be biomarkers for ICS therapeutic responsiveness in specific asthma subgroups for precision medicine in asthma.

INHALED β2-ADRENERGIC RECEPTOR AGONISTS

Adverse Responses as a Rationale for Pharmacogenetic Studies of β-Agonists

SABA (albuterol, levalbuterol, and salbutamol) are the most commonly prescribed medications for asthma. LABA (salmeterol and formoterol) and ultralong-acting β2-agonists (vilanterol and indacaterol) are prescribed with an ICS when asthma is not controlled with ICS therapy. β2-agonists bind to the β2-adrenergic receptor to regulate bronchial smooth muscle relaxation or bronchodilation. This class of drugs has been shrouded in controversy for over 50 years related to associated increases in asthma-related mortality.

In the 1960s, there was an increase in asthma mortality associated with a high-dose SABA, isoproterenol, followed by a second mortality epidemic in the 1970s attributed to a potent, less selective SABA, fenoterol.[4-8] A surveillance safety study in the United Kingdom in 1993 and the Salmeterol Asthma Multicenter Research Trial (SMART) in the United States in 2005 have suggested a small increase in asthma-related deaths in asthma subjects treated with salmeterol.[9,10] The SMART and metaanalyses incorporating these data led to a review by the U.S. Food and Drug Administration (FDA) in 2005 and a boxed warning for all LABAs and LABA-containing compound preparations.[39]

Numerous clinical trials, including recent large LABA safety studies mandated by the FDA, have shown that ICS and LABA combination therapy has beneficial effects on asthma control and risk of exacerbation without an increased risk of serious asthma-related adverse events.[40-42] Thus, LABAs are safe in the vast majority of asthma patients, and life-threatening adverse responses are most likely rare occurring in a small, at-risk subgroup, which could be identified with pharmacogenetic studies of β-agonist response (see Table 9.2). In addition, an increase in asthma-related life-threatening events and death in the SMART was only found in African-Americans with asthma while Africans-Americans

were more likely to experience treatment failures during LABA therapy compared with whites in clinical trials from the NHLBI Asthma Clinical Research Network (ACRN) suggesting that ethnic-specific variation could determine β-agonist response.[3,10]

Pharmacogenetic Studies of the β2-Adrenergic Receptor Gene

The most intensively studied candidate gene in asthma pharmacogenetics is the *ADRB2*, which contains more than 49 different genetic variants in multiethnic asthma cohorts.[43-45] The most well-studied variant is a common coding SNP, Gly[16]Arg, associated with altered receptor downregulation in response to SABA, in vitro.[46] Early studies have consistently shown that Arg[16] homozygotes had greater bronchodilator response to a one-time treatment with SABA compared with Gly[16] homozygotes in different racial and ethnic groups, including an ethnic-specific association in Puerto Rican asthma subjects not found in Mexican Americans.[47,48]

Subsequent analyses of two independent trial cohorts treated with chronic, regular albuterol therapy demonstrated that Arg[16] homozygotes had a decline in peak expiratory flow rate (PEFR) during regular albuterol use while Gly[16] homozygotes had an unchanged PEFR during regular albuterol use.[49,50] These studies led to the ACRN Beta Agonists Response by Genotype (BARGE) trial, a prospective genotype-stratified, crossover study of Gly[16]Arg homozygote genotypes.[16] During regular albuterol treatment in the BARGE trial, Gly[16] homozygotes had an increased PEFR, improved asthma symptoms scores, and decreased rescue inhaler use (ipratropium was used as a rescue to minimize additional β-agonist exposure) with regular albuterol therapy. In contrast, Arg[16] homozygotes did not show an improvement in PEFR and had increased symptoms and rescue inhaler use.[16] These studies do not apply to current asthma management guidelines, which recommend SABA as rescue therapy only, but paved the way for pharmacogenetic studies of chronic LABA treatment.

The earliest pharmacogenetic study of LABA response consisted of small subgroups from two ACRN trials that showed that Arg[16] homozygotes experienced a decline in PEFR and a deterioration of symptoms during LABA treatment.[51] Multiple, subsequent studies in LABA-treated asthma trial cohorts have shown no difference in PEFR between Gly[16]Arg genotypes including two prospective, genotype-stratified studies and analyses of three large clinical trial cohorts consisting of nearly 2000 asthma subjects.[52-55] In a secondary analysis of the ACRN Long-Acting β-Agonist Response by Genotype (LARGE), methacholine PC20 doubled in

TABLE 9.2
β2-Adrenergic Receptor Agonist Pharmacogenetic Candidate Genes

Gene	Associated Loci	Study Design	Response Phenotype
CRHR2	rs255100, rs7783837, rs2284220, rs2267716, rs2267715	Candidate gene study	Bronchodilator response
ADCY9	Ile^{772}Met (rs2230739)	Candidate gene study	Bronchodilator response, FEV1 response
ADRB2	Gly^{16}Arg (rs1042713), Thr^{164}Ile (rs1800888), −376 Insertion-Deletion	Candidate gene study	Bronchodilator response, bronchial hyperresponsiveness, exacerbations
ARG1	rs2781659	Candidate gene study	Bronchodilator response
ARG2	rs7140310 and rs10483801	Candidate gene study	Bronchodilator response
NOS3	Asp^{298}Glu (rs1799983)	Candidate gene study	FEV1 response
THRB	rs892940	Candidate gene study	Bronchodilator response
CHRM2	rs8191992, rs6962027, rs6967953	Candidate gene study	Symptom control
HSP8A	rs1461496	Candidate gene study	FEV1 response
SLC24A4	rs77441273	GWAS	Bronchodilator response
IGF2R	rs8191725	GWAS	Bronchodilator response
PAPPA2	rs77977790	GWAS	Bronchodilator response
SPON1	rs77149876	GWAS	Bronchodilator response
NCOA3	115501901	GWAS	Bronchodilator response
SPATS2L	rs295137	GWAS	Bronchodilator response
ASB3/SOCS	rs350729, rs1840321, rs1384918	GWAS	Bronchodilator response
SPATA13-AS1		GWAS	Bronchodilator response

FEV1, forced expiratory volume in 1 s; *GWAS*, genome-wide association study.
Genes are listed by gene symbol, associated genetic variant (single nucleotide polymorphism rs number and coding change, if applicable), genetic study design, and response phenotype for which a pharmacogenetic association has been described.

Gly^{16} subjects during LABA and ICS therapy consistent with a bronchoprotective effect not observed in Arg^{16} homozygotes, a bronchoprotective effect also seen in a prior study.[54,56]

The Gly^{16}Arg variant is a common SNP, with an allele frequency of 40%–50% in different ancestral or ethnic groups and likely only has a small effect on the rare and severe adverse LABA responses observed in the SMART cohort. Thus, these adverse responses related to LABA therapy could be related to rare variants with a strong biologic effect (see Fig. 9.2). Thr^{164}Ile is a rare coding variant found most commonly in non-Hispanic whites, which results in a significant reduction of G-protein signaling and ligand binding affinity in response to different SABAs and LABAs, in vitro.[43,44,57,58] Thr^{164}Ile in non-Hispanic

whites and a 25-base-pair promoter insertion variant in African-American asthma subjects were associated with severe exacerbations requiring hospitalization, an association observed in only LABA-treated subjects.[44] These rare *ADRB2* variant effects must be confirmed in multiethnic LABA-treated trial cohorts and examples of rare variants with ethnic-specific, infrequently strong effects on LABA response.

Biologic Pathway Candidate Gene Studies of β-Agonist Response

Candidate gene studies have also been performed with genes in the G protein–coupled β2-adrenergic receptor pathway. A coding variant in the gene encoding adenylyl cyclase type 9 (Ile^{772}Met in *ADCY9*) was associated with SABA bronchodilator response in

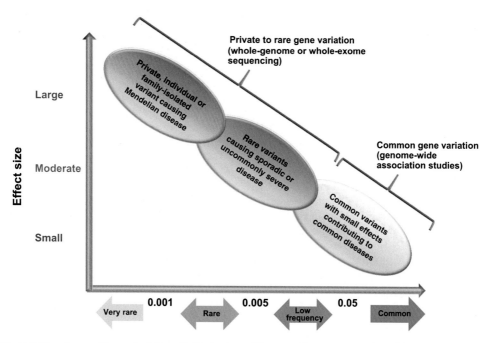

FIG. 9.2 **Spectrum of Impact of Genetic Variants on Disease.** Common genetic variants have a small to modest effect size. Multiple common variants contribute cumulatively to common disease susceptibility and therapeutic responsiveness. Rare genetic variants contribute to disease susceptibility and therapeutic responsiveness with a large effect size. (Adapted from Tsuji S, et al. *Hum Mol Genet.* 2010;19(R1):R67; with permission.)

the presence of glucocorticoid therapy in CAMP and LABA lung function response in a Korean pediatric trial cohort.[59,60] Studies of the gene encoding the corticotropin-releasing hormone receptor 2 (*CRHR2*), a G protein–coupled receptor that regulates relaxation of smooth muscle, also identified five SNPs associated with SABA bronchodilator response in three independent cohorts.[61]

In the nitric oxide pathway, arginases metabolize L-arginine, which is synthesized to nitric oxide by nitric oxide synthase to regulate smooth muscle relaxation. The genes that encode for arginase-1 (ARG1) and arginase-2 (*ARG2*) contain SNPs associated with bronchodilator response in independent European white cohorts (rs2781659 in *ARG1*, rs7140310 and rs10483801 in *ARG2*).[62,63] A pathway-related coding variant in the nitric oxide synthase gene (Asp[298]Glu in *NOS3*) was associated with lung function response to ICS/LABA combination therapy in a small pediatric cohort.[64]

Few biologic candidate gene studies have identified loci associated with therapeutic response to

LABA but have been informative of the plausible biologic mechanisms underlying the pharmacogenetics of LABA therapy.[23] Three SNPs in a muscarinic cholinergic receptor gene (rs8191992, rs6962027, and rs6967953 in *CHRM2*) and rs1461496 in a heat-shock protein gene (*HSPA8*) were associated with asthma control questionnaire scores and lung function, respectively, during LABA and ICS combination therapy.[23] Muscarinic cholinergic receptors inhibit β-agonist-induced bronchodilation while *HSP8* encodes for a heat-shock protein that acts as a chaperone protein in the glucocorticoid receptor pathway, a pathway known to regulate β2-adrenergic receptor expression.[65,66]

Genome-Wide Association Studies and Integrative Genomics Identify Novel β-Agonist Pharmacogenetic Loci

A small number of GWAS has also been used to identify novel loci for SABA bronchodilator response in asthma subjects. A GWAS performed in non-Hispanic white asthma subjects from six clinical trial cohorts was the first to identify and replicate a SNP (rs295137) association with acute SABA bronchodilator response near the *SPATS2L* gene.[67] mRNA knockdown of *SPATS2L* in airway smooth muscle cells resulted in increased β2-adrenergic receptor expression supporting a role for this locus in regulating the β2-adrenergic receptor pathway. Subsequent GWAS have identified SNPs adjacent to multiple plausible biologic candidate genes for SABA response, including genes encoding protein kinase C theta (*PRKCQ*), interleukin receptors (*IL15RA, IL2RA*), and two genes (*ASB3* [ankyrin repeat] and *SOCS* [suppressor of cytokine signaling box-containing protein 3]) hypothesized to determine smooth muscle proliferation.[68,69] Finally, integrative approaches identified differentially expressed transcription factor genes in epithelial and smooth muscle cells in response to a SABA, isoproterenol, in vitro, for the identification of novel pharmacogenetic loci. This analysis of differentially expression transcription factors led to the discovery of a SNP (rs892940) in *THRB* (thyroid hormone receptor β) gene, which was associated with SABA bronchodilator response in an asthma cohort.[70]

Pharmacogenetic Studies in Diverse, Multiethnic Cohorts Identify Ethnic-Specific Loci

The majority of pharmacogenetic studies for asthma therapies have included non-Hispanic whites. Thus, recent GWAS chip genotyping in multiethnic cohorts have demonstrated the importance of evaluating diverse clinical trial cohorts for the identification of unique, ethnic-specific pharmacogenetic loci using a combination of methods, including GWAS and whole-genome admixture mapping. In contrast to GWAS, which compares allele frequencies with a phenotype, admixture mapping estimates ancestry at each SNP and tests for association between ancestry and phenotype.[71]

In Mexican and Puerto Rican Latino children with asthma, admixture mapping in combination with GWAS identified novel, ethnic-specific genetic loci associated with SABA bronchodilator response, including rare variants. Three SNPs were found in Puerto Ricans, including rs77977790 in *PAPPA2*, rs77149876 in *SPON1*, and rs115501901 in *NCOA3* while two SNPs were found in both ethnic groups, rs8191725 in *IGF2R* and rs77441273 in *SLC24A4*. Additional known candidate genes also had rare exonic variants associated with albuterol response in Latinos, including variants in *ADCY9, CHHR2, SPATS2L,* and *THRB,*

suggesting that ethnic-specific, rare variation could influence interethnic differences in drug response phenotypes.[72] A GWAS in African-Americans also identified novel variation on *SPATA13-AS1* associated with SABA response in controls and replicated in African-American and white asthma cohorts. This region contains a gene (*SPATA13*) encoding Asef2 that hypothetically activates Rho-family GTPases to influence smooth muscle contraction.[73]

Gene-Gene Interactions and Genetic Profiles for Precision Medicine

As pharmacogenetic studies continue to identify novel loci, it will be critical to consider gene-gene interactions of interrelated pathway genes that diminish or magnify pharmacogenetic effects. In Puerto Ricans with asthma, the Gly^{16}Arg variant in *ADRB2* interacts with variants in the S-nitrosoglutathione reductase, a gene in the nitric oxide biosynthetic pathway, to additively influence bronchodilator response to albuterol.[74] A Bayesian analysis or a systems biology approach has used whole-genome genotyping chip data to identify novel gene-gene interactions between SNPs in 15 different genes, which predicted SABA bronchodilation more accurately than each individual locus.[75] Systems biology approaches are an example of how the cumulative effects of an expanding catalogue of variation from biologic candidate gene studies, GWAS, and admixture mapping will be developed into individualized genetic profiles for precision medicine in asthma.

LEUKOTRIENE MODIFIERS
Candidate Genes Studies of the Leukotriene Biosynthetic and Signaling Pathways

Leukotriene modifying drugs are available as two classes of therapies: 5-lipooxygenase (5-LO) inhibitors (zileuton) and cysteinyl leukotriene receptor 1 antagonists (montelukast, zafirlukast). Such as is the case of ICS responsiveness, there is substantial interindividual variability in therapeutic response to leukotriene-modifying drugs, with a significant proportion of nonresponders, suggesting that there is a genetic basis.[19] Pharmacogenetic studies of LTM therapy have mostly investigated candidate genes in leukotriene biosynthetic and signaling pathways (see Table 9.3).

The first biologic candidate gene study for LTMs in asthma evaluated a tandem repeat polymorphism in the regulatory promoter region of the gene encoding 5-lipooxygenase (*ALOX5*) associated with therapeutic

TABLE 9.3
Leukotriene Modifier Pharmacogenetic Candidate Genes

Gene	Associated Loci	Study Design	Response Phenotype
ALOX5	rsrs4987105, rs4986832, rs2115819	Candidate gene study	PEFR, FEV1 response
LTC4S	rs730012	Candidate gene study	Exacerbations
LTA4H	rs2660845	Candidate gene study	Exacerbations
MRPI	rs119774	Candidate gene study	FEV1 response
SLCO2B1	Arg312Gln (rs12422149)	Candidate gene study	Symptom control
HDAC2	rs3757016	Candidate gene study	FEV1 response
CRHR1	rs1876828, rs739645, rs1876831, rs1876829	Candidate gene study	FEV1 response
MRPP3	rs12436663	GWAS	FEV1 response
GLT1D1	rs517020	GWAS	FEV1 response

FEV1, forced expiratory volume in 1 s; *PEFR*, peak expiratory flow rate.
Genes are listed by gene symbol, associated genetic variant (single nucleotide polymorphism rs number and coding change, if applicable), genetic study design, and response phenotype for which a pharmacogenetic association has been described.

response to a 5-LO inhibitor.[76] A subsequent study showed that subjects treated with montelukast who had the wild-type allele of this repeat (five tandem repeats) had higher FEV1, less exacerbations, and less albuterol usage compared with subjects who were homozygous for the minor allele (four tandem repeats).[77] Subsequent candidate gene studies have identified SNPs in *ALOX5* that affect response to LTM, including different SNPs in *ALOX5* (rs4987105 and rs4986832, see Table 9.3) that were associated with lung function change in clinical trial cohorts treated with montelukast and zileuton.[78–80]

Additional candidate gene studies of the leukotriene pathway have confirmed the role of *ALOX5* variation on response to montelukast while identifying novel pathway variation.[80] These studies have found pharmacogenetic associations (see Table 9.3) between SNPs in *ALOX5* (rs2115819) (see Fig. 9.3), the genes encoding leukotriene A4 hydrolase (rs2660845 on *LTA4H*) and leukotriene C4 synthase (rs730012 on *LTC4S*), and *MRP1* (rs119774), which encodes for multidrug resistance protein 1, a transmembrane transport protein that transports leukotriene C4 to the extracellular space. One candidate gene study in a trial cohort treated with ICS, ICS and LABA, or LTM therapy identified three SNPs in *CRHR1* (rs739645, rs1876831, and rs1876829) and a SNP in *HDAC2* (rs3757016) associated with opposing therapeutic effects on lung function between ICS and montelukast treatments.[23] Finally, a study of a pharmacokinetic

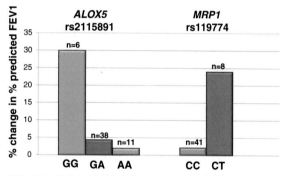

FIG. 9.3 Retrospective Pharmacogenetic Analysis of Leukotriene Pathway Genes. Twenty-eight single nucleotide polymorphisms were genotyped in genes throughout the pathway using DNA from 61 non-Hispanic white participants with poorly controlled, mild to moderate, persistent asthma randomized to treatment with montelukast. Subjects homozygote for the minor allele from *ALOX5* rs2115891 and from *MRP1* rs119774 had an improved forced expiratory volume in 1 s (FEV1) compared with subjects with the major allele. (Adapted from Lima JJ, Zhang S, Grant A, et al. Influence of leukotriene pathway polymorphisms on response to montelukast in asthma. *Am J Respir Crit Care Med*. February 15, 2006;173(4):379–385; with permission.)

gene locus coding for a solute carrier organic anion transporter family member 2B1 gene (*SLCO2B1*) identified a coding variant (Arg312Gln, rs12422149) associated with montelukast levels and symptom control in a small clinical trial cohort.[81]

Genome-Wide Association Studies of Zileuton Response Identifies a Novel Pharmacogenetic Locus

Only one GWAS has evaluated LTM therapeutic responsiveness in two zileuton-treated clinical trial discovery cohorts, a zileuton-treated replication trial cohort, and two montelukast-treated replication trial cohorts.[82] A SNP in an intron of *MRPP3* (rs12436663) reached genome-wide significance and replicated. Homozygotes for the minor allele of a SNP had the lowest change in FEV1, even a negative change in FEV1, during zileuton treatment. *MRPP3* is a gene involved in transfer RNA processing and maturation that resides in a cluster of genes on chromosome14q implicated in IgE-related phenotypes and autoimmune disease. Another SNP in the gene encoding for a glycosyl transferring protein (rs517020 on *GLT1D1*) was associated with reduction in FEV1 with the minor allele after both zileuton and montelukast treatment.

Pharmacogenetic studies of LTM responsiveness in asthma have identified multiple related pathway genes with the potential to be biomarkers for future precision profiles to identify an appropriate subgroup of responders to this commonly used therapy. Future studies with particular emphasis on focusing on drug metabolism may be valuable to identify additional novel variation for LTM responsiveness.

DEVELOPMENT OF BIOLOGIC THERAPIES

Pharmacogenetic studies will be a critical for the evaluation of targeted biologic therapies currently under development to treat a subgroup of eosinophilic, severe asthma patients refractory to usual management. As of early 2017, two drugs that target the IL-5 pathway are approved for eosinophilic asthma.[83,84] Additional biologic therapy targeting the Th2 lymphocyte inflammatory pathways by binding interleukin (IL)-4 and IL-13 and the IL-4α receptor subunit (encoded by *IL4RA*) have shown promise for the management of uncontrolled, persistent eosinophilic asthma and are under development.[85]

Pitrakinra: A Case Scenario

A pharmacogenetic study of a molecular inhibitor of IL-4α receptor subunit, pitrakinra, offers a glimpse into how pharmacogenetic approaches may be incorporated into future biologic therapy development for clinical use. A phase2b safety clinical trial of pitrakinra did not show a significant difference in asthma exacerbations between pitrakinra and placebo-treated subjects. However, a candidate study of the gene encoding the IL-4α receptor subunit (*IL4RA*) in this trial cohort found that homozygotes for the major allele of an SNP, rs8832, in *IL4RA* had a significant reduction in asthma exacerbations and asthma symptoms during treatment with pitrakinra compared with heterozygotes or homozygotes for the alternative, minor allele who showed no response to this drug[86] (see Fig. 9.4). This study demonstrates that pharmacogenetics approaches can identify a responsive subgroup to a drug even when the whole trial cohort does not show a response, an approach that can be applied to the development of expensive biologic therapies where it has been critical to identify the most responsive subgroups based on molecular phenotypes.

LIMITATIONS OF CURRENT PHARMACOGENETIC STUDIES

Inability to Consistently Replicate Loci

Despite the significant progress of the field of asthma pharmacogenetics, the genetic loci discovered to date account for only a small percentage of the total variability in treatment response, and pharmacogenetic loci from earlier studies have been inconsistently replicated in subsequent cohorts. These limitations possibly result from multiple factors including small, underpowered sample sizes, an inability to narrow down causative SNPs with a given GWAS chip platform, the identification of an appropriate asthma subgroup for a specific pharmacogenetic locus (adult vs. pediatric asthma for *GLCCI1*), the inability to completely account for environmental (including drug-drug interactions) or epigenetic factors, and the study of populations with varying degrees of genetic diversity with different patterns of LD between SNPs.

Inclusion of Ethnically Diverse Cohorts (and Genomes) in Pharmacogenetic Studies

An important limitation of current pharmacogenetic studies is the inclusion of genetically diverse ethnic groups such as African-Americans and Hispanics. The diverse genomes of these modern racial or ethnic groups largely resulted from racial admixture during the European colonization of the Americas over the past 500 years.[87,88] Because of the human origins in Africa, individuals of African descent have had a greater number of recombination events over many generations, resulting in fewer coinherited polymorphisms within genomic regions and shorter regions of LD (i.e., greater genetic diversity) compared with European whites.[89] Thus in white populations, fewer SNPs need to be genotyped to "tag" genetic regions compared with populations of significant African descent (i.e., African-Americans

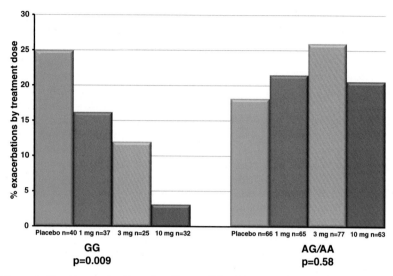

FIG. 9.4 **Exacerbation Frequency Based on Dose of Pitrakinra and Stratified by *IL4RA* Single Nucleotide Polymorphism (SNP) rs8832.** Pitrakinra is an IL-4/IL-13 pathway antagonist. Nineteen SNPs from *IL4RA* were genotyped in 407 non-Hispanic white subjects. Subjects homozygous for the major G allele from rs8832 randomized to pitrakinra had decreased frequency of asthma exacerbations compared with subjects with the minor allele. (Adapted from Slager RE, Otulana BA, Hawkins GA, et al. IL-4 receptor polymorphisms predict reduction in asthma exacerbations during response to an anti-IL-4 receptor α antagonist. *J Allergy Clin Immunol.* August 2012;130(2):516.e4–522.e4; with permission.)

and Puerto Ricans). In addition, allele frequencies of polymorphisms differ between ancestral populations, and rare variants (allele frequency <0.05) are more frequently found in African-Americans than in European Americans.[89,90] Thus, some SNPs do not replicate in different ethnic groups (for instance, Gly[16]Arg has been associated with SABA response in Puerto Ricans but not in Mexican Americans) while some pharmacogenetic studies have identified novel variants that are only present in specific ethnic groups.[43,44,48,72]

The inclusion of multiethnic trial cohorts requires careful selection of genetic variants because of varying allele frequencies between ancestral or ethnic populations and the consideration of common socioeconomic, cultural, and environmental factors.[71] Pharmacogenetic studies of multiethnic populations that account for interethnic differences in genetic diversity and rare variation will become increasingly possible as ongoing next-generation whole-exome and whole-genome sequencing projects such as the NHLBI GO Exome Sequencing Program, NHLBI Trans-Omics for Precision Medicine (TopMed) Program, the 1000 Human Genomes Project, and the Consortium on Asthma in African Ancestry Populations (CAAPA) have identified and continue to identify an expanding catalogue of common and rare genetic variation from diverse racial and ethnic populations.[90,91]

Evaluating Appropriate Outcomes in the Appropriate Asthma Subgroup

Additional limitations that might affect the ability to identify causal variants in current pharmacogenetic studies are the selected endpoints to define therapeutic response. For example, when evaluating the life-threatening adverse responses in LABA therapy, using severe asthma exacerbations that require hospitalization as a surrogate outcome measurement, as was done by the FDA for the LABA safety study, might be more appropriate than using change in lung function. In addition, selecting the subgroup of patients with more severe asthma and a history of frequent asthma-related healthcare utilization as a study cohort might better elucidate pharmacogenetic loci that affect severe adverse outcomes with LABA therapy.

HOW WILL PHARMACOGENETIC PROFILES BE APPLIED FOR PRECISION MEDICINE IN ASTHMA?

Important Components of Future Pharmacogenetic Profiles for Precision Medicine

Precision medicine is a new model of healthcare research and delivery that focuses on prevention and treatment strategies based on an individual's unique characteristics.[92] Ultimately, the goal of pharmacogenetics research is to develop genetic profiles that can help guide clinicians' treatment decisions for their asthma patients that will be the most effective with minimal adverse effects. Any future genetic profile that will be used in the clinical setting to guide treatment decisions will need to have five components. First, it would need to include common and rare variants that predict therapeutic responsiveness to different treatment options taking into account a patient's ancestral background or ethnic group. The catalogue of pharmacogenetic variation will expand as whole-genome genotyping, and next-generation sequencing is completed on larger multiethnic trial cohorts for pharmacogenetic studies.

Second, genetic profiles will include variants that predict unintended adverse responses. For example, rare variants that cause an adverse response to LABA therapy could be identified on a patient's genetic profile, which would prompt the clinician to choose an alternative step-up therapy for an asthma patient such as a muscarinic antagonist. Third, genetic profiles will need to account for gene-gene and gene-environment interactions, particularly as multiple drugs are used in combination. For example, treatment with LABA and ICS combination therapy may cause gene-gene pathway interactions that enhance or diminish the genetic effects of pharmacogenetic variants on therapeutic response because of altered biologic interactions between the β2-adrenergic and glucocorticoid receptor pathways.[65,66] Fourth, variation that determines drug pharmacokinetics will need to be included in a genetic profile as this may affect effective drug dosing and prevent drug toxicity. *CYP3A4* and *SLCO2B1* are loci that may affect drug pharmacokinetics and response to ICS and LTM therapy, respectively.[28,81] Eventually, these pharmacogenetic profiles will need to be implemented on a large scale for clinical care providers and accessed through an integrated electronic medical record (EMR).

The Expansion of the Electronic Medical Record and Pharmacogenetic Profiles

With the recent expansion of the EMR in clinical practice, large general populations with EMR data have made large-scale genetic studies possible to confirm asthma risk genes and identify potentially novel genetic risk factors in a "real-world" setting.[93] This recent expansion of the EMR has coincided with a significant drop in the costs of whole-genome genotyping and sequencing.[94] This historic convergence has resulted in new initiatives for the advancement of precision medicine through large-scale EMR-based genomics research, including the Precision Medicine Initiative, which allocated $215 million for the whole-genome sequencing in more than 1 million people in EMR-based clinical networks throughout the United States. This initiative demonstrates the promise of the EMR for pharmacogenomics research as medication use and compliance data are integrated to optimally enable studies of longitudinal asthma phenotypes.[94]

Implementing pharmacogenetic profiles in the clinical setting through the EMR requires several changes to the current healthcare system.[95] Institution-wide strategies need to be in place for the large-scale collection, isolation, and whole-genome or pharmacogenetic variant genotyping of DNA from clinic patients. EMRs currently flag drug-drug interactions and could be updated to include flagging of potential gene-drug associations to assist clinicians with making the best individualized decisions. Pharmacogenetic profiles will be complicated by a number of factors, including the ethnic group, sex, severity of disease, and use of concomitant medications, each of which is important to consider for the interpretation of an individual patient's profile for the delivery of appropriate therapy. Finally, the cost of genetic tests and genetic-based prescribing will need to be taken into account before third-party payers will consider coverage. Genetic-based prescribing will need to be cost-effective for it to be adopted and implemented on a large scale.

CONCLUSIONS

Asthma pharmacogenetics is a field in rapid development. The studies published to date rely mostly on candidate gene studies and GWAS to identify potentially important loci. The pharmacogenetic loci identified thus far would have a low accuracy in predicting individual responsiveness to specific therapy if they were used in a genetic profile. As the cost of high-throughput genotyping and next-generation sequencing continues to decrease, additional data will be available for analysis in more ethnically diverse populations. These data combined with newer analytic techniques, including systems biology approaches, will rapidly expand the field of knowledge in asthma pharmacogenetics and made strides toward the development of precision medicine approaches by identifying multiple genes for expanding pharmacogenetic profiles. A continued collaborative effort to integrate the comprehensive characterization of ethnically diverse asthma clinical trial populations with analytical methods that account for a rapidly increasing library of genetic variation will be required to translate pharmacogenetic discoveries into clinical practice.

REFERENCES

1. Proceedings of the ATS workshop on refractory asthma: current understanding, recommendations, and unanswered questions. American Thoracic Society. *Am J Respir Crit Care Med.* 2000;162(6):2341–2351.
2. Chan MT, Leung DY, Szefler SJ, Spahn JD. Difficult-to-control asthma: clinical characteristics of steroid-insensitive asthma. *J Allergy Clin Immunol.* 1998;101(5):594–601.
3. Wechsler ME, Castro M, Lehman E, et al. Impact of race on asthma treatment failures in the asthma clinical research network. *Am J Respir Crit Care Med.* 2011;184(11):1247–1253.
4. Grainger J, Woodman K, Pearce N, et al. Prescribed fenoterol and death from asthma in New Zealand, 1981-7: a further case-control study. *Thorax.* 1991;46(2):105–111.
5. Crane J, Pearce N, Burgess C, Jackson R, Beasley R. End of New Zealand asthma epidemic. *Lancet.* 1995;345(8955):984–985.
6. Pearce N, Grainger J, Atkinson M, et al. Case-control study of prescribed fenoterol and death from asthma in New Zealand, 1977-81. *Thorax.* 1990;45(3):170–175.
7. Pearce N, Burgess C, Crane J, Beasley R. Fenoterol, asthma deaths, and asthma severity. *Chest.* 1997;112(4):1148–1150.
8. Stolley PD. Asthma mortality. Why the United States was spared an epidemic of deaths due to asthma. *Am Rev Respir Dis.* 1972;105(6):883–890.
9. Castle W, Fuller R, Hall J, Palmer J. Serevent nationwide surveillance study: comparison of salmeterol with salbutamol in asthmatic patients who require regular bronchodilator treatment. *BMJ.* 1993;306(6884):1034–1037.
10. Nelson HS, Weiss ST, Bleecker ER, Yancey SW, Dorinsky PM, Group SS. The Salmeterol Multicenter Asthma Research Trial: a comparison of usual pharmacotherapy for asthma or usual pharmacotherapy plus salmeterol. *Chest.* 2006;129(1):15–26.
11. Drazen JM, Silverman EK, Lee TH. Heterogeneity of therapeutic responses in asthma. *Br Med Bull.* 2000;56(4):1054–1070.
12. Kalow W, Tang BK, Endrenyi L. Hypothesis: comparisons of inter- and intra-individual variations can substitute for twin studies in drug research. *Pharmacogenetics.* 1998;8(4):283–289.
13. Meyers DA, Postma DS, Stine OC, et al. Genome screen for asthma and bronchial hyperresponsiveness: interactions with passive smoke exposure. *J Allergy Clin Immunol.* 2005;115(6):1169–1175.
14. Daniels SE, Bhattacharrya S, James A, et al. A genome-wide search for quantitative trait loci underlying asthma. *Nature.* 1996;383(6597):247–250.
15. Van Eerdewegh P, Little RD, Dupuis J, et al. Association of the ADAM33 gene with asthma and bronchial hyperresponsiveness. *Nature.* 2002;418(6896):426–430.
16. Israel E, Chinchilli VM, Ford JG, et al. Use of regularly scheduled albuterol treatment in asthma: genotype-stratified, randomised, placebo-controlled cross-over trial. *Lancet.* 2004;364(9444):1505–1512.
17. Peters SP, Anthonisen N, Castro M, et al. Randomized comparison of strategies for reducing treatment in mild persistent asthma. *N Engl J Med.* 2007;356(20):2027–2039.
18. Sorkness CA, Lemanske RF, Mauger DT, et al. Long-term comparison of 3 controller regimens for mild-moderate persistent childhood asthma: the Pediatric Asthma Controller Trial. *J Allergy Clin Immunol.* 2007;119(1):64–72.
19. Szefler SJ, Phillips BR, Martinez FD, et al. Characterization of within-subject responses to fluticasone and montelukast in childhood asthma. *J Allergy Clin Immunol.* 2005;115(2):233–242.
20. Inglis GC, Ingram MC, Holloway CD, et al. Familial pattern of corticosteroids and their metabolism in adult human subjects–the Scottish Adult Twin Study. *J Clin Endocrinol Metab.* 1999;84(11):4132–4137.
21. Tantisira KG, Lake S, Silverman ES, et al. Corticosteroid pharmacogenetics: association of sequence variants in CRHR1 with improved lung function in asthmatics treated with inhaled corticosteroids. *Hum Mol Genet.* 2004;13(13):1353–1359.
22. Tantisira KG, Lazarus R, Litonjua AA, Klanderman B, Weiss ST. Chromosome 17: association of a large inversion polymorphism with corticosteroid response in asthma. *Pharmacogenet Genomics.* 2008;18(8):733–737.
23. Mougey EB, Chen C, Tantisira KG, et al. Pharmacogenetics of asthma controller treatment. *Pharmacogenomics J.* 2013;13(3):242–250.
24. Hawkins GA, Lazarus R, Smith RS, et al. The glucocorticoid receptor heterocomplex gene STIP1 is associated with improved lung function in asthmatic subjects treated with inhaled corticosteroids. *J Allergy Clin Immunol.* 2009;123(6):1376–1383.e1377.
25. Tantisira KG, Hwang ES, Raby BA, et al. TBX21: a functional variant predicts improvement in asthma with the use of inhaled corticosteroids. *Proc Natl Acad Sci USA.* 2004;101(52):18099–18104.
26. Ye YM, Lee HY, Kim SH, et al. Pharmacogenetic study of the effects of NK2R G231E G>A and TBX21 H33Q C>G polymorphisms on asthma control with inhaled corticosteroid treatment. *J Clin Pharm Ther.* 2009;34(6):693–701.
27. Kim MH, Kim SH, Kim YK, et al. A polymorphism in the histone deacetylase 1 gene is associated with the response to corticosteroids in asthmatics. *Korean J Intern Med.* 2013;28(6):708–714.
28. Stockmann C, Fassl B, Gaedigk R, et al. Fluticasone propionate pharmacogenetics: CYP3A4*22 polymorphism and pediatric asthma control. *J Pediatr.* 2013;162(6):1222–1227. 1227.e1221-e1222.

29. Perin P, Potočnik U. Polymorphisms in recent GWA identified asthma genes CA10, SGK493, and CTNNA3 are associated with disease severity and treatment response in childhood asthma. *Immunogenetics*. 2014;66(3): 143–151.

30. Bernstein DI, Kashon M, Lummus ZL, et al. CTNNA3 (alpha-catenin) gene variants are associated with diisocyanate asthma: a replication study in a Caucasian worker population. *Toxicol Sci*. 2013;131(1):242–246.

31. McGeachie MJ, Wu AC, Tse SM, et al. CTNNA3 and SEMA3D: promising loci for asthma exacerbation identified through multiple genome-wide association studies. *J Allergy Clin Immunol*. 2015;136(6):1503–1510.

32. Tantisira KG, Lasky-Su J, Harada M, et al. Genomewide association between GLCCI1 and response to glucocorticoid therapy in asthma. *N Engl J Med*. 2011;365(13): 1173–1183.

33. Hosking L, Bleecker E, Ghosh S, et al. GLCCI1 rs37973 does not influence treatment response to inhaled corticosteroids in white subjects with asthma. *J Allergy Clin Immunol*. 2014;133(2):587–589.

34. Tantisira KG, Damask A, Szefler SJ, et al. Genome-wide association identifies the T gene as a novel asthma pharmacogenetic locus. *Am J Respir Crit Care Med*. 2012;185(12): 1286–1291.

35. Park HW, Dahlin A, Tse S, et al. Genetic predictors associated with improvement of asthma symptoms in response to inhaled corticosteroids. *J Allergy Clin Immunol*. 2014;133(3):664–669.e665.

36. Wang Y, Tong C, Wang Z, et al. Pharmacodynamic genome-wide association study identifies new responsive loci for glucocorticoid intervention in asthma. *Pharmacogenomics J*. 2015;15(5):422–429.

37. Himes BE, Jiang X, Wagner P, et al. RNA-Seq transcriptome profiling identifies CRISPLD2 as a glucocorticoid responsive gene that modulates cytokine function in airway smooth muscle cells. *PLoS One*. 2014;9(6): e99625.

38. Qiu W, Rogers AJ, Damask A, et al. Pharmacogenomics: novel loci identification via integrating gene differential analysis and eQTL analysis. *Hum Mol Genet*. 2014;23(18):5017–5024.

39. US Food and Drug Administration. FDA Drug Safety Communication: FDA requires post-market safety trials for long-acting beta-agonists (LABAs). https://www.fda.gov/Drugs/DrugSafety/ucm251512.htm.

40. Peters SP, Prenner BM, Mezzanotte WS, Martin P, O'Brien CD. Long-term safety and asthma control with budesonide/formoterol versus budesonide pressurized metered-dose inhaler in asthma patients. *Allergy Asthma Proc*. 2008;29(5):499–516.

41. Stempel DA, Raphiou IH, Kral KM, et al. Serious asthma events with fluticasone plus salmeterol versus fluticasone alone. *N Engl J Med*. 2016;374(19):1822–1830.

42. Peters SP, Bleecker ER, Canonica GW, et al. Serious asthma events with budesonide plus formoterol vs. budesonide alone. *N Engl J Med*. 2016;375(9):850–860.

43. Hawkins GA, Tantisira K, Meyers DA, et al. Sequence, haplotype, and association analysis of ADRbeta2 in a multiethnic asthma case-control study. *Am J Respir Crit Care Med*. 2006;174(10):1101–1109.

44. Ortega VE, Hawkins GA, Moore WC, et al. Effect of rare variants in ADRB2 on risk of severe exacerbations and symptom control during longacting β agonist treatment in a multiethnic asthma population: a genetic study. *Lancet Respir Med*. 2014;2(3):204–213.

45. Drysdale CM, McGraw DW, Stack CB, et al. Complex promoter and coding region beta 2-adrenergic receptor haplotypes alter receptor expression and predict in vivo responsiveness. *Proc Natl Acad Sci USA*. 2000;97(19):10483–10488.

46. Green SA, Turki J, Bejarano P, Hall IP, Liggett SB. Influence of beta 2-adrenergic receptor genotypes on signal transduction in human airway smooth muscle cells. *Am J Respir Cell Mol Biol*. 1995;13(1):25–33.

47. Lima JJ, Thomason DB, Mohamed MH, Eberle LV, Self TH, Johnson JA. Impact of genetic polymorphisms of the beta2-adrenergic receptor on albuterol bronchodilator pharmacodynamics. *Clin Pharmacol Ther*. 1999;65(5): 519–525.

48. Choudhry S, Ung N, Avila PC, et al. Pharmacogenetic differences in response to albuterol between Puerto Ricans and Mexicans with asthma. *Am J Respir Crit Care Med*. 2005;171(6):563–570.

49. Israel E, Drazen JM, Liggett SB, et al. The effect of polymorphisms of the beta(2)-adrenergic receptor on the response to regular use of albuterol in asthma. *Am J Respir Crit Care Med*. 2000;162(1):75–80.

50. Taylor DR, Drazen JM, Herbison GP, Yandava CN, Hancox RJ, Town GI. Asthma exacerbations during long term beta agonist use: influence of beta(2) adrenoceptor polymorphism. *Thorax*. 2000;55(9):762–767.

51. Wechsler ME, Israel E. beta-adrenergic receptor genotype and response to salmeterol. *J Allergy Clin Immunol*. 2007;120(1):218–219. author reply 219–220.

52. Bleecker ER, Yancey SW, Baitinger LA, et al. Salmeterol response is not affected by beta2-adrenergic receptor genotype in subjects with persistent asthma. *J Allergy Clin Immunol*. 2006;118(4):809–816.

53. Bleecker ER, Postma DS, Lawrance RM, Meyers DA, Ambrose HJ, Goldman M. Effect of ADRB2 polymorphisms on response to longacting beta2-agonist therapy: a pharmacogenetic analysis of two randomised studies. *Lancet*. 2007;370(9605):2118–2125.

54. Wechsler ME, Kunselman SJ, Chinchilli VM, et al. Effect of beta2-adrenergic receptor polymorphism on response to longacting beta2 agonist in asthma (LARGE trial): a genotype-stratified, randomised, placebo-controlled, crossover trial. *Lancet*. 2009;374(9703): 1754–1764.

55. Bleecker ER, Nelson HS, Kraft M, et al. Beta2-receptor polymorphisms in patients receiving salmeterol with or without fluticasone propionate. *Am J Respir Crit Care Med*. 2010;181(7):676–687.

56. Lee DK, Currie GP, Hall IP, Lima JJ, Lipworth BJ. The arginine-16 beta2-adrenoceptor polymorphism predisposes to bronchoprotective subsensitivity in patients treated with formoterol and salmeterol. *Br J Clin Pharmacol.* 2004;57(1):68–75.

57. Green SA, Cole G, Jacinto M, Innis M, Liggett SB. A polymorphism of the human beta 2-adrenergic receptor within the fourth transmembrane domain alters ligand binding and functional properties of the receptor. *J Biol Chem.* 1993;268(31):23116–23121.

58. Green SA, Rathz DA, Schuster AJ, Liggett SB. The Ile164 beta(2)-adrenoceptor polymorphism alters salmeterol exosite binding and conventional agonist coupling to G(s). *Eur J Pharmacol.* 2001;421(3):141–147.

59. Tantisira KG, Small KM, Litonjua AA, Weiss ST, Liggett SB. Molecular properties and pharmacogenetics of a polymorphism of adenylyl cyclase type 9 in asthma: interaction between beta-agonist and corticosteroid pathways. *Hum Mol Genet.* 2005;14(12):1671–1677.

60. Kim SH, Ye YM, Lee HY, Sin HJ, Park HS. Combined pharmacogenetic effect of ADCY9 and ADRB2 gene polymorphisms on the bronchodilator response to inhaled combination therapy. *J Clin Pharm Ther.* 2011;36(3):399–405.

61. Poon AH, Tantisira KG, Litonjua AA, et al. Association of corticotropin-releasing hormone receptor-2 genetic variants with acute bronchodilator response in asthma. *Pharmacogenet Genomics.* 2008;18(5):373–382.

62. Litonjua AA, Lasky-Su J, Schneiter K, et al. ARG1 is a novel bronchodilator response gene: screening and replication in four asthma cohorts. *Am J Respir Crit Care Med.* 2008;178(7):688–694.

63. Vonk JM, Postma DS, Maarsingh H, Bruinenberg M, Koppelman GH, Meurs H. Arginase 1 and arginase 2 variations associate with asthma, asthma severity and beta2 agonist and steroid response. *Pharmacogenet Genomics.* 2010;20(3):179–186.

64. Iordanidou M, Paraskakis E, Tavridou A, Paschou P, Chatzimichael A, Manolopoulos VG. G894T polymorphism of eNOS gene is a predictor of response to combination of inhaled corticosteroids with long-lasting β2-agonists in asthmatic children. *Pharmacogenomics.* 2012;13(12):1363–1372.

65. Profita M, Gagliardo R, Di Giorgi R, et al. Biochemical interaction between effects of beclomethasone dipropionate and salbutamol or formoterol in sputum cells from mild to moderate asthmatics. *Allergy.* 2005;60(3):323–329.

66. Usmani OS, Ito K, Maneechotesuwan K, et al. Glucocorticoid receptor nuclear translocation in airway cells after inhaled combination therapy. *Am J Respir Crit Care Med.* 2005;172(6):704–712.

67. Himes BE, Jiang X, Hu R, et al. Genome-wide association analysis in asthma subjects identifies SPATS2L as a novel bronchodilator response gene. *PLoS Genet.* 2012;8(7):e1002824.

68. Duan QL, Lasky-Su J, Himes BE, et al. A genome-wide association study of bronchodilator response in asthmatics. *Pharmacogenomics J.* 2014;14(1):41–47.

69. Israel E, Lasky-Su J, Markezich A, et al. Genome-wide association study of short-acting β2-agonists. A novel genome-wide significant locus on chromosome 2 near ASB3. *Am J Respir Crit Care Med.* 2015;191(5):530–537.

70. Duan QL, Du R, Lasky-Su J, et al. A polymorphism in the thyroid hormone receptor gene is associated with bronchodilator response in asthmatics. *Pharmacogenomics J.* 2013; 13(2):130–136.

71. Ortega VE, Meyers DA. Pharmacogenetics: implications of race and ethnicity on defining genetic profiles for personalized medicine. *J Allergy Clin Immunol.* 2014;133(1):16–26.

72. Drake KA, Torgerson DG, Gignoux CR, et al. A genome-wide association study of bronchodilator response in Latinos implicates rare variants. *J Allergy Clin Immunol.* 2014;133(2):370–378.

73. Padhukasahasram B, Yang JJ, Levin AM, et al. Gene-based association identifies SPATA13-AS1 as a pharmacogenomic predictor of inhaled short-acting beta-agonist response in multiple population groups. *Pharmacogenomics J.* 2014;14(4):365–371.

74. Choudhry S, Que LG, Yang Z, et al. GSNO reductase and beta2-adrenergic receptor gene-gene interaction: bronchodilator responsiveness to albuterol. *Pharmacogenet Genomics.* 2010;20(6):351–358.

75. Himes BE, Wu AC, Duan QL, et al. Predicting response to short-acting bronchodilator medication using Bayesian networks. *Pharmacogenomics.* 2009;10(9):1393–1412.

76. Drazen JM, Yandava CN, Dube L, et al. Pharmacogenetic association between ALOX5 promoter genotype and the response to anti-asthma treatment. *Nat Genet.* 1999;22(2):168–170.

77. Telleria JJ, Blanco-Quiros A, Varillas D, et al. ALOX5 promoter genotype and response to montelukast in moderate persistent asthma. *Respir Med.* 2008;102(6):857–861.

78. Klotsman M, York TP, Pillai SG, et al. Pharmacogenetics of the 5-lipoxygenase biosynthetic pathway and variable clinical response to montelukast. *Pharmacogenet Genomics.* 2007;17(3):189–196.

79. Tantisira KG, Lima J, Sylvia J, Klanderman B, Weiss ST. 5-lipoxygenase pharmacogenetics in asthma: overlap with Cys-leukotriene receptor antagonist loci. *Pharmacogenet Genomics.* 2009;19(3):244–247.

80. Lima JJ, Zhang S, Grant A, et al. Influence of leukotriene pathway polymorphisms on response to montelukast in asthma. *Am J Respir Crit Care Med.* 2006;173(4): 379–385.

81. Mougey EB, Feng H, Castro M, Irvin CG, Lima JJ. Absorption of montelukast is transporter mediated: a common variant of OATP2B1 is associated with reduced plasma concentrations and poor response. *Pharmacogenet Genomics.* 2009;19(2):129–138.

82. Dahlin A, Litonjua A, Irvin CG, et al. Genome-wide association study of leukotriene modifier response in asthma. *Pharmacogenomics J.* 2016;16(2):151–157.

83. Ortega HG, Liu MC, Pavord ID, et al. Mepolizumab treatment in patients with severe eosinophilic asthma. *N Engl J Med.* 2014;371(13):1198–1207.

84. Bjermer L, Lemiere C, Maspero J, Weiss S, Zangrilli J, Germinaro M. Reslizumab for inadequately controlled asthma with elevated blood eosinophil levels: a randomized phase 3 study. *Chest.* 2016;150(4):789–798.

85. Wenzel S, Castro M, Corren J, et al. Dupilumab efficacy and safety in adults with uncontrolled persistent asthma despite use of medium-to-high-dose inhaled corticosteroids plus a long-acting beta2 agonist: a randomised double-blind placebo-controlled pivotal phase 2b dose-ranging trial. *Lancet.* 2016;388(10039):31–44.

86. Slager RE, Otulana BA, Hawkins GA, et al. IL-4 receptor polymorphisms predict reduction in asthma exacerbations during response to an anti-IL-4 receptor α antagonist. *J Allergy Clin Immunol.* 2012;130(2):516–522.e514.

87. Choudhry S, Burchard EG, Borrell LN, et al. Ancestry-environment interactions and asthma risk among Puerto Ricans. *Am J Respir Crit Care Med.* 2006;174(10):1088–1093.

88. Kumar R, Seibold MA, Aldrich MC, et al. Genetic ancestry in lung-function predictions. *N Engl J Med.* 2010;363(4):321–330.

89. Marth G, Schuler G, Yeh R, et al. Sequence variations in the public human genome data reflect a bottlenecked population history. *Proc Natl Acad Sci USA.* 2003;100(1):376–381.

90. Genomes Project C, Abecasis GR, Auton A, et al. An integrated map of genetic variation from 1,092 human genomes. *Nature.* 2012;491(7422):56–65.

91. Exome Variant Server. *NHLBI Exome Sequencing Project (ESP)*; 2012. http://evs.gs.washington.edu/EVS/.

92. Collins FS, Varmus H. A new initiative on precision medicine. *N Engl J Med.* 2015;372(9):793–795.

93. Almoguera B, Vazquez L, Mentch F, et al. Identification of four novel loci in asthma in European American and African American populations. *Am J Respir Crit Care Med.* 2017;195(4):456–463.

94. Ortega VE, Torgerson DG. On a collision course: the electronic medical record and genetic studies of asthma. *Am J Respir Crit Care Med.* 2017;195(4):412–414.

95. McCarty CA, Wilke RA. Biobanking and pharmacogenomics. *Pharmacogenomics.* 2010;11(5):637–641.

CHAPTER 10

Environmental Assessment and Control

PERDITA PERMAUL, MD • WANDA PHIPATANAKUL, MD, MS

IMPORTANCE OF ENVIRONMENTAL CONTROL

Asthma affects a high proportion of children in the United States, accounting for over 14million missed school days per year[1] and costing billions of dollars in healthcare utilization.[2] Furthermore, asthma morbidity disproportionately affects minorities and low-income groups in urban neighborhoods.[3] Exposure to allergens, and in particular indoor allergens, plays a significant part in the pathogenesis of atopic diseases, including asthma, allergic rhinitis, and atopic dermatitis. The biologic function of allergens may enhance immunoglobulin E (IgE) responses and play a direct role in causing allergic inflammation. The degree of exposure to environmental allergens, in addition to the atopic genetic predisposition of the individual, influences the development of IgE (sensitization) and Th2 responses. It is difficult to know, however, whether environmental control methods have a role in the primary prevention of asthma; the results of several primary prevention trials have been mixed.[46] Despite these findings, a Cochrane metaanalysis estimated that environmental control practices reduced the risk of current asthma by approximately 30%50% in children.[7]

Childhood asthma is more closely linked to allergic sensitization and allergen exposure than adult asthma. Studies indicate that more than 80% of school age children with asthma are sensitized to at least one indoor allergen and that allergic sensitization is a strong predictor of disease persistence in later life.[6,8] The timing of sensitization is also an important factor; Rubner and colleagues demonstrated that aeroallergen sensitization at younger ages was associated with an increased risk of asthma in later childhood.[9] Children are likely to become sensitized to the allergen that predominates in their local environment. Therefore, the effects of these individual allergens will vary depending on the socioeconomic status, weather, and geographical location, among the many factors. The common indoor allergens include house-dust mites, cockroaches, rodents, furry pets such as cats and dogs, and molds. Previous studies identified unique urban allergen exposures in homes and schools as important risk factors for asthma morbidity,[6,10–12] namely mouse and cockroach allergens, and demonstrated that interventions to reduce home exposure improve asthma outcomes.[13] As such, several studies have investigated the effects of multifaceted intervention regimens, which include education, thorough cleaning, use of high-efficiency particulate arrestance (HEPA) air filters, integrated pest management (IPM), and maintenance of these practices.[13–15] The term multifaceted has been used to describe interventions directed toward more than one asthma trigger or interventions with more than one component.

It is important that patients with asthma take all the essential actions recommended to reduce their exposure to indoor environmental asthma triggers.[16] A priority message from the National Asthma Education and Prevention Program (NAEPP) Expert Panel Report 3 guidelines for the management of asthma is that for any patient with persistent asthma, the clinician should (1) identify allergen exposures; (2) use skin testing or in vitro testing to assess specific sensitivities to indoor allergens; and (3) implement environmental controls to reduce exposure to relevant allergens.[17] Strategies for allergen avoidance should include a comprehensive targeted environmental control strategy that takes into account the patient's sensitizations and exposures. It should be considered the first line of therapy for patients with indoor allergen sensitivities.

PRIORITY STEPS IN IMPLEMENTING ENVIRONMENTAL CONTROL MEASURES: WHAT EVERY CLINICIAN SHOULD KNOW

Few patients with asthma actually take the steps needed to reduce their exposure to indoor environmental triggers. Healthcare providers have a responsibility to ask about environmental exposures and to ensure that patients have the knowledge and resources to implement environmental control measures. Those with written asthma action plans are more likely to take actions to reduce exposures; however, less than half of children with asthma are actually given one.[18] Although the home environment is important, consideration should also be given to other places where the patient spends time such as school, day care, and the workplace. Once environmental exposures are identified, an allergy referral should be placed for skin testing to define exposure risk. In vitro testing for allergens can be considered before allergy referral, but false positives occur. Low-cost environmental interventions are a reasonable first start with costly interventions reserved for postallergy consultation. Environmental control measures can and should supplement good medical care. The healthcare provider may refer to the comprehensive practice parameters published for the management of house-dust mites,[19] cockroaches,[20] rodents,[21] furry pets,[22] and molds[23] (see Table 10.1).

It is essential that primary care providers have good communication skills when dealing with patients, families, and the community for environmental control measures to be effective. Some environmental interventions involve highly sensitive issues such as smoking, and cockroach and mouse infestation. Developing proficiency in asking these sensitive questions to families will more likely yield honest answers and the possibility of an intervention in homes of those who might otherwise have been unreceptive. Furthermore, adherence to certain interventions remains a special challenge for the healthcare provider, such as smoking cessation or removal of pets from the home. There should be good lines of communication between the primary care provider and asthma specialist/allergist for the implementation of environmental control measures to be fruitful.

ASSESSMENT AND IMPLEMENTATION
Home
Assessment first begins in the primary care provider's office. Providers should identify children and/or adults with at-risk asthma (asthma-related hospitalizations and/or emergency department visits, poor medication adherence, concomitant allergen sensitization) and in need for asthma intervention services. A thorough environmental history should be obtained to identify potential environmental exposures in the home that are known to trigger asthma symptoms and exacerbations, including allergens and pollutants (see the NEEF's

Asthma Environmental History Form at https://www.neefusa.org/resource/asthma-environmental-history-form).[24] This would include questions regarding the presence of pets or pests, conditions favoring dust mite breeding, presence of smokers in the home, and the use of gas stoves. In addition to making a local specialist referral (allergy, pulmonary) for expert evaluations and care and providing recommendations regarding specific control measures (see Table 10.1), a referral to a community asthma program is beneficial.

Employing community health workers as members of the underserved racial and ethnic communities in which they work is one evidence-based strategy for providing culturally competent care. Community health workers have been legitimized for their cultural and linguistic proficiency and their ability to form trusting relationships with patients and act as mediators between healthcare providers and their patients. A home visit and environmental assessment to identify and reduce asthma triggers in the home might be performed by the community health worker. A successful home visit includes asthma education, assessment of health literacy, medication adherence, and environmental assessment making note of common asthma triggers such as molds, pests, clutter/dust, smoking, harsh cleaning products and air fresheners, and pets. Educational material may be given including smoking cessation literature and referral forms to a smoking quit line. This is also an opportune time to review the patient's asthma action plan.

Indoor allergen exposure in inner-city homes has garnered a great deal of attention since children living in these areas have greater asthma severity, decreased asthma control, and greater healthcare use.[25] In the late 1990s, the National Cooperative Inner-City Asthma Study showed highly detectable levels of cockroach allergen in inner-city homes and demonstrated that children with asthma who were both sensitized and exposed to high levels of cockroach allergen had increased asthma morbidity.[10] Mouse allergen is also prevalent in inner-city homes,[26] and exposure is associated with increased asthma morbidity.[12,14,27] Based on these findings, home intervention strategies to reduce pest allergen levels have been studied. IPM is a multidisciplinary approach that uses a range of pest control methods. There are four fundamental IPM principles: (1) monitoring pest populations with sticky traps to find out where they are living and hiding (reservoirs); (2) blocking pest access and entryways; (3) eliminating food and water (facilitating factors); and (4) selectively applying low-toxicity pesticides. The provision

TABLE 10.1
Environmental Control of Allergens and Mold

	Dust Mites	Cockroach	Mouse	Cat/Dog	Pollens	Mold
Allergenic proteins	Der p 1 Der f 1	Bla g 1 Bla g 2	Mus m 1 Mus m 2	Fel d 1 (cat) Can f 1 (dog)	Varies by tree, grass, weed species	Varies by mold species
Information	• Requires moisture for survival • Feeds off dead skin cells and micro organisms	• Bla g 1 is in feces • Bla g 2 is an aspartic protease • Infestation associated with inner-cities, low SES, populated areas	• Allergen found in mouse urine, dander, and fur hair follicles • Infestation associated with inner-cities, low SES, populated areas	• Allergen found in saliva, skin, dander, and fur • Allergen carried on small particles, remains airborne, and adherent to surfaces • After removal, the decline in Fel d 1 is slow • Reservoirs include bedding, furniture, and carpeting	• Spread by wind, highest levels on dry, windy day	• A wide variety of indoor and outdoor molds • Common indoor molds are *Aspergillus* and *Penicillium* species • Common outdoor molds are *Cladosporium*, *Alternaria*, *Epicoccum* • Depends on moisture for growth
Control measures	• Encase mattresses, pillows, and box springs • Wash bedding in hot water and dry in high heat every 1–2 weeks • Remove reservoirs such as stuffed toys, carpets, and upholstered furniture • Vacuum carpets with HEPA filtration regularly • Keep indoor humidity levels below 50%, use of a humidity gauge is helpful • Acaricides, tannic acid, and air filters with limited or unproven benefit	• Home extermination of occupant and neighbors, but not effective alone • IPM → combined use of insecticide, professional cleaning, occupant education • Remove reservoirs such as carpeting, bedding, or other areas containing allergen • Roach traps • Repair holes in walls and points of entry • Eliminate food sources, wash dirty dishes, cover trash cans, close food containers	• Home extermination of occupant and neighbors, but not effective alone • IPM → combined use of insecticide, professional cleaning, occupant education • Remove reservoirs such as carpeting, bedding, or other areas containing allergen • Mouse traps • Repair holes in walls and points of entry • Eliminate food sources, wash dirty dishes, cover trash cans, close food containers	• First line → removal of pet, followed by cleaning to remove reservoirs • If unwilling to remove: • Keep pet out of bedroom • Encase mattress and pillows • HEPA air filter, especially in the bedroom • Remove carpeting • Cat/dog immersion washing, must be frequent to be effective • No scientific evidence to support "hypoallergenic" pets	• Keep house and car windows closed • Run air conditioner • Avoid lawn mowing • Shower, wash hair, and change clothes after being outside for prolonged period • Flush eyes out periodically with chilled artificial tears before medicated drops • Consider nasal rinse • Consider face mask	• Use of air conditioner in the summer • Use of dehumidifier in the basement • Repair of leaks • Removal of water-damaged materials • Run vent in bathroom and kitchen • Clean moldy areas with a fungicide → cleaning agents containing hypochlorite are effective

HEPA, high-efficiency particulate arrestance; *IPM*, integrated pest management; *SES*, socioeconomic status.

of IPM supplies such as HEPA vacuum cleaners, dust mite proof bedding encasements, and plastic storage bins to decrease clutter and reduce reservoirs for pests is important for families who cannot afford them. In a landmark study, Morgan and colleagues revealed that among inner-city children with atopic asthma, an individualized, home-based, multifaceted environmental intervention decreased exposure to indoor allergens, including cockroach and dust-mite allergens, leading to decreased asthma morbidity.[13]

Environmental intervention studies are investigating new ways to implement therapeutic intervention strategies tailored to the individual. A randomized controlled trial evaluating the effect of individualized multifaceted allergen reduction in the home on the ability to reduce asthma controller therapy concluded that despite a significant reduction in measured allergen levels in the intervention group, it did not result in a reduction in asthma controller therapy.[28] Another study compared a year-long IPM intervention plus pest management education versus pest management education alone among mouse-sensitized and exposed children; both groups had a reduction in mouse allergen levels and there was no significant difference in maximal asthma symptom days between the two groups.[29] In most situations, IPM is cost-prohibitive and difficult to implement. Rabito et al. demonstrated that a single low-cost intervention to reduce cockroach exposure, the strategic placement of insecticidal bait in the homes of children with asthma, resulted in significant cockroach reduction and improved asthma outcomes when compared with the no intervention control group.[30] Researchers are currently studying the effects of environmental interventions on modifiable epigenetic mechanisms. Changes in methylation and gene expression profiles found in nasal and/or oral samples might serve as a biomarker for asthma outcomes in response to changes in exposure over time (see Chapter 14: Systems Biology Approach to Asthma Management).

In the era of personalized medicine, the implementation of an individualized tailored environmental intervention strategy based on a patient's sensitization status and home exposures is ideal. Home allergen sampling is used in clinical research by measuring allergen levels in dust samples collected by vacuuming settled dust or gathering airborne dust from filtered air within a room. After collection, fine dust is then extracted and sent to a laboratory for quantification of allergens. These methods are not feasible for patients. The development of in-home test kits to measure allergen levels is being evaluated.

School

Although years of previous research have demonstrated the association between environmental exposures in the inner-city home environment and significant childhood asthma morbidity,[10,31–33] many of these allergens and pollutants are also present in the inner-city school environments.[34–36] This is noteworthy because children spend 7-12h per day in school settings, representing an occupational model for children. The environment outside of the home, especially in the United States, is less well understood, in part because of the challenges of community outreach and buy-in. Literature reviews have discussed the limited school-based environmental intervention studies to date in the United States and highlight the dire need for them.[37,38] As a consequence, successful home-based strategies currently serve as the prototype for school-based environmental interventions.

Prior studies found cockroach and mouse allergens highly prevalent in school environments.[34,39] The School Inner-City Asthma Study (SICAS) is a National Institute of Health (NIH) and National Institute of Allergy and Infectious Disease (NIAID) funded, comprehensive, prospective study of inner-city school and classroom-specific exposures and asthma morbidity among inner-city students in the Northeastern United States, adjusting for home exposures.[40] The SICAS results demonstrated substantial levels of mouse allergen in school classrooms compared with the same students' homes,[35] with exposure to mouse allergen in schools associated with increased asthma symptoms and decreased lung function.[11] Interestingly, cat and dog allergen levels were lower in these inner-city schools when compared with European school-based studies showing higher levels, likely due to passive transfer from students who owned pets in their homes.[41] This highlights how geographic, climatic, and cultural differences might influence the prevalence of allergens in varying environments.

A feasible school-based environmental intervention is IPM. Given the SICAS findings of high mouse allergen levels in school classrooms, a NIH/NIAID SICAS Intervention Study, using environmental control strategies modeled from successful home-based interventions, is under way with health outcomes results pending. Pilot data from this study showed that a classroom-based air cleaner intervention led to significant reductions in particulate matter (PM) with a diameter of <2.5m and black carbon.[42] In another study, dedicated school clothing and banning pet ownership in Swedish schools showed that airborne cat allergen levels were on average four to six times lower in classes with school clothing or pet ownership ban compared with control classes.[43]

A multicenter prospective study in Europe found high levels of molds in schools, particularly those with moisture damage.[44] These mold findings corroborate results from SICAS, which found elevated mold levels in settled dust and airborne concentrations in inner-city schools.[45] One pilot study showed that HEPA air filters reduce mold spore counts in day-care centers.[46] These results show promise for the implementation of multifaceted intervention strategies in school and day-care settings.

School-based health centers (SBHCs) provide an ideal setting in which to incorporate environmental components into existing chronic disease programs (see Chapter 13: School-Centered Asthma Programs). There are over 2000 SBHCs throughout the country serving an ethnically diverse population of more than 2 million children, primarily in low-income areas. A large number of these centers offer asthma management. SBHC staff members can play a role in maintaining healthy indoor environments in school by increasing awareness, facilitating an indoor air quality assessment, or implementing specific interventions to address molds, dust mites, pests, pets, and ventilation.

The U.S. Environmental Protection Agency (EPA) created the Indoor Air Quality Tools for Schools Program, with the aim of improving environmental conditions in schools. It provides recommended actions for teachers, facilities staff, and school officials, such as keeping ventilation units in classrooms free of clutter, reducing the number of items made of cloth in the classroom, removing classroom pets that cause allergic reactions or trigger asthma attacks in students, and reporting maintenance problems in classrooms immediately. These measures should be taken until more widespread multifaceted intervention strategies are implemented. Additionally, the School-Based Asthma Management Program[47] and the Centers for Disease Control and Prevention (CDC) Healthy Schools Program offer toolkits to schools. These toolkits help to develop asthma-friendly schools that provide appropriate school health services for students with asthma and a safe and healthy school environment to reduce asthma triggers.

Air

A growing body of work is demonstrating that concentrations of many pollutants are higher indoors than outdoors[48] and higher in urban homes as compared with rural homes.[49] Exposure to indoor pollutants is independently associated with increased respiratory symptoms and rescue asthma medication usage in urban children with asthma.[50] The best studied indoor pollutants include airborne PM, nitrogen dioxide (NO_2), and environmental tobacco smoke (ETS).

Airborne PM is measured in different size fractions; fine PM has an aerodynamic diameter of 2.5 m or less ($PM_{2.5}$), and coarse PM has an aerodynamic diameter greater than 2.5 m and up to 10 m ($PM_{2.5\text{-}10}$). Both fine and course PM comprise PM_{10}. Smoking, sweeping, and stove use contribute significantly to both indoor $PM_{2.5}$ and PM_{10} levels.[50] Indoor PM exposures are associated with worsening asthma symptoms in inner-city children with asthma.[50] NO_2 is a pollutant gas produced from high-temperature combustion. Indoor combustion sources include gas stoves, heaters, and poorly vented furnaces and fireplaces and produce high indoor NO_2 concentrations. Belanger and colleagues showed that children with asthma exposed to indoor NO_2 levels well below the EPA outdoor standard (53 ppb) were at risk for increased frequency of wheeze, night symptoms, and use of rescue medication.[51] Interestingly, newer data suggest that overweight and obese individuals are more affected by air pollutant exposure with increased asthma symptoms.[52] The use of HEPA air filters to reduce indoor PM is currently being studied as an effective long-term strategy to reduce indoor air pollution, but more studies are needed.[42]

ETS is known to exacerbate asthma. Tobacco smoke contains solid particles and semivolatile and volatile organic compounds, which function as respiratory irritants. Halterman and colleagues reported that 50% of inner-city children with asthma are exposed to ETS, and more than 60% of those children have a mother or caregiver who smokes.[53] In a cross-sectional study, using NHANES data of 2250 youths with asthma, 17.3% reported using tobacco smoke products, and of the nonsmokers, 53.2% were exposed to second-hand smoke in their homes.[54] The measurement of cotinine levels has become a useful tool for determining passive smoke exposure with higher levels in urine, serum, and saliva associated with a higher risk for severe asthma. There have been a few intervention trials targeting smoking cessation and reduction of second-hand smoke exposure in the home.[55,56] However, a Cochrane review found that most intervention studies aimed at reducing children's ETS exposure were ineffective.[57] Evidence suggests that HEPA air filters might be useful, especially for children who are not able to avoid second-hand smoke. In a double-blind randomized control trial of children with asthma and known second-hand ETS exposure, the use of HEPA air filters resulted in a reduction in the number of unscheduled asthma visits and fewer airborne nicotine particles in the intervention group when compared with the control group.[56] Nevertheless, the most effective measure to control ETS is avoidance of second-hand exposure.

Recent attention has been given to third-hand smoke (THS) exposure in children. THS denotes smoke pollutants remaining in the indoor environment and on surfaces after active smoking has stopped. These pollutants can persist for weeks to months and pose a potential health hazard for crawling children and infants/toddlers eating nonfood items.

In addition to the implementation of better cook stoves, ventilation-related strategies, and avoidance of second-hand smoke exposure, green housing is being studied as a method to improve health outcomes in the asthma population. Green housing uses low-impact materials with the goal of energy efficiency and improved health outcomes. In a low-income population, green housing had lower concentrations of $PM_{2.5}$, NO_2, nicotine, and decreased mold and pest infestation.[58] It should also be noted that while energy efficiency is desirable, levels of indoor air pollutants may increase because of limiting leakage of air between the indoor and outdoor environments. Efforts should be taken to increase air exchange such as exhaust fans.

Outdoor allergen exposures include multiple sources such as tree, grass, and weed pollens as well as fungal spores. These particles are released into the air by wind, rain, and mechanical disturbances and can travel widely, making source control unfeasible. To avoid outdoor allergen exposure, recommendations are made to stay indoors on days when pollen and mold counts are high and to keep windows closed. Lawn mowing should be avoided or kept to a minimum and the use of a face mask and goggles is advised. After being outside, it is important that individuals wash their hands and face, change their clothes, and wash hair daily. It is noteworthy that an increased incidence of asthma exacerbations is observed at the beginning of thunderstorms during pollen season (thunderstorm asthma). Thunderstorms cause pollen grains to rupture by osmotic shock thereby releasing very small particles (0.52m) into the atmosphere that can reach lower airways and induce asthma symptoms in patients with known asthma.[59] Outdoor mold control may be accomplished by removing leaves and other debris that can enhance mold growth.

GEOGRAPHIC INFORMATION SYSTEM

In recent years, the ability to locate residences in space and obtain geocodable health data, coupled with the use of geographic information system (GIS), has given researchers the enhanced ability to link exposure information to individual addresses. GIS is a computerized system for input, storage, management, display, and analysis of data that can be precisely linked to a geographic location. GIS tools are being used to manipulate asthma data with spatial zip code data, with resulting data presented on a geographical map. The resulting output has become valuable for asthma research planning and helping to guide strategic decisions by healthcare agencies, healthcare providers, and the general public.

Most environmental exposure and health studies in patients with asthma use exposures averaged over the course of a day and do not take into account the spatial/temporal variability that likely occurs as a person moves from home, into transportation, and then into school and work microenvironments. For instance, schools are typically centrally located within a community in close proximity to highways, heavy traffic routes, and commercial and industrial buildings. School locations also serve as a site for drop-off/pickup, idling of cars, bus stops, potentially contributing to an increase in ambient air pollution. Kingsley et al. showed that 3.2million (6.5%) children across the United States attended schools located within 100m of a major roadway defined by the United States Census Bureau.[60] Air pollutants that are found near busy roads as a product of traffic exhaust, such as NO_2 and PM, have been shown to be associated with respiratory illness in children,[61,62] and the use of GIS has provided evidence that living in proximity to traffic increases the incidence of asthma[63] and risk of exacerbations in both children and adults.[64]

Asthma is complex and linked to a number of factors such as healthcare access, crime and violence, stress, environmental allergens, and pollutants. In an urban environment, Clougherty and colleagues used a GIS-based approach to demonstrate a significant association between violent crime and asthma emergency department visits, while crowding and poor access to resources modified the association between area-level NO_2 and asthma emergency department visits.[65] The use of GIS has enabled quantification of complex spatial patterning and confounding between contextual exposures and its interaction with air pollution on asthma. We now have an understanding of asthma prevalence and its associated triggers in a dimension that could not have been possible before the availability of GIS. These results will help in making further decisions regarding planning for asthma research and studying the separate and combined effects of multiple urban exposures.

PUBLIC HEALTH

Asthma is a chronic respiratory disease increasingly prevalent in the United States, particularly among children in the inner-city environment. The evidence-based NAEPP Expert Panel Report 3 guidelines for managing and treating asthma encourage activities that may be conducted at the public health level, such as asthma education and self-management, coordination of care across various settings, institutional changes to improve quality of care, and the reduction of indoor and outdoor asthma triggers.[17] Effective public health programs can provide this education and support. Unfortunately, start-up funding is needed to get these community programs under way. Historically, these funds have come from public health agency grants, institutional funding, the NIH, and private funders. Long-term sustainable care redesign requires ongoing funding from public and private payers, which is more difficult to attain.

Public health agencies have a critical role in helping to reduce environmental factors affecting asthma and the human and financial burden of the disease. In 1999, the CDC created the National Asthma Control Program (NACP), which provides funding to state and local partners to carry out public health interventions with the ultimate goal of helping patients with asthma manage their asthma appropriately and, thereby, reduce the burden of asthma symptoms and costs. The NACP has been successful in funding various state asthma programs to improve asthma on a population level in diverse sectors such as state public health agencies, schools, homes, and in healthcare. A recent study showed that asthma self-management education and home-based interventions can improve asthma control and prevent exacerbations with most programs showing a positive return on investment.[66] Families need help establishing priorities for environmental control measures that will be suitable for their own and/or their child's asthma while taking into consideration family and socioeconomic circumstances. In keeping with these needs, the U.S. Department of Housing and Urban Development developed the Healthy Homes Initiative to protect children with asthma and their families from housing-related health and safety hazards.

Health payment reform can offer opportunities to apply population health approaches to tackling asthma morbidity (see Chapter 2: Population Health Management: A Systematic Approach to Asthma Care in a Pediatric Network of Care).[67] Our current reimbursement model is fee-for-service where the provider is paid for the medical service provided, i.e., well-child visit, emergency department visit. Few healthcare payers have invested in environmental interventions for asthma, such as community worker home visits, smoking cessation programs, and home remediation, to name a few. For this to occur, a paradigm shift needs to occur to reward better health outcomes rather than focusing on the volume of services. Medicaid, the public insurer for half of all low-income children in the United States, is starting to move in the direction of enhanced fee-for-service and bundled payment programs. Under this payment model, participating states will reimburse for preventive services recommended by a physician. For healthcare systems to move toward a population health management approach, providers and hospitals will need to demonstrate cost savings in the form of reduced asthma-related emergency department visits, hospitalizations, and medication use, to get buy-in from public and private insurers. It is important that healthcare providers keep abreast of these new emerging payment models for environmental interventions.

ADVOCACY

Advocacy and public policy work are important for protecting the health and safety of those with asthma, especially in vulnerable populations. For children and adults without access to quality healthcare, education on the environmental triggers of asthma is impossible or severely limited. Emergency rooms or urgent care facilities may serve as the only source of primary care for this population and should be included in the chronic disease management services that are essential to reducing the severity and frequency of exacerbations. Thus, advocacy requires partnerships within the medical community, as well as the collaborative effort of family, relatives and neighbors, school, and the community.

An assessment of environmental exposures in the community is a first step in asthma advocacy to reduce health disparities. Identifying root causes of social inequalities, identifying environmental health hazards, and connecting all of these to public health outcomes are critical. Although exposures in the home environment are significant, working with school officials to identify potential environmental asthma triggers in schools is also vital for advocacy work centered on prevention strategies. Advocacy issues have included increasing funding for research and clinical trials, reducing emissions of outdoor air pollutants, promoting tobacco-free workplaces and schools, and establishing policy within the U.S. Department of Housing and Urban Development to require all federally funded public housing to be smoke-free. In line with this, the Patient-Centered

Outcomes Research Institute is a new independent, nonprofit, nongovernmental organization created to fund patient-centered research that will improve health outcomes for patients with high-burden conditions, such as asthma. Environmental risk factors must be communicated to community members, school board members, political groups, legislative bodies, and other stakeholders. Collaborations must then be birthed for change to occur.

Healthcare providers have an important proactive role to play in working with the community to prevent certain environmental exposures. Developing networks of community groups and public officials can enhance a provider's effectiveness in accomplishing goals. Providers should also become aware of community resources, such as smoking cessation programs and community asthma initiatives, to which they can refer patients.

CONCLUSIONS

Environmental allergen and pollutant exposures are risk factors for the development of asthma. Assessment of both the home and school environments of patients with asthma is essential. Healthcare providers have a responsibility to ask about environmental exposures and to ensure that patients have the resources to implement control measures. Advocacy and public policy work must continue to reduce the disparities that exist in urban environments and involve partnerships between health professionals, patients, healthy policy makers, public agency groups, and researchers.

REFERENCES

1. (CDC) CfDCaP. Vital signs: asthma prevalence, disease characteristics, and self-management education: United States, 2001-2009. *MMWR Morb Mortal Wkly Rep*. 2011; 60(17):547–552.
2. Hasegawa K, Tsugawa Y, Brown DF, Camargo CA. Childhood asthma hospitalizations in the United States, 2000-2009. *J Pediatr*. 2013;163(4):1127–1133.e1123.
3. Beck AF, Huang B, Simmons JM, et al. Role of financial and social hardships in asthma racial disparities. *Pediatrics*. 2014;133(3):431–439.
4. Woodcock A, Lowe LA, Murray CS, et al. Early life environmental control: effect on symptoms, sensitization, and lung function at age 3 years. *Am J Respir Crit Care Med*. 2004;170(4):433–439.
5. Toelle BG, Garden FL, Ng KK, et al. Outcomes of the childhood asthma prevention study at 11.5 years. *J Allergy Clin Immunol*. 2013;132(5):1220–1222.e1223.
6. Sporik R, Holgate ST, Platts-Mills TA, Cogswell JJ. Exposure to house-dust mite allergen (Der p I) and the development of asthma in childhood. A prospective study. *N Engl J Med*. 1990;323(8):502–507.
7. Maas T, Kaper J, Sheikh A, et al. Mono and multifaceted inhalant and/or food allergen reduction interventions for preventing asthma in children at high risk of developing asthma. *Cochrane Database Syst Rev*. 2009;(3). http://dx.doi.org/10.1002/14651858. CD006480.
8. Illi S, von Mutius E, Lau S, et al. Perennial allergen sensitisation early in life and chronic asthma in children: a birth cohort study. *Lancet*. 2006;368(9537):763–770.
9. Rubner FJ, Jackson DJ, Evans MD, et al. Early life rhinovirus wheezing, allergic sensitization, and asthma risk at adolescence. *J Allergy Clin Immunol*. 2017;139(2):501–507.
10. Rosenstreich DL, Eggleston P, Kattan M, et al. The role of cockroach allergy and exposure to cockroach allergen in causing morbidity among inner-city children with asthma. *N Engl J Med*. 1997;336(19):1356–1363.
11. Sheehan WJ, Permaul P, Petty CR, et al. Association between allergen exposure in inner-city schools and asthma morbidity among students. *JAMA Pediatr*. 2017;171(1): 31–38.
12. Grant T, Aloe C, Perzanowski M, et al. Mouse sensitization and exposure are associated with asthma severity in urban children. *J Allergy Clin Immunol Pract*. 2016. http://dx.doi.org/10.1016/j.jaip.2016.10.020.
13. Morgan WJ, Crain EF, Gruchalla RS, et al. Results of a home-based environmental intervention among urban children with asthma. *N Engl J Med*. 2004;351(11): 1068–1080.
14. Pongracic JA, Visness CM, Gruchalla RS, Evans R, Mitchell HE. Effect of mouse allergen and rodent environmental intervention on asthma in inner-city children. *Ann Allergy Asthma Immunol*. 2008;101(1):35–41.
15. Phipatanakul W, Cronin B, Wood RA, et al. Effect of environmental intervention on mouse allergen levels in homes of inner-city Boston children with asthma. *Ann Allergy Asthma Immunol*. 2004;92(4):420–425.
16. Matsui EC, Abramson SL, Sandel MT, IMMUNOLOGY SOAA, HEALTH COE. Indoor environmental control practices and asthma management. *Pediatrics*. 2016;138(5).
17. Program NAEaP. Expert Panel Report 3 (EPR-3): guidelines for the diagnosis and management of asthma-summary Report 2007. *J Allergy Clin Immunol*. 2007;120 (suppl 5):S94–S138.
18. Simon AE, Akinbami LJ. Asthma action plan receipt among children with asthma 2-17 Years of age, United States, 2002-2013. *J Pediatr*. 2016;171:283–289.e281.
19. Portnoy J, Miller JD, Williams PB, et al. Environmental assessment and exposure control of dust mites: a practice parameter. *Ann Allergy Asthma Immunol*. 2013;111(6): 465–507.
20. Portnoy J, Chew GL, Phipatanakul W, et al. Environmental assessment and exposure reduction of cockroaches: a practice parameter. *J Allergy Clin Immunol*. 2013;132(4): 802–808. e801–e825.

21. Phipatanakul W, Matsui E, Portnoy J, et al. Environmental assessment and exposure reduction of rodents: a practice parameter. *Ann Allergy Asthma Immunol.* 2012;109(6):375–387.

22. Portnoy J, Kennedy K, Sublett J, et al. Environmental assessment and exposure control: a practice parameter—furry animals. *Ann Allergy Asthma Immunol.* 2012; 108(4):223. e221–e215.

23. Larenas-Linnemann D, Baxi S, Phipatanakul W, Portnoy JM, Workgroup EA. Clinical evaluation and management of patients with suspected fungus sensitivity. *J Allergy Clin Immunol Pract.* 2016;4(3):405–414.

24. Environmental management of pediatric asthma. *Guidelines for Health Care Providers.* Washington, DC: National Environmental Education and Training Foundation (NEETF); August 2005; Reaffirmed in 2013.

25. Szefler SJ, Gergen PJ, Mitchell H, Morgan W. Achieving asthma control in the inner city: do the National Institutes of Health Asthma Guidelines really work? *J Allergy Clin Immunol.* 2010;125(3):521–526; quiz 527–528.

26. Phipatanakul W, Eggleston PA, Wright EC, Wood RA. Mouse allergen. I. The prevalence of mouse allergen in inner-city homes. The National Cooperative Inner-City Asthma Study. *J Allergy Clin Immunol.* 2000;106(6):1070–1074.

27. Ahluwalia SK, Peng RD, Breysse PN, et al. Mouse allergen is the major allergen of public health relevance in Baltimore City. *J Allergy Clin Immunol.* 2013;132(4):830–835. e831–e832.

28. DiMango E, Serebrisky D, Narula S, et al. Individualized household allergen intervention lowers allergen level but not asthma medication use: a randomized controlled trial. *J Allergy Clin Immunol Pract.* 2016;4(4):671–679.e674.

29. Matsui EC, Perzanowski M, Peng RD, et al. Effect of an integrated pest management intervention on asthma symptoms among mouse-sensitized children and adolescents with asthma: a randomized clinical trial. *JAMA.* 2017;317(10):1027–1036.

30. Rabito FA, Carlson JC, He H, Werthmann D, Schal C. A single intervention for cockroach control reduces cockroach exposure and asthma morbidity in children. *J Allergy Clin Immunol.* 2017. http://dx.doi.org/10.1016/j.jaci.2016.10.019.

31. Eggleston PA, Rosenstreich D, Lynn H, et al. Relationship of indoor allergen exposure to skin test sensitivity in inner-city children with asthma. *J Allergy Clin Immunol.* 1998;102(4 Pt 1):563–570.

32. Kattan M, Mitchell H, Eggleston P, et al. Characteristics of inner-city children with asthma: the national cooperative inner-city asthma study. *Pediatr Pulmonol.* 1997;24(4):253–262.

33. Crain EF, Walter M, O'Connor GT, et al. Home and allergic characteristics of children with asthma in seven U.S. urban communities and design of an environmental intervention: the Inner-City Asthma Study. *Environ Health Perspect.* 2002;110(9):939–945.

34. Chew GL, Correa JC, Perzanowski MS. Mouse and cockroach allergens in the dust and air in northeastern United States inner-city public high schools. *Indoor Air.* 2005;15(4):228–234.

35. Permaul P, Hoffman E, Fu C, et al. Allergens in urban schools and homes of children with asthma. *Pediatr Allergy Immunol.* 2012;23(6):543–549.

36. Salo PM, Sever ML, Zeldin DC. Indoor allergens in school and day care environments. *J Allergy Clin Immunol.* 2009;124(2):185–192, 192.e181–e189; quiz 193–184.

37. Huffaker M, Phipatanakul W. Introducing an environmental assessment and intervention program in inner-city schools. *J Allergy Clin Immunol.* 2014;134(6): 1232–1237.

38. Hauptman M, Phipatanakul W. Recent advances in environmental controls outside the home setting. *Curr Opin Allergy Clin Immunol.* 2016;16(2):135–141.

39. Sarpong SB, Wood RA, Karrison T, Eggleston PA. Cockroach allergen (Bla g 1) in school dust. *J Allergy Clin Immunol.* 1997;99(4):486–492.

40. Phipatanakul W, Bailey A, Hoffman EB, et al. The school inner-city asthma study: design, methods, and lessons learned. *J Asthma.* 2011;48(10):1007–1014.

41. Perzanowski MS, Rönmark E, Nold B, Lundbck B, Platts-Mills TA. Relevance of allergens from cats and dogs to asthma in the northernmost province of Sweden: schools as a major site of exposure. *J Allergy Clin Immunol.* 1999;103(6):1018–1024.

42. Jhun I, Gaffin JM, Coull BA, et al. School environmental intervention to reduce particulate pollutant exposures for children with asthma. *J Allergy Clin Immunol Pract.* 2017;5(1):154–159.e153.

43. Karlsson AS, Andersson B, Renström A, Svedmyr J, Larsson K, Borres MP. Airborne cat allergen reduction in classrooms that use special school clothing or ban pet ownership. *J Allergy Clin Immunol.* 2004;113(6):1172–1177.

44. Borràs-Santos A, Jacobs JH, Täubel M, et al. Dampness and mould in schools and respiratory symptoms in children: the HITEA study. *Occup Environ Med.* 2013;70(10): 681–687.

45. Baxi SN, Muilenberg ML, Rogers CA, et al. Exposures to molds in school classrooms of children with asthma. *Pediatr Allergy Immunol.* 2013;24(7):697–703.

46. Bernstein JA, Levin L, Crandall MS, Perez A, Lanphear B. A pilot study to investigate the effects of combined dehumidification and HEPA filtration on dew point and airborne mold spore counts in day care centers. *Indoor Air.* 2005;15(6):402–407.

47. Lemanske RF, Kakumanu S, Shanovich K, et al. Creation and implementation of SAMPRO: a school-based asthma management program. *J Allergy Clin Immunol.* 2016;138(3):711–723.

48. Matsui EC. Environmental exposures and asthma morbidity in children living in urban neighborhoods. *Allergy.* 2014;69(5):553–558.

49. Hulin M, Caillaud D, Annesi-Maesano I. Indoor air pollution and childhood asthma: variations between urban and rural areas. *Indoor Air.* 2010;20(6):502–514.

50. McCormack MC, Breysse PN, Matsui EC, et al. In-home particle concentrations and childhood asthma morbidity. *Environ Health Perspect.* 2009;117(2):294–298.

51. Belanger K, Holford TR, Gent JF, Hill ME, Kezik JM, Leaderer BP. Household levels of nitrogen dioxide and pediatric asthma severity. *Epidemiology.* 2013;24(2): 320–330.

52. Lu KD, Breysse PN, Diette GB, et al. Being overweight increases susceptibility to indoor pollutants among urban children with asthma. *J Allergy Clin Immunol.* 2013;131(4):1017–1023, 1023.e1011–e1013.

53. Halterman JS, Borrelli B, Tremblay P, et al. Screening for environmental tobacco smoke exposure among inner-city children with asthma. *Pediatrics.* 2008;122(6):1277–1283.

54. Kit BK, Simon AE, Brody DJ, Akinbami LJ. US prevalence and trends in tobacco smoke exposure among children and adolescents with asthma. *Pediatrics.* 2013;131(3): 407–414.

55. Butz AM, Matsui EC, Breysse P, et al. A randomized trial of air cleaners and a health coach to improve indoor air quality for inner-city children with asthma and secondhand smoke exposure. *Arch Pediatr Adolesc Med.* 2011;165(8):741–748.

56. Lanphear BP, Hornung RW, Khoury J, Yolton K, Lierl M, Kalkbrenner A. Effects of HEPA air cleaners on unscheduled asthma visits and asthma symptoms for children exposed to secondhand tobacco smoke. *Pediatrics.* 2011;127(1):93–101.

57. Priest N, Roseby R, Waters E, et al. Family and carer smoking control programmes for reducing children's exposure to environmental tobacco smoke. *Cochrane Database Syst Rev.* 2008;(4):CD001746. http://dx.doi.org/10.1002/14651858. CD001746.

58. Colton MD, MacNaughton P, Vallarino J, et al. Indoor air quality in green vs conventional multifamily low-income housing. *Environ Sci Technol.* 2014;48(14):7833–7841.

59. D'Amato G, Liccardi G, Frenguelli G. Thunderstorm-asthma and pollen allergy. *Allergy.* 2007;62(1):11–16.

60. Kingsley SL, Eliot MN, Carlson L, et al. Proximity of US schools to major roadways: a nationwide assessment. *J Expo Sci Environ Epidemiol.* 2014;24(3):253–259.

61. Rabinovitch N, Strand M, Gelfand EW. Particulate levels are associated with early asthma worsening in children with persistent disease. *Am J Respir Crit Care Med.* 2006;173(10):1098–1105.

62. Cakmak S, Mahmud M, Grgicak-Mannion A, Dales RE. The influence of neighborhood traffic density on the respiratory health of elementary schoolchildren. *Environ Int.* 2012;39(1):128–132.

63. Khreis H, Kelly C, Tate J, Parslow R, Lucas K, Nieuwenhuijsen M. Exposure to traffic-related air pollution and risk of development of childhood asthma: a systematic review and meta-analysis. *Environ Int.* 2017;100:1–31.

64. Lindgren P, Johnson J, Williams A, Yawn B, Pratt GC. Asthma exacerbations and traffic: examining relationships using link-based traffic metrics and a comprehensive patient database. *Environ Health.* 2016;15(1):102.

65. Shmool JL, Kubzansky LD, Newman OD, Spengler J, Shepard P, Clougherty JE. Social stressors and air pollution across New York City communities: a spatial approach for assessing correlations among multiple exposures. *Environ Health.* 2014;13:91.

66. Hsu J, Wilhelm N, Lewis L, Herman E. Economic evidence for US asthma self-management education and home-based interventions. *J Allergy Clin Immunol Pract.* 2016;4(6):1123–1134.e1127.

67. Tschudy MM, Sharfstein J, Matsui E, et al. Something new in the air: paying for community-based environmental approaches to asthma prevention and control: work group Report of the practice, diagnostics and therapeutics committee of the American academy of allergy, asthma & immunology. *J Allergy Clin Immunol.* 2017. http://dx.doi.org/10.1016/j.jaci.2016.12.975.

CHAPTER 11

Phenotype and Genotype Determinants of Asthma Treatments

FERNANDO HOLGUIN, MD, MPH

INTRODUCTION

Asthma Phenotypes, the Evolution of a Concept Into Clinical Practice

The multitude of mechanisms and risk factors causing bronchial hyperresponsiveness, coupled with a high degree of treatment response heterogeneity, strongly suggest asthma is a complex syndrome, rather than a single disease. This idea is not entirely new, but its uptake in clinical practice has been rather slow until the recent availability of precise biologic therapies that only work on a subset of patients. These newer treatment strategies have encouraged clinicians to think beyond the "one-disease one-treatment" concept. Previously classified as being "extrinsic" or "intrinsic," depending on whether environmental trigger factors were readily recognizable or not, the concept of defining different types of "asthma" has evolved from simple arbitrary classifications into unbiased groups that more closely represent the different types of patients encountered in daily practice.

In the last decade, multiple cross-sectional studies have used sophisticated mathematical and machine-learning algorithms to organize large sets of clinical variables into asthma clusters, which are each characterized by a constellation of observable clinical and demographic traits that make a unique phenotype.[1-4] Although there is some degree of variability in the results generated by these techniques, patterns such as those determined by the timing of asthma onset have clearly emerged. The early-onset asthma phenotype (diagnosed during childhood) is primarily driven by allergic inflammation, usually has elevated eosinophils and IgE levels, and may be either mild or severe; in contrast, later-onset (after childhood) asthmatics represent a more heterogeneous group that includes phenotypes with less preponderance of T2-related biomarkers, may be associated with obesity or female gender, and have features of chronic airway obstruction. The late-onset eosinophilic types are usually more severe and associated with chronic rhinosinusitis with or without polyps. Those with aspirin-associated respiratory disease (AERD) also fall in this category.

Although the results of nonbiased grouping techniques have generated enormous enthusiasm and broadened our understanding of the clinical manifestations of this disease, there is a general lack of knowledge and consensus as to how different asthma phenotypes, beyond IgE or eosinophil levels, can guide treatment strategies. To complicate matters even further, although phenotypes are clinically relevant, they do not necessarily relate to a unique underlying disease process. In fact, more than one specific disease mechanism or endotype can be present in a given phenotype and vice versa, and multiple phenotypes can have the same endotype.[5] This may potentially explain why asthma therapy is not universally effective, even when prescribed to those otherwise meeting specific treatment criteria. Therefore while still in its infancy, using phenotypic and endotypic data to develop precision-based treatment algorithms has the potential to improve outcomes and minimize morbidity from exposure to unnecessary glucocorticoids. This chapter will discuss how using specific phenotypical information—clinical, demographic, genetic, or biomarker levels—can help understand treatment response heterogeneity and inform clinical therapeutic reasoning to achieve a personalized asthma treatment with greater efficacy and better safety.

Using Asthma Phenotypes to Guide Therapeutic Decision-Making

After confirming the diagnosis and before initiating therapy, it is important to determine a patient's asthma phenotype. Although it is impractical to expect that patients will meet all of the observable characteristics described in the cluster studies, some are easily ascertained and key to determining the likelihood of therapeutic success. These include (1) biomarkers of T2-related inflammation (i.e., peripheral blood

TABLE 11.1
Phenotype Determinants of Asthma Therapy

	Clinical Characteristics	Preferential Treatment Response
EOSINOPHILIC ASTHMA		
Allergic asthma Early onset (childhood)	Mild to severe Elevated FeNO Peripheral eosinophilia Elevated IgE Skin prick test	Inhaled glucocorticoids Anti-IgE
Persistent eosinophilic Late onset	Severe Peripheral eosinophilia Elevated FeNO Often with severe rhinosinusitis with or without nasal polyps can have aspirin sensitivity (AERD)	Poorly responsive to inhaled glucocorticoids Systemic glucocorticoids 5-Lipoxygenase inhibitor Anti-IL-5 If AERD, aspirin desensitization
ABPM Late onset	Severe Long duration, mucus production Peripheral eosinophilia Markedly elevated IgE, specific IgE Bronchiectasis	Systemic glucocorticoids Antifungals Omalizumab
NONEOSINOPHILIC ASTHMA		
Neutrophilic predominant asthma	Severe Fixed airway obstruction ± smoking related	LAMA Possibly macrolides
Obese, late onset	Female predominant Low or normal FeNO Very symptomatic but less airway obstruction	Poorly responsive to inhaled glucocorticoids LAMA Weight loss

ABPM, Allergic bronchopulmonary mycoses; *AERD*, Aspirin-exacerbated respiratory disease; *LAMA*, long-acting muscarinic antagonist.

eosinophils, exhaled nitric oxide [eNO]), (2) allergic inflammation (IgE levels), (3) lung function (degree of airway obstruction and bronchodilation response), (4) clinical factors (age of asthma onset), (5) demographic (race, ethnicity, obesity). Phenotypic characteristics associated with disease severity or asthma control that do not directly determine response to treatment have been purposely left out. Also, to facilitate the understanding of phenotypes and their relation to asthma therapy, these have been divided into eosinophilic and noneosinophilic categories. Specific asthma endotypes will be discussed within each of these groups.

Eosinophilic and Early-Onset Asthma Phenotype

Eosinophilic asthma (≥2% sputum eosinophils or ≥200 k/μL in peripheral blood) constitutes roughly ~50% of the asthmatic population and encompasses mild to moderate and severe allergic early-onset asthma, allergic bronchopulmonary mycoses (ABPM), and severe

late-onset with or without AERD (See Table 11.1).[6,7] Asthmatics with elevated eosinophils, whether in sputum or peripherally, have long been recognized to be more responsive to inhaled or systemic glucocorticoids. In 1958, Morrow Brown observed that of 90 asthmatics treated with oral glucocorticoids, 5 mg three times per week, 100% of those with eosinophilic sputum achieved complete or partial relief of respiratory symptoms in contrast to only 14% of those without sputum eosinophils.[8] These findings have been replicated in more recent studies of inhaled and systemic glucocorticoids. Compared with placebo, 8 weeks of inhaled mometasone in symptomatic asthmatics with sputum eosinophils >1.9% led to a doubling concentration in methacholine and a significant improvement in Juniper asthma quality of life questionnaire scores; whereas in the less eosinophilic group, mometasone was not different from placebo.[9] A recent Severe Asthma Research Program (SARP) study of 526 adult and 188 children severe and nonsevere asthmatics evaluated the clinical response to systemic glucocorticoids by comparing the before and after changes after a single IM dose of 40 mg triamcinolone; while only 20% of adults and 22% of children with severe asthma achieved a significant response in FEV_1 (≥10% change), adults with elevated blood or sputum eosinophils were twice as likely to do so. Interestingly, elevated eNO (>20 ppb) and greater baseline bronchodilator response provided the best sensitivity and specificity in predicting response to triamcinolone.[7]

These results, which are consistent with findings from other studies, suggest that phenotypes characterized by increased Th2 inflammation have improved response to glucocorticoids. This was clearly shown in a post hoc analysis of Vitamin D in Asthma (VIDA) study participants during which participants were treated with 20 mg of oral prednisone/day for 1-week before randomization.[1] The primary outcome, which was defined as achieving at least a 5% increase in FEV_1, was subsequently compared across different asthma clusters using the same methodology as the original SARP cluster study. Nearly 40% of participants in the early-onset and highly atopic phenotype achieved the primary outcome in contrast to only 11% in the late-onset obese cluster. Analysis of SARP-derived asthma clusters in 611 children from three CARE clinical trials also showed significant differences in the response to glucocorticoids. In the studies, which examined step 2 therapy, the early-onset (mean 2.2 years) and late-onset (mean 5.9 years) normal lung function clusters had the greatest fluticasone-related % change in FEV1. For step 3, the early-onset/severe lung function cluster (mean 1.8 years) had the greatest % FEV_1 change in response to inhaled glucocorticoids and long-acting β-agonist combination.[10]

Together, results from these studies argue that the likelihood of response to corticosteroids can in part be determined by phenotypical factors associated with the degree of T2 inflammation, and recent studies using functional genomics suggest that this response may also be genetically determined. In a landmark study, the airway epithelial gene expression of periostin, CLCA1, and Serpinb2 clearly separated asthmatics into two: a high and low group.[11] The high group also had higher levels of IL-13 and IL-5 (T2 cytokines) and had a significantly increased FEV_1 after 6 weeks of inhaled glucocorticoids; in contrast, the low group had much lower T2-related cytokines and did not respond to inhaled glucocorticoids. The fact that the expression of these genes can be quantified using induced sputum has the potential to identify steroid responders and further personalize the treatment of asthma.[12] For a further discussion on genetic determinants of corticosteroid responsiveness,

please see Chapter 9, Pharmacogenomics and Applications to Asthma Management.

Severe Eosinophilic Asthma Phenotypes

Eosinophilic asthmatics with more severe disease who fail to improve with GINA (Global Initiative for Asthma) or EPR (Expert Report Panel) step 4 therapies need additional medications to achieve control and minimize exposure to systemic glucocorticoids (see Table 11.1). Those with severe allergic asthma with elevated IgE and evidence of atopy can benefit from omalizumab (monoclonal anti-IgE antibody), particularly if the intent is to reduce the frequency of asthma exacerbations.[13] Elevated biomarker levels of T2-related inflammation, such as FeNO, periostin, and peripheral eosinophilia, predict a better response to this type of biologic therapy.[14] Many of these patients will also meet criteria for mepolizumab, an anti-IL-5 monoclonal antibody; however, there are no comparative studies or expert guidelines suggesting which approach to use first. To improve lung function, reduce systemic glucocorticoids, and enhance asthma-related quality of life, in addition to reducing exacerbation rate, IL-5 monoclonal antibodies could be a preferable option for those with eosinoiphilia.[15–17] For late-onset asthma phenotypes with persistent eosinophilia and significant rhinosinusitis with or without nasal polyps, treatment alternatives include 5-lipoxygenase inhibitors and anti-IL-5 monoclonal antibodies; for those that additionally have aspirin sensitivity and therefore meet criteria for aspirin-exacerbated respiratory disease (AERD), allergic desensitization can be beneficial.[18] Patients with severe asthma and markedly elevated IgE levels should be evaluated for ABPM (central bronchiectasis, sensitization to aspergillus fumigatus, fleeting infiltrates); these patients could benefit from a 4- to 6-month trial of antifungals, anti-IgE, and, for refractory cases, even additional anti-IL-5.[19–21] For an in-depth discussion on treatment of severe asthma, please see Chapter 3, Management of Severe Asthma in Adults.

Noneosinophilic Asthma

Approximately 50% of the asthmatic adult and pediatric population do not have significantly elevated airway or peripheral eosinophils. These patients are more likely to have late-onset (after childhood) disease and be part of a heterogeneous group of phenotypes that include (1) obesity-related asthma with a high female preponderance and low atopy, (2) chronic obstructive pulmonary disease–like asthma with paucigranulocytic airway inflammation and/or predominantly airway smooth muscle cell involvement, and (3) neutrophilic airway inflammation.[22] Noneosinophilic phenotypes can benefit from treatment with short-acting β-agonists yet are less likely to increase FEV1 and/or improve level of asthma control when treated with inhaled glucocorticoids. Long-acting muscarinic antagonists (LAMA) can be effective in this group. An open-label 4-week study of 17 adult asthmatics on moderate- to high-dose inhaled glucocorticoids treated with tiotropium showed a significant inverse correlation between the % of sputum eosinophils at baseline with the % change in FEV_1 after treatment, suggesting that noneosinophilic asthmatics benefit more from LAMAs.[23] However, post hoc analyses of large randomized clinical trials have not replicated this finding. In the PrimoTinA-Asthma clinical trial, which randomized 912 poorly controlled asthmatics on inhaled glucocorticoids and long-acting β-agonists to tiotropium versus placebo, there was no significant difference in exacerbations or FEV_1 change between those with baseline peripheral eosinophils above or below $0.6 \times 10^9/L$.[24] Also, a multicenter study that randomized 215 poorly controlled asthmatics on low-dose inhaled glucocorticoids to the addition of salmeterol, versus doubling inhaled glucocorticoids or tiotropium, failed to show baseline peripheral eosinophils as being predictive of LAMA response. However, those with greater airway obstruction and lower resting heart rate (greater cholinergic tone) were more likely to benefit.[25]

Additional therapeutic options with potential benefits are macrolide antibiotics. These drugs in addition to being antimicrobial agents have multiple antiinflammatory effects, including reducing IL-8 levels and decreasing neutrophilic airway inflammation.[26] Although existing evidence does not show macrolides to be better than placebo for the majority of clinical outcomes,[27] two subgroup analyses suggest that they could be beneficial in noneosinophilic asthma phenotypes. The AZISAST clinical trial randomized moderate to severe asthmatics with a history of prior exacerbations on high-dose inhaled glucocorticoids with or without long-acting β-agonists to 250 mg of azithromycin three times per week for 26 weeks.[28] Although azithromycin was no different from placebo in the overall study population, it significantly reduced the rate of exacerbations in those with baseline peripheral eosinophils <200/μL (33% vs. 62%, RR 0.54 [95%C.I. 0.29–0.98]). Clarithromycin, on the other hand, has been shown in a placebo-controlled study of refractory asthmatics treated with 500 mg/day for 8 weeks to reduce neutrophilic airway inflammation and IL-8 protein and expression, lower MMP-9, and improve asthma-related quality of life.[29] Interestingly, those

with noneosinophilic asthma benefited the most. In addition to macrolides, neutrophilic airway inflammation associated with cigarette smoking can potentially benefit from leukotriene modifiers.[30]

Obesity asthma phenotype
Nearly 40% of asthmatics in the United States are obese, which is greater than the prevalence in the general population.[31] Widely recognized as an asthma comorbidity, it has been associated with greater morbidity and reduced treatment efficacy to either inhaled glucocorticoids or leukotriene modifiers.[32] The relationship between these chronic diseases is complex, bidirectional, and potentially affecting any child or adult asthma phenotype. Given that the pathophysiology is poorly understood, there are no drug interventions that specifically benefit obese asthmatics. However, diet- and lifestyle-induced weight loss has the potential of being beneficial because it has been associated with improved outcomes particularly when the weight reduction is at least 10%.[33] In obese asthmatics undergoing bariatric surgery, those with a normal IgE seem to benefit more from this intervention when compared with those with higher levels, suggesting that obesity's effect on asthma varies depending on the underlying asthma phenotype.[34]

Race and ethnicity as determinants of asthma treatment efficacy and safety
Asthma is well known to disproportionately affect some racial and ethnic groups more than others. For example, relative to whites, blacks have greater rates of asthma morbidity and mortality, and Puerto Rican Hispanics have the greatest asthma severity.[35] There are multiple factors, stemming from social determinants of health to genetic risks, which potentially explain these health disparities.[36] Although an extensive review on asthma, race, and ethnicity is beyond the scope of this chapter, there are some phenotype and genotype characteristics that can potentially determine treatment response and safety. In contrast to whites, IgE independently predicts asthma severity in blacks[37] and could explain why anti-IgE has been shown to be highly effective in reducing asthma morbidity in predominantly African-American inner-city populations.[38] Whether or not blacks respond better to different concentrations of inhaled glucocorticoids with and without long-acting β-agonists is unknown; however, the ongoing NIH AsthmaNet's BARD (Best African American Response to Asthma Drugs) study will provide much needed answers to this important question. Compared with Mexicans, Puerto Ricans have more severe airway

obstruction, greater rates of severe asthma exacerbation, and poor asthma control.[39] Some of these differences can be partly explained by the fact that Puerto Ricans have on average more than 7% lower bronchodilator reversibility when compared with those of Mexican descent.[40] Interestingly, although Puerto Ricans have earlier asthma onset and longer disease duration than Mexican asthmatics, there are no differences regarding IgE levels. Having a reduced bronchodilator response is an important clinical finding, considering that short-acting β-agonists are one of the main treatments in acute exacerbations.

The Salmeterol Multicenter Asthma Research Trial (SMART) study was terminated early after an interim analysis in 26,335 patients found a significant increase in respiratory and asthma-related deaths in salmeterol-randomized participants; these outcomes were respectively four and nearly five times greater in African-Americans.[41] Although it had been hypothesized that ADRB2 (β-2 adrenergic receptor) polymorphisms could explain why this race group had greater mortality when treated with salmeterol, results from several studies have refuted this possibility. However, one study demonstrated greater airway hyperresponsiveness to methacholine in blacks harboring the ADRB2 arg/arg genotype despite the use of salmeterol[42]; it is also conceivable that ADB2R rare variants could explain the higher rates of adverse outcomes in salmeterol-treated patients. This hypothesis was tested in a study in which sequencing of the ADRB2 identified six rare variants whose frequency was more common in African-Americans. Among these, two were associated with increased asthma exacerbation rates in those treated with LABA.[43] These findings suggest alterations in the therapeutic response to LABA in these asthma genetic subpopulations resulting from rare ADRB2 variants. For more details on ADRB2 polymorphisms and pharmacogenomics, please see Chapter 9, Pharmacogenomics and Applications to Asthma Management.

In summary, asthma is a highly heterogeneous disease in which response to asthma therapy varies widely across patients. The collection of observable characteristics or traits that make a unique clinical phenotype can be readily obtained through the clinical history, physical examination, lung function testing, and basic laboratories. These factors can help determine the likelihood of response to corticosteroids or alternative treatments. For more severe asthmatics requiring additional biologic therapies, careful phenotypical evaluation is necessary to ensure adequate treatment response. The availability of these newer therapeutic options, which only work in a subset of patients, is shifting the care

of asthma away from one-treatment, one-disease mentality, toward a more comprehensive approach and a better understanding of this complex airway syndrome. Just as providing a diagnosis of "anemia" or "arthritis" to a patient without further characterization would be considered completely inadequate and insufficient to determine the best therapeutic options, it should be no different for asthma.

REFERENCES

1. Moore WK, King TS, Bleecker ER, Meyers DA, Peters SP, Wenzel SE. SARP clinical clusters predict steroid responsiveness and risk of asthma exacerbations in the asthmanet VIDA (Vitamin D in asthma) trial. *Am J Respir Crit Care Med*. 2015;191.
2. Sutherland ER, Goleva E, King TS, et al. Cluster analysis of obesity and asthma phenotypes. *PLoS One*. 2012;7:e36631.
3. Haldar P, Pavord ID, Shaw DE, et al. Cluster analysis and clinical asthma phenotypes. *Am J Respir Crit Care Med*. 2008;178:218–224.
4. Moore WC. The natural history of asthma phenotypes identified by cluster analysis. Looking for chutes and ladders. *Am J Respir Crit Care Med*. 2013;188:521–522.
5. Lotvall J, Akdis CA, Bacharier LB, et al. Asthma endotypes: a new approach to classification of disease entities within the asthma syndrome. *J Allergy Clin Immunol*. 2011;127:355–360.
6. McGrath KW, Icitovic N, Boushey HA, et al. A large subgroup of mild-to-moderate asthma is persistently noneosinophilic. *Am J Respir Crit Care Med*. 2012;185:612–619.
7. Phipatanakul W, Mauger DT, Sorkness RL, et al. Effects of age and disease severity on systemic corticosteroid responses in asthma. *Am J Respir Crit Care Med*. 2016. http://dx.doi.org/10.1164/rccm.201607-1453OC.
8. Brown HM. Treatment of chronic asthma with prednisolone; significance of eosinophils in the sputum. *Lancet*. 1958;2:1245–1247.
9. Berry M, Morgan A, Shaw DE, et al. Pathological features and inhaled corticosteroid response of eosinophilic and non-eosinophilic asthma. *Thorax*. 2007;62:1043–1049.
10. Fitzpatrick AM, Teague WG, Meyers DA, et al. Heterogeneity of severe asthma in childhood: confirmation by cluster analysis of children in the national institutes of health/ national heart, lung, and blood institute severe asthma Research Program. *J Allergy Clin Immunol*. 2011;127:382–389. e381–e313.
11. Woodruff PG, Modrek B, Choy DF, et al. T-helper type 2-driven inflammation defines major subphenotypes of asthma. *Am J Respir Crit Care Med*. 2009;180:388–395.
12. Peters MC, Mekonnen ZK, Yuan S, Bhakta NR, Woodruff PG, Fahy JV. Measures of gene expression in sputum cells can identify TH2-high and TH2-low subtypes of asthma. *J Allergy Clin Immunol*. 2014;133:388–394.
13. Strunk RC, Bloomberg GR. Omalizumab for asthma. *N Engl J Med*. 2006;354:2689–2695.

14. Hanania NA, Wenzel S, Rosen K, et al. Exploring the effects of omalizumab in allergic asthma: an analysis of biomarkers in the EXTRA study. *Am J Respir Crit Care Med.* 2013;187:804–811.

15. Bel EH, Ortega HG, Pavord ID. Glucocorticoids and mepolizumab in eosinophilic asthma. *N Engl J Med.* 2014;371:2434.

16. Bel EH, Wenzel SE, Thompson PJ, et al. Oral glucocorticoid-sparing effect of mepolizumab in eosinophilic asthma. *N Engl J Med.* 2014;371:1189–1197.

17. Ortega HG, Liu MC, Pavord ID, et al. Mepolizumab treatment in patients with severe eosinophilic asthma. *N Engl J Med.* 2014;371:1198–1207.

18. Ledford DK, Wenzel SE, Lockey RF. Aspirin or other nonsteroidal inflammatory agent exacerbated asthma. *J Allergy Clin Immunol Pract.* 2014;2:653–657.

19. Altman MC, Lenington J, Bronson S, Ayars AG. Combination omalizumab and mepolizumab therapy for refractory allergic bronchopulmonary aspergillosis. *J Allergy Clin Immunol Pract.* 2017;5(4).

20. Li JX, Fan LC, Li MH, Cao WJ, Xu JF. Beneficial effects of Omalizumab therapy in allergic bronchopulmonary aspergillosis: a synthesis review of published literature. *Respir Med.* 2017;122:33–42.

21. Stevens DA, Schwartz HJ, Lee JY, et al. A randomized trial of itraconazole in allergic bronchopulmonary aspergillosis. *N Engl J Med.* 2000;342:756–762.

22. Wenzel SE. Asthma phenotypes: the evolution from clinical to molecular approaches. *Nat Med.* 18:716–725.

23. Iwamoto H, Yokoyama A, Shiota N, et al. Tiotropium bromide is effective for severe asthma with noneosinophilic phenotype. *Eur Respir J.* 2008;31:1379–1380.

24. Kerstjens HA, Engel M, Dahl R, et al. Tiotropium in asthma poorly controlled with standard combination therapy. *N Engl J Med.* 2012;367:1198–1207.

25. Peters SP, Bleecker ER, Kunselman SJ, et al. Predictors of response to tiotropium versus salmeterol in asthmatic adults. *J Allergy Clin Immunol.* 2013;132:1068–1074. e1061.

26. Wong EH, Porter JD, Edwards MR, Johnston SL. The role of macrolides in asthma: current evidence and future directions. *Lancet Respir Med.* 2014;2:657–670.

27. Kew KM, Undela K, Kotortsi I, Ferrara G. Macrolides for chronic asthma. *Cochrane Database Syst Rev.* 2015. http://dx.doi.org/10.1002/14651858.CD002997.pub4.

28. Brusselle GG, Vanderstichele C, Jordens P, et al. Azithromycin for prevention of exacerbations in severe asthma (AZISAST): a multicentre randomised double-blind placebo-controlled trial. *Thorax.* 2013;68:322–329.

29. Simpson JL, Powell H, Boyle MJ, Scott RJ, Gibson PG. Clarithromycin targets neutrophilic airway inflammation in refractory asthma. *Am J Respir Crit Care Med.* 2008;177:148–155.

30. Lazarus SC, Chinchilli VM, Rollings NJ, et al. Smoking affects response to inhaled corticosteroids or leukotriene receptor antagonists in asthma. *Am J Respir Crit Care Med.* 2007;175:783–790.

31. Prevention CfDCa. Asthma and obesity. 2017. Available from: https://www.cdc.gov/asthma/asthma_stats/asthma_obesity.htm; 2013.

32. Dixon AE, Holguin F, Sood A, et al. An official American Thoracic Society Workshop report: obesity and asthma. *Proc Am Thorac Soc.* 7:325–335.

33. Ma J, Strub P, Xiao L, et al. Behavioral weight loss and physical activity intervention in obese adults with asthma. A randomized trial. *Ann Am Thorac Soc.* 2015;12:1–11.

34. Dixon AE, Pratley RE, Forgione PM, et al. Effects of obesity and bariatric surgery on airway hyperresponsiveness, asthma control, and inflammation. *J Allergy Clin Immunol.* 128:508–515. e502.

35. Crocker D, Brown C, Moolenaar R, et al. Racial and ethnic disparities in asthma medication usage and health-care utilization: data from the national asthma survey. *Chest.* 2009;136:1063–1071.

36. Gold DR, Wright R. Population disparities in asthma. *Annu Rev Public Health.* 2005;26:89–113.

37. Gamble C, Talbott E, Youk A, et al. Racial differences in biologic predictors of severe asthma: data from the severe asthma Research Program. *J Allergy Clin Immunol.* 2010;126:1149–1156. e1141.

38. Busse WW, Morgan WJ, Gergen PJ, et al. Randomized trial of omalizumab (anti-IgE) for asthma in inner-city children. *N Engl J Med.* 2011;364:1005–1015.

39. Rosser FJ, Forno E, Cooper PJ, Celedon JC. Asthma in Hispanics. An 8-year update. *Am J Respir Crit Care Med.* 2014;189:1316–1327.

40. Burchard EG, Avila PC, Nazario S, et al. Lower bronchodilator responsiveness in Puerto Rican than in Mexican subjects with asthma. *Am J Respir Crit Care Med.* 2004;169:386–392.

41. Nelson HS, Weiss ST, Bleecker ER, Yancey SW, Dorinsky PM, Group SS. The Salmeterol Multicenter Asthma Research Trial: a comparison of usual pharmacotherapy for asthma or usual pharmacotherapy plus salmeterol. *Chest.* 2006;129:15–26.

42. Wechsler ME, Kunselman SJ, Chinchilli VM, et al. Effect of beta2-adrenergic receptor polymorphism on response to longacting beta2 agonist in asthma (LARGE trial): a genotype-stratified, randomised, placebo-controlled, crossover trial. *Lancet.* 2009;374:1754–1764.

43. Ortega VE, Hawkins GA, Moore WC, et al. Effect of rare variants in ADRB2 on risk of severe exacerbations and symptom control during longacting beta agonist treatment in a multiethnic asthma population: a genetic study. *Lancet Respir Med.* 2014;2:204–213.

CHAPTER 12

Predicting and Preventing Asthma Exacerbations

DR. HEATHER HOCH, MD, MSCS • DR. ANDREW H. LIU, MD

INTRODUCTION

There is much to be gained by accurate prediction and effective prevention of asthma exacerbations. For asthma patients, this would reduce a major risk of asthma and improve safety and quality of life. There is a large societal cost to asthma exacerbations. For example, in the United States in 2007, the total annual cost of asthma was estimated to be $56 billion due to hospital costs (~1.8 million emergency room visits and 0.4 million hospitalizations), missed school days, and missed parental and patient work days.[1-3] Exacerbation-prone asthmatics have higher total and asthma-related healthcare costs ($9223 vs. $5011 per year) than those who do not exacerbate.[4] Over time, asthma exacerbations may contribute to progressive lung function decline,[5-8] reduced lung growth,[9] and significant long-term physiologic impairment due to sporadic events. Accordingly, asthma exacerbations are a target of asthma research and personalized care, aiming for rigorous prediction and prevention of asthma exacerbations to revolutionize the status quo.

Defining Exacerbations

In asthma research and care, asthma exacerbations have a variety of definitions. Although this can complicate comparisons of clinical investigations and trials that use exacerbations as an outcome,[10] they relate to fundamental distinctions in severity, physiology, and risk and cost burden. The consistent theme of exacerbation definitions is discrete events that require medical intervention. The US National Institutes of Health National Heart, Lung, and Blood Institute (NIH NHLBI) Expert Panel Report defined an exacerbation as "…acute or subacute episodes of progressively worsening shortness of breath, cough, wheezing, and chest tightness, or some combination of these symptoms.[11]" Exacerbations can be further characterized by severity as mild, moderate, and severe (with life-threatening subset) (Table 12.1).[11,12] The frequently used exacerbation criteria to assess asthma risk

when classifying asthma severity and control is simply: "Exacerbation requiring oral or systemic corticosteroids.[11]" The international "Global Initiative for Asthma" guidelines similarly defines asthma exacerbations as "…a progressive increase in symptoms of shortness of breath, cough, wheezing or chest tightness and progressive decrease in lung function, i.e., they represent a change from the patient's usual status that is sufficient to require a change in treatment," and it also similarly classifies exacerbation severity as a risk parameter for classification of asthma severity and control.[13] Further distinctions in asthma exacerbations include two distinct phenotypes of near-fatal events: (1) abrupt onset, with loss of consciousness or respiratory arrest associated with extremely high $PaCO_2$ and recovery within hours or (2) gradual worsening, increased work of breathing over days, near-normal $PaCO_2$, and gradual recovery over weeks.[14,15]

PREDICTING EXACERBATIONS (TABLE 12.2)

A variety of demographic and clinical factors have been evaluated for exacerbation prediction.[16,17] Asthma exacerbations demonstrate significant demographic disparities: in the United States, children (especially young children), women, black/African-American and Puerto Rican race/ethnicities, and the economically disadvantaged have higher rates of asthma exacerbations, hospitalizations, and deaths.[3] Obesity is a moderate risk factor for asthma exacerbations in adolescents and adults but has not been consistently validated in children.[18-21]

A recent (within the last 3–12 months) severe asthma exacerbation is a relatively strong and consistent predictor of future exacerbations,[22-25] indicating an exacerbation-prone phenotype, deserving of enhanced management to prevent recurrent events. Regarding severe exacerbations in children, prior asthma hospitalization increased the likelihood of subsequent asthma hospitalizations, such that the probability of

TABLE 12.1
Asthma Exacerbation Definitions by Severity

	Symptoms and Signs	Initial PEF (or FEV1)	Clinical Course
Mild	Dyspnea only with activity (assess tachypnea in young children)	PEF ≥70% predicted or personal best	• Usually cared for at home • Prompt relief with inhaled SABA • Possible short course of oral systemic corticosteroids
Moderate	Dyspnea interferes with or limits usual activity	PEF 40%–69% predicted or personal best	• Usually requires office or ED visit • Relief from frequent inhaled SABA • Oral systemic corticosteroids; some symptoms last for 1–2 days after treatment has begun
Severe	Dyspnea at rest; interferes with conversation	PEF <40% predicted or personal best	• Usually requires ED visit and likely hospitalization • Partial relief from frequently inhaled SABA • Oral systemic corticosteroids; some symptoms last tor >3 days after treatment is begun • Adjunctive therapies are helpful
Subset: life-threatening	Too dyspneic to speak; perspiring	PEF <25% predicted or personal best	• Requires ED/hospitalization; possible intensive care unit • Minimal or no relief from frequent inhaled SABA • Intravenous corticosteroids • Adjunctive therapies are helpful

ED, emergency department; *FEV1*, forced expiratory volume in 1 s; *PEF*, peak expiratory flow; *SABA*, short-acting β-agonist.
Note: Patients are instructed to use quick-relief medications if symptoms occur or if PEF drops below 80% predicted or personal best. If PEF is 50%–79%, the patient should monitor response to quick-relief medication carefully and consider contacting a clinician. If PEF is below 50%, immediate medical care is usually required. In the urgent *or* emergency care setting, the following parameters describe the severity and likely clinical course of an exacerbation.
From National Asthma Education and Prevention Program. Expert panel report 3 (EPR-3): guidelines for the diagnosis and management of asthma-summary report 2007. *J Allergy Clin Immunol*. 2007;120(suppl 5):S94–138; with permission.

TABLE 12.2
Factors Associated With Asthma Exacerbations

Demographic	History	Lung Function	Biomarkers	Environmental
Children/young children	Previous exacerbation(s)	Spirometry: FEV1 FEV1/FVC FEF 25–75	Eosinophils: Peripheral blood Sputum	Indoor allergens with sensitization
Women	Poor asthma control	Bronchodilator response	Number of inhalant allergen sensitizations	Outdoor allergens with sensitization
Black and Puerto Rican race/ethnicity	SABA inhaler prescription refills	Bronchial hyperrespon-siveness to methacholine	Exhaled nitric oxide	Viral infections
Economically disadvantaged	Difficult-to-Control asthma	Impulse Oscillometry		Smoking/smoke exposure status
Overweight	Poor controller medication adherence			

FEF, forced expiratory flow; *FEV1*, forced expiratory volume in 1 s; *FVC*, forced vital capacity; *SABA*, short-acting β-agonist.

a subsequent asthma hospitalization increased from 30% after a first admission, to 46% after a second, and 59% after a third.[26] Differential predictors may exist to predict the immediate risk of an exacerbation versus long-term risk.[27]

Poor asthma control has been associated with exacerbations. Asthmatic children who are difficult to control while receiving guidelines-based care have more asthma exacerbations.[28] Loss of asthma control in young children, especially daytime cough/wheeze and nighttime albuterol use, is a good predictor of next-day exacerbations.[27] The widely used Asthma Control Test (ACT) has been modestly predictive of asthma exacerbations,[29,30] as have the Asthma Control Questionnaire[31] and Asthma Therapy Assessment Questionnaire (ATAQ).[25,32] In a Kaiser health systems study, an ACT score ≤ 15, indicating very poor control, increased the 12-month risk of emergency hospital care for asthma (OR 2.5).[33]

Short-acting β-agonist (SABA) used to treat asthma symptoms can be a surrogate indicator of poor asthma control, and SABA pharmacy dispensing has been associated with fatal and near-fatal asthma exacerbations[34,35] *SABA prescription dispensing* have been a useful predictor of severe asthma exacerbations.[25,36] Using a large Medicaid and commercial insurance database, use of three or more albuterol canisters over 12 months was most predictive of subsequent asthma exacerbations, with each additional SABA canister increasing exacerbation risk by 8%–14% and 14%–18% in children and adults, respectively.[37] Similarly, ≥4 SABA canister prescriptions over 3 months was associated with an ICU hospitalization for asthma.[38]

Conventional biomarkers have been extensively evaluated for their ability to predict asthma exacerbations. Studies to evaluate the predictive ability of lung function measures on asthma exacerbations have shown that decreases in peak expiratory flow rates can predict future exacerbations.[39] Spirometric lung function parameters including FEV1% predicted, forced expiratory flow (FEF) 25%–75% predicted, forced expiratory volume in 1 s/forced vital capacity (FEV1/FVC) ratio, and impulse oscillometry airway resistance have been associated with exacerbation risk.[40–42] One study showed that FEV1 <60% predicted was a significant predictor of exacerbation risk in the following 4 months.[43] Bronchial hyperresponsiveness (BHR) to methacholine has been associated with asthma exacerbations.[44]

Inflammatory biomarkers have been considered as asthma exacerbation predictors. Increases in the slope of daily fractional exhaled nitric oxide (FeNO)

measurements have been noted in the time immediately preceding an asthma exacerbation[45]; however, data on predictive ability of FeNO alone in managed children have been mixed.[46–48] Elevated peripheral blood eosinophils (e.g., >300–400 cells/μL) have been shown to be predictive in some evaluations of both adults and children.[41,47–49]

Analyses to discern at-risk asthmatics have identified specific *asthma phenotypes* with greater asthma severity and exacerbation risk.[50] In United States inner-city children who experience a disparately high burden of asthma exacerbations, children receiving guidelines-based asthma management, and those who were difficult-to-control had a high burden of exacerbations.[28] Additional analyses of these children revealed a cluster phenotype with the highest exacerbation rates and high levels of allergy indicated by a high number of allergen sensitizations (mean 14 of 22 [64%] positive allergen sensitization tested) and high total serum immunoglobulin E (IgE) (mean 616 IU/L).[50] Cluster analyses to distinguish severe asthma phenotypes in adults, performed in the NIH NHLBI–sponsored Severe Asthma Research Program, identified two severe asthma phenotypic clusters with higher exacerbation rates.[51] These phenotypes were also distinguished by earlier age of onset (i.e., in childhood), lower baseline lung function, and greater bronchodilator responses. However, follow-up of these SARP participants did not find greater 3-year exacerbation rates or poorer asthma control in any one particular phenotype.[52]

Predictors of asthma exacerbations can differ from predictors of symptoms or control. In a post hoc study of children with asthma in the Childhood Asthma Management Program (CAMP), not being treated with inhaled corticosteroids, lower FEV1/FVC ratio, and greater BHR to methacholine predicted poor control; in comparison younger age, history of exacerbation in the prior year, >3 days of prednisone use in the past 3 months, and higher total eosinophil counts as well as lower FEV1/FVC ratio and greater BHR to methacholine predicted exacerbations.[44]

Exacerbation predictors in children may differ from those in adults. In one study, tobacco smoking, low lung function, African-American ethnicity, and history of severe asthma were associated with asthma exacerbations in adults, but only history of severe asthma was associated with asthma exacerbations in children <10 years of age.[53] Significant differences may even exist between children and adolescents; in another study, recent exacerbations, SABA use, and low lung function were predictors of exacerbations in both children and adolescents/adults; however, asthma control as measured by the ATAQ was predictive only in the asthmatic adolescent/adult populations.[54]

Composite exacerbation scoring indices have also been developed to determine if combinations of predictors can strengthen exacerbation prediction.[41,47,48,55] Composite indices may offer an effective way to predict an individual's risk for exacerbations; however, few have been validated or implemented to our knowledge. In children, a *Seasonal Asthma Exacerbation Index* that evaluates predictors by season was developed and validated (Fig. 12.1A–B).[47,48] This index was comprised of season-specific exacerbation risk factors: eosinophils, IgE, allergen skin test positivity, FEV1/FVC ratio, FeNO, age, treatment step, and exacerbation in the previous 3 months (Table 12.3). Each risk factor was given a score of 0–2 (low/medium/high) that were summed for a total score. In two studies, high composite index scores were associated with increased exacerbation rates in each of the four seasons (Fig. 12.1A–B). Such composite indices should be tested for predictive accuracy and considered for integration into the electronic health record for provider decision support in the clinical setting.

ENVIRONMENTAL EXPOSURES AND EXACERBATION RISK

There is substantial evidence that common environmental exposures underlie and trigger asthma exacerbations, especially in those who are susceptible. More than 80% of asthma exacerbations in children have been associated with a respiratory viral infection, mostly human rhinovirus,[56] and are strongly associated with the high prevalence of asthma exacerbations after the return to school in the fall season.[57] In children, respiratory virus infection associations with exacerbations range from 36% to 92%,[58,59] and 41%–78% in adults.[41]

A critical assessment of the evidence for the role of indoor environmental exposures and asthma exacerbations conducted by the Institute of Medicine,[60] with a recent update,[61] concluded sufficient evidence to establish causation or association between the following exposures and asthma exacerbations:

- Causation: dust mite, cat, and cockroach allergens in sensitized individuals; tobacco smoke
- Association: dog and fungal allergens in sensitized individuals; dampness; nitrogen dioxide

There is also strong evidence for indoor mouse allergen exposure in homes and schools and worsened asthma symptoms in sensitized children.[62–64]

There is limited or suggestive evidence for numerous other indoor exposures associated with asthma

exacerbations, including birds, cows, horses, endotoxin, formaldehydes, and fragrances. Associations between peak pollen levels and emergency department (ED) visits for asthma exacerbations exist,[65] and the association seems to be particularly high in asthmatic children.[66] Additionally, asthma exacerbation levels can increase dramatically after thunderstorms and have been associated with increased, electrostatically fractured pollen and fungal allergen exposures in sensitized patients.[67]

Accordingly, national and international guidelines strongly state the importance of evaluating and addressing environmental triggers that can make asthma worse and trigger exacerbations; for example, in the US NIH asthma management guidelines, identifying and addressing indoor allergens in sensitized individuals are considered Evidence Category A (supported by randomized, controlled trials with rich body of supportive data), and tobacco smoke, wood-burning fireplaces, and strong odors are considered Evidence Category C.[11,13] Although allergen exposures in sensitized individuals can trigger asthma exacerbations, a recent study demonstrated a mechanism linking IgE to innate antiviral responses to rhinovirus in exacerbation-prone asthmatic children, thereby revealing another mechanism for allergen exposures in sensitized individuals to render susceptibility to asthma exacerbations.[68] Considering the extent to which specific environmental exposures have an established role in asthma exacerbations, it is notable that these exposure measures have rarely been included with other risk factors to strengthen exacerbation prediction.

PREVENTING EXACERBATIONS (TABLE 12.4)

A major reason for identifying which patients are at risk for an asthma exacerbation is for intervention to prevent the exacerbation(s) from occurring. A main objective of asthma controller therapies is to reduce exacerbation risk.

Inhaled Corticosteroids and the Importance of Adherence in Preventing Exacerbations

Inhaled corticosteroid (ICS) controller therapy remains a mainstay of treatment for the prevention of asthma exacerbations. In the NHLBI-sponsored CAMP study of children with mild to moderate persistent asthma (enrolled at ages 6–11 years)[69] and the Prevention of Early Asthma in Kids study of preschool children at high risk for persistent asthma (enrolled at ages 2–3 years),[69,70] daily ICS use was associated with a ~40% reduction in the rate of asthma exacerbations over the course of multiple years.

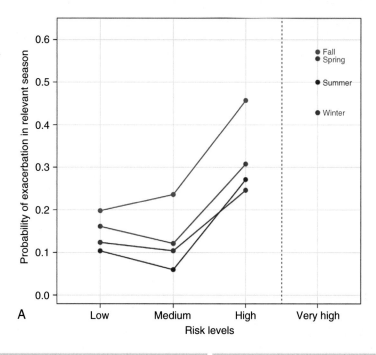

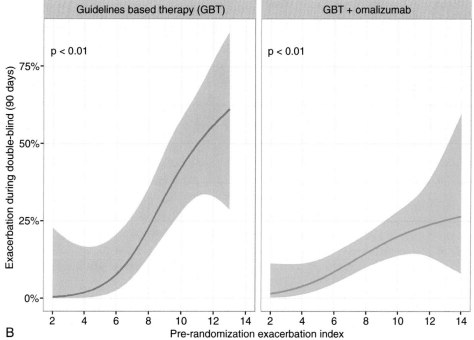

FIG. 12.1 **(A)** Seasonal Exacerbation Predictive index for prediction of asthma exacerbations in children. **(B)** Validation of a seasonal predictive index for asthma exacerbations. ((A) From Teach SJ, Gergen PJ, Szefler S, et al. Seasonal risk factors for asthma exacerbations among inner-city children. *J Allergy Clin Immunol*. 2015;135(6):1465–73; with permission. (B) From Hoch HE, Calatroni A, West JB, et al. Can We predict fall asthma exacerbations? Validation of the seasonal asthma exacerbation index. *J Allergy Clin Immunol*. 2017; with permission.)

TABLE 12.3
Scoring Schema for Derivation of the Seasonal Prediction Index

Variable	Baseline/Seasonal	Low (0 Points)	Medium (1 Point)	High (2 Points)
Age at recruitment (years)	Baseline characteristic	13–20		6–12
Total IgE (kU/L)	Baseline characteristic	0–100	100–300	>300
Allergen skin tests (positive results of 14)	Baseline characteristic	0–4	5–7	8–14
Blood eosinophils (%)	Baseline characteristic	0–2	2–6	6–22
Exacerbation in previous season	Previous season	No		Yes
ICS (treatment steps)	Previous season	Steps 0–3	Steps 4–5	Step 6
FEV1/FVC ratio (×100)	Previous season	>85	75–85	<75
FeNO (ppb)	Previous season	0–15	15–40	>40

ICS, inhaled corticosteroid; IgE, immunoglobulin E; FEV1, forced expiratory volume in 1 s; FVC, forced vital capacity.
From Teach SJ, Gergen PJ, Szefler S, et al. Seasonal risk factors for asthma exacerbations among inner-city children. *J Allergy Clin Immunol* 2015;135(6):1465–73; with permission.

TABLE 12.4
Interventions to Reduce Asthma Exacerbations and Mitigate Their Severity

Preventive Therapy	Avoidance of Environmental Triggers	Mitigating Exacerbation Severity	Others
Inhaled corticosteroid controller therapy (adherence is key)	Allergens in sensitized	Early administration of oral corticosteroids	Weight loss (in adults)
Biologic therapies • anti-IgE • anti-IL-5 (eosinophils)	Tobacco smoke exposure	Azithromycin (young children)	
	Mold/dampness		
	Viral infections		
	Air quality (indoor and outdoor)		

In conventional asthma management, adherence to ICS controller therapy is essential to reduction in exacerbation risk. Up to 24% of asthma exacerbations may be attributable to ICS nonadherence,[71] and adherence to asthma ICS has been shown to decrease the risk of asthma exacerbations.[72] Reasons for ICS nonadherence can range from forgetting and competing demands,[73] to perceived medication reactions,[74] to attitudes and beliefs about medications and asthma itself.[75] Determining medication adherence is a key to determining treatment failure when making decisions about stepped-up care.

There is evidence that the addition of long-acting β-agonist (LABA) therapy to ICS controller therapy in fixed-dose combination inhalers increases adherence to medication,[76,77] which could potentially account for improved outcomes in those treated with ICS-LABA combination controller medication.[78]

Conventional strategies to improve adherence have included traditional, behavioral, and technologic interventions (Table 12.5). Clinicians often rely on self-reported, subjective measures of adherence; however, these have shown to significantly overestimate the true levels of ICS controller adherence.[79] FeNO has been investigated as a method to assess ICS controller adherence.[80,81] New technologies offer the opportunity to objectively measure ICS adherence as well.[82] For example, a study of high-risk asthmatic children using text messaging for medication reminders based on digital ascertainment of ICS usage is ongoing.[83] Using

TABLE 12.5
Strategies to Improve Adherence to Daily Asthma Medications

Traditional	• Sticky notes/reminders • Medication placement/linking to established routines (i.e., near the toothbrush) • Calendar (sticker charts)
Behavioral	• Addressing barriers to adherence • Education • Self-evaluation and goal setting • Motivational interviewing/readiness to change • Rewards
Technology	• Monitoring devices • Cell phone reminders

Data from Dean A, Walters J, Hall T. A systematic review of interventions to enhance medication adherence in children and adolescents with chronic illness. *Arch Dis Child*. 2010; and Ruppar TM, Dobbels F, Lewek P, et al. Systematic review of clinical practice guidelines for the improvement of medication adherence. *Int J Behav Med*. 2015;22(6):699–708.

TABLE 12.6
Conceptual Approach to Asthma Medication Adherence and Asthma Control

	Adherent	**Non-adherent**
Controlled	• Continue to monitor for control and or medication side effects • Consider stepping down therapy after 3 months of adequate control	• Reassess if the patient is on the correct medication step • Reassess if the diagnosis is correct • Assess reasons for nonadherence • Consider stepping down therapy after 3 months of adequate control
Not controlled	• Consider stepping up therapy • Consider alternative diagnoses • Evaluate the validity of adherence assessments (i.e., using pharmacy fill records or technology to track rather than relying on self-reported adherence)	• Assess reasons for nonadherence • Motivational interviewing for ability to change behavior • Consider enhanced/tech strategies to track adherence • Close follow-up • Consider engaging multiple providers including primary care providers, school nurses, specialists

objective methods of adherence monitoring, patients can be divided into four groups, using adherence and asthma control to guide management (Table 12.6). Objective assessment of ICS controller adherence can distinguish true treatment failure for stepped-up care such as subspecialist evaluation and immunomodulatory therapy.

Immunomodulatory biologic therapies

For severe asthmatics, an advancement in personalized care has been the advent of immunomodulatory "biologic" therapies. The anti-IgE monoclonal antibody omalizumab was the first FDA-approved biologic therapy for severe asthma and has been shown to reduce risk of asthma exacerbations in adults[84] and children,[68,85,86]

including exacerbation-prone children receiving guidelines-based care.[55,82] Allergen sensitization when combined with viral infection results in increased risk for asthma exacerbation in both adults and children,[87] likely for any number of reasons including allergic inhibition of normal innate antiviral responses, to increased airway inflammation in viral infections.[41,88] The monoclonal antibody to IgE omalizumab has been shown to reduce asthma exacerbations by improving interferon-alpha responses to viruses,[68] making it a key potential therapeutic option for viral-induced asthma exacerbations, possibly due to cross-linking of IgE by allergens, which can inhibit innate antiviral responses. However, even at-risk children do not experience an exacerbation with every viral infection, suggesting that the interaction of various cofactors for exacerbations requires further study.

Recently, anti-IL-5, antieosinophilic agents including mepolizumab[89,90] and reslizumab[91] have also been FDA-approved and shown to be effective in reducing exacerbation frequency. However, it is important to be able to identify the characteristics that define those asthmatics most likely to benefit from the various types of immunomodulatory therapy.[47] For example, in severe asthmatics, mepolizumab significantly reduced exacerbation rates by 52% in those with peripheral blood eosinophils >150 cells/mcl, and by 70% in those with peripheral blood eosinophils >500 cells/mcl.[92] Further studies to develop a systematized approach to elucidate the specific asthma phenotypes most likely to benefit from each type of therapy are the next step in the personalization of asthma care. In clinical practice, it is possible that injectable immunomodulators' effectiveness in reducing exacerbations is in part related to the assured adherence of in-clinic administration and improvements in management resulting from routine clinic appointments for these injectable therapies (e.g., every 2–4 weeks).

Reducing exacerbation triggers

Although some of the key environmental trigger factors are known, effectively reducing these exposures to reduce asthma exacerbation risk can be difficult. Schools remain a key locale of viral transmission in children, and a significant decrease in asthma exacerbations is seen during school closures.[93] One attempt to reduce respiratory virus–triggered exacerbations in schools with a hand hygiene program was not successful, although the findings were confounded by an influenza outbreak.[94]

Intervention studies to reduce allergen exposure in sensitized asthmatics have had mixed results. A large randomized controlled multifaceted intervention to reduce home allergen exposures in inner-city asthmatic children significantly reduced cockroach, dust mite, and cat allergen exposures and reduced asthma symptom days and nights, while having a significant but modest effect on asthma exacerbations.[95] A cockroach-specific intervention with insecticide bait had a similar reduction in asthma severity, with a modest effect on exacerbations.[96] In one study, allergen-impermeable bedding covers to reduce dust mite exposure did not significantly improve asthma.[97] However, a recent 12-month randomized intervention with dust mite–impermeable bed covers in asthmatic children demonstrated no difference in exacerbations but a significant reduction in severe exacerbations indicated

by hospitalization.[98] A randomized controlled trial in asthmatic children of home remediation of dampness and mold demonstrated a significant reduction in exacerbations postremediation.[99] To our knowledge, there is only one small study of pet removal in pet-allergic asthmatics, demonstrating significant improvement in methacholine-induced BHR, an effect that was largely attributable to reduction in pet rodent or ferret exposure, not cats or dogs.[100]

Tobacco smoke exposure is a significant contributor to asthma exacerbations, both in chronic and acute exposure states.[61,101] It is important to note that self-reported tobacco exposure has been shown less sensitive than objectively measured nicotine biomarkers for predicting exacerbations,[102] with as many as 70% of children having positive testing for salivary cotinine in families who claimed no smoke exposure; therefore, it is important not to take all denials of environmental tobacco exposure at face value, and utilizing objective measures such as cotinine may be a better predictor of the effect of tobacco smoke on exacerbations.[102] Unfortunately, evidence for the effectiveness of counseling interventions aimed at reducing environmental tobacco smoke exposure in kids is lacking[103]; however, there is some evidence that legislation to ban indoor smoking in public places may be associated with a decrease in asthma exacerbations on a population level.[104] Poor air quality, both indoor and outdoor, has also been positively associated with exacerbations[101,105,106] and should be considered as possibly modifiable factors in the prevention of them.

In adults, weight loss may be a key way to prevent asthma exacerbations, e.g., one study found risk of asthma exacerbation was cut in half after bariatric surgery in adult asthmatics.[107]

Reducing exacerbation severity

Once an exacerbation occurs, it is possible to intervene early to keep exacerbations from becoming severe/life-threatening and to reduce their duration. Early administration of systemic corticosteroids remains a mainstay of the treatment of asthma exacerbations.[11,13] Early administration (within 75 minutes of admission) of oral corticosteroids in the ED setting has been shown to decrease the risk of inpatient admission for asthmatic children.[108] Although some studies support the early administration of oral corticosteroids for exacerbations by patients and parents/caregivers at home as well, rigorous randomized controlled trials supporting home administration of oral corticosteroids is lacking,[109] in part because of its wide practice in severe, exacerbation-prone asthmatics.

Because bacterial infection may be an important cofactor in asthma exacerbations, azithromycin has been studied in clinical trials as an exacerbation intervention. In adult asthmatics, azithromycin did not shorten the duration or reduce the severity of exacerbations.[110] However, in young asthmatics, mostly preschool age children with asthmalike conditions, azithromycin reduced the duration and progression of exacerbations.[111,112] In a small study of infants hospitalized with bronchiolitis, an azithromycin course was associated with less subsequent recurrent wheezing episodes.[113] This suggests that in young, preschool children with recurrent, severe asthmalike episodes, azithromycin may improve exacerbation outcomes when administered early in the course of an exacerbation; validation studies would help to determine if this practice should become standard of care.

SUMMARY AND NEXT STEPS

Much is already known about asthma exacerbation risk and prevention. Currently, medical history, biomarkers, environmental assessments, and technology have allowed for more personalization of asthma care for the prevention of asthma exacerbations than ever before. Further study into the underlying mechanisms for asthma exacerbations and gene-environmental interactions will provide for further personalization in the future. Future steps to further personalize asthma therapy includes the further elucidation of genetic-environmental interaction risk factors for exacerbations including the role of the human rhinovirus receptor in asthma exacerbations,[114] proteomics,[115] and metabolomic[116] and microbiome[117,118] evaluations. This expanding understanding of exacerbation risk could be harnessed into more precise, and possibly even real-time exacerbation prediction, as has been envisioned.[119] However, in the meantime, providers can utilize currently available information to predict asthma exacerbations, including demographic information, asthma history (especially recent severe exacerbation), markers of lung function, biomarkers including allergen sensitization, FeNO and eosinophils, and indoor and outdoor environmental exposures.

The clinician already has several tools at his/her disposal to personalize therapy, including accurate clinical phenotyping and adherence assessments, to provide the best possible therapy to reduce asthma exacerbations. The next step is utilizing a systematized approach to predicting and preventing asthma exacerbations in individual patients to create the most personalized approach possible. This process begins by finding appropriate ways to measure medication adherence, as well as obtaining relevant predictive biomarkers and lung function markers in all high-risk patients. Evaluating risks in individuals by seasonal risk is a component of personalization in asthma care because of the seasonality of severity in most patients. Utilizing physician decision support tools and means to monitor clinical effectiveness is the future of exacerbation prevention and rate reduction in population health.

REFERENCES

1. CDC Vital Signs-Asthma. https://www.cdc.gov/vitalsigns/asthma/.
2. Barnett SB, Nurmagambetov TA. Costs of asthma in the United States: 2002-2007. *J Allergy Clin Immunol.* 2011;127(1):145–152.
3. Moorman JE, Akinbami LJ, Bailey CM, et al. National surveillance of asthma: United States, 2001-2010. *Vital Health Stat 3.* 2012;35:1–58.
4. Ivanova JI, Bergman R, Birnbaum HG, Colice GL, Silverman RA, McLaurin K. Effect of asthma exacerbations on health care costs among asthmatic patients with moderate and severe persistent asthma. *J Allergy Clin Immunol.* 2012;129(5):1229–1235.
5. Calhoun WJ, Haselkorn T, Miller DP, Omachi TA. Asthma exacerbations and lung function in patients with severe or difficult-to-treat asthma. *J Allergy Clin Immunol.* 2015;136(4):1125–1127. e1124.
6. O'Byrne PM, Pedersen S, Lamm CJ, Tan WC, Busse WW. Severe exacerbations and decline in lung function in asthma. *Am J Respir Crit Care Med.* 2009;179(1):19–24.
7. Bai TR, Vonk JM, Postma DS, Boezen HM. Severe exacerbations predict excess lung function decline in asthma. *Eur Respir J.* 2007;30(3):452–456.
8. Belgrave DC, Buchan I, Bishop C, Lowe L, Simpson A, Custovic A. Trajectories of lung function during childhood. *Am J Respir Crit Care Med.* 2014;189(9):1101–1109.
9. McGeachie MJ, Yates KP, Zhou X, et al. Patterns of growth and decline in lung function in persistent childhood asthma. *N Engl J Med.* 2016;374(19):1842–1852.
10. Torvinen S, Rémuzat C, Mzoughi O, Plich A, Toumi M. PRS7-Comparative effectiveness analysis of mab In Asthma: The Importance Of Exacerbation Definition. *Value in Health.* 2015;18(7):A495.
11. National Heart, Lung, Blood Institute. *National Asthma Education and Prevention Program Expert Panel Report 3: Guidelines for the Diagnosis and Management of Asthma: Full Report 2007*; 2007. https://www.nhlbi.nih.gov/health-pro/guidelines/current/asthma-guidelines/full-report.
12. Expert Panel Report 3 (EPR-3). Guidelines for the Diagnosis and management of asthma-summary Report 2007. *J Allergy Clin Immunol.* 2007;120(5 suppl):S94–S138.

13. *Global Strategy for Asthma Management and Prevention-Updated 2017*; 2017. http://ginasthma.org/2017-gina-report-global-strategy-for-asthma-management-and-prevention/.

14. Wasserfallen JB, Schaller MD, Feihl F, Perret CH. Sudden asphyxic asthma: a distinct entity? *Am Rev Respir Dis.* 1990;142(1):108–111.

15. Plaza V, Serrano J, Picado C, Sanchis J. Frequency and clinical characteristics of rapid-onset fatal and near-fatal asthma. *Eur Respir J.* 2002;19(5):846–852.

16. Forno E, Celedon JC. Predicting asthma exacerbations in children. *Curr Opin Pulm Med.* 2012;18(1):63–69.

17. Puranik S, Forno E, Bush A, Celedon JC. Predicting severe asthma exacerbations in children. *Am J Respir Crit Care Med.* 2017;195(7):854–859.

18. Kattan M, Kumar R, Bloomberg GR, et al. Asthma control, adiposity, and adipokines among inner-city adolescents. *J Allergy Clin Immunol.* 2010;125(3):584–592.

19. Schatz M, Zeiger RS, Zhang F, Chen W, Yang SJ, Camargo Jr CA. Overweight/obesity and risk of seasonal asthma exacerbations. *J Allergy Clin Immunol Pract.* 2013;1(6):618–622.

20. Strunk RC, Colvin R, Bacharier LB, et al. Airway obstruction worsens in young adults with asthma who become obese. *J Allergy Clin Immunol Pract.* 2015;3(5):765–771. e762.

21. Lang JE, Hossain J, Smith K, Lima JJ. Asthma severity, exacerbation risk, and controller treatment burden in underweight and obese children. *J Asthma.* 2012;49(5):456–463.

22. Covar RA, Szefler SJ, Zeiger RS, et al. Factors associated with asthma exacerbations during a long-term clinical trial of controller medications in children. *J Allergy Clin Immunol.* 2008;122(4):741–747.e744.

23. Haselkorn T, Zeiger RS, Chipps BE, et al. Recent asthma exacerbations predict future exacerbations in children with severe or difficult-to-treat asthma. *J Allergy Clin Immunol.* 2009;124(5):921–927.

24. Miller MK, Lee JH, Miller DP, Wenzel SE, Group TS. Recent asthma exacerbations: a key predictor of future exacerbations. *Respir Med.* 2007;101(3):481–489.

25. Chipps BE, Zeiger RS, Dorenbaum A, et al. Assessment of asthma control and asthma exacerbations in the epidemiology and natural history of asthma: outcomes and treatment regimens (TENOR) observational cohort. *Curr Respir Care Rep.* 2012;1(4):259–269.

26. Bloomberg GR, Trinkaus KM, Fisher Jr EB, Musick JR, Strunk RC. Hospital readmissions for childhood asthma: a 10-year metropolitan study. *Am J Respir Crit Care Med.* 2003;167(8):1068–1076.

27. Swern AS, Tozzi CA, Knorr B, Bisgaard H. Predicting an asthma exacerbation in children 2 to 5 years of age. *Ann Allergy Asthma Immunol.* 2008;101(6):626–630.

28. Pongracic JA, Krouse RZ, Babineau DC, et al. Distinguishing characteristics of difficult-to-control asthma in inner-city children and adolescents. *J Allergy Clin Immunol.* 2016;138(4):1030–1041.

29. Cajigal S, Wells KE, Peterson EL, et al. Predictive properties of the asthma control test and its component questions for severe asthma exacerbations. *J Allergy Clin Immunol Pract.* 2017;5(1):121–127. e122.

30. Ko FW, Hui DS, Leung TF, et al. Evaluation of the asthma control test: a reliable determinant of disease stability and a predictor of future exacerbations. *Respirology.* 2012;17(2):370–378.

31. Bateman ED, Reddel HK, Eriksson G, et al. Overall asthma control: the relationship between current control and future risk. *J Allergy Clin Immunol.* 2010;125(3):600–608. 608.e601-608.e606.

32. Sullivan SD, Wenzel SE, Bresnahan BW, et al. Association of control and risk of severe asthma-related events in severe or difficult-to-treat asthma patients. *Allergy.* 2007;62(6):655–660.

33. Schatz M, Zeiger RS, Drane A, et al. Reliability and predictive validity of the Asthma Control Test administered by telephone calls using speech recognition technology. *J Allergy Clin Immunol.* 2007;119(2):336–343.

34. Spitzer WO, Suissa S, Ernst P, et al. The use of beta-agonists and the risk of death and near death from asthma. *N Engl J Med.* 1992;326(8):501–506.

35. Suissa S, Blais L, Ernst P. Patterns of increasing beta-agonist use and the risk of fatal or near-fatal asthma. *Eur Respir J.* 1994;7(9):1602–1609.

36. Schatz M, Zeiger RS, Vollmer WM, et al. Validation of a beta-agonist long-term asthma control scale derived from computerized pharmacy data. *J Allergy Clin Immunol.* 2006;117(5):995–1000.

37. Stanford RH, Shah MB, D'Souza AO, Dhamane AD, Schatz M. Short-acting beta-agonist use and its ability to predict future asthma-related outcomes. *Ann Allergy Asthma Immunol.* 2012;109(6):403–407.

38. Eisner MD, Lieu TA, Chi F, et al. Beta agonists, inhaled steroids, and the risk of intensive care unit admission for asthma. *Eur Respir J.* 2001;17(2):233–240.

39. Thamrin C, Zindel J, Nydegger R, et al. Predicting future risk of asthma exacerbations using individual conditional probabilities. *J Allergy Clin Immunol.* 2011;127(6):1494–1502. e1493.

40. Rao DR, Gaffin JM, Baxi SN, Sheehan WJ, Hoffman EB, Phipatanakul W. The utility of forced expiratory flow between 25% and 75% of vital capacity in predicting childhood asthma morbidity and severity. *J Asthma.* 2012;49(6):586–592.

41. Greenberg S. Asthma exacerbations: predisposing factors and prediction rules. *Curr Opin Allergy Clin Immunol.* 2013;13(3):225–236.

42. Schulze J, Biedebach S, Christmann M, Herrmann E, Voss S, Zielen S. Impulse oscillometry as a predictor of asthma exacerbations in young children. *Respiration.* 2016;91(2):107–114.

43. Fuhlbrigge AL, Weiss ST, Kuntz KM, Paltiel AD. Forced expiratory volume in 1 second percentage improves the classification of severity among children with asthma. *Pediatrics.* 2006;118(2):e347–355.

44. Wu AC, Tantisira K, Li L, et al. Predictors of symptoms are different from predictors of severe exacerbations from asthma in children. *Chest.* 2011;140(1):100–107.

45. van der Valk RJ, Baraldi E, Stern G, Frey U, de Jongste JC. Daily exhaled nitric oxide measurements and asthma exacerbations in children. *Allergy.* 2012;67(2):265–271.

46. van Vliet D, Alonso A, Rijkers G, et al. Prediction of asthma exacerbations in children by innovative exhaled inflammatory markers: results of a longitudinal study. *PLoS One.* 2015;10(3):e0119434.

47. Hoch HE, Calatroni A, West JB, et al. Can we predict fall asthma Exacerbations? Validation of the seasonal asthma exacerbation index. *J Allergy Clin Immunol.* 2017. http://dx.doi.org/10.1016/j.jaci.2017.01.026.

48. Teach SJ, Gergen PJ, Szefler SJ, et al. Seasonal risk factors for asthma exacerbations among inner-city children. *J Allergy Clin Immunol.* 2015;135(6):1465–1473. e1465.

49. Price D, Wilson AM, Chisholm A, et al. Predicting frequent asthma exacerbations using blood eosinophil count and other patient data routinely available in clinical practice. *J Asthma Allergy.* 2016;9:1–12.

50. Zoratti EM, Krouse RZ, Babineau DC, et al. Asthma phenotypes in inner-city children. *J Allergy Clin Immunol.* 2016;138(4):1016–1029.

51. Moore WC, Meyers DA, Wenzel SE, et al. Identification of asthma phenotypes using cluster analysis in the Severe Asthma Research Program. *Am J Respir Crit Care Med.* 2010;181(4):315–323.

52. Bourdin A, Molinari N, Vachier I, et al. Prognostic value of cluster analysis of severe asthma phenotypes. *J Allergy Clin Immunol.* 2014;134(5):1043–1050.

53. McCoy K, Shade DM, Irvin CG, et al. Predicting episodes of poor asthma control in treated patients with asthma. *J Allergy Clin Immunol.* 2006;118(6):1226–1233.

54. Zeiger RS, Yegin A, Simons FE, et al. Evaluation of the National Heart, Lung, and Blood Institute guidelines impairment domain for classifying asthma control and predicting asthma exacerbations. *Ann Allergy Asthma Immunol.* 2012;108(2):81–87.

55. Forno E, Fuhlbrigge A, Soto-Quiros ME, et al. Risk factors and predictive clinical scores for asthma exacerbations in childhood. *Chest.* 2010;138(5):1156–1165.

56. Johnston SL, Pattemore PK, Sanderson G, et al. Community study of role of viral infections in exacerbations of asthma in 9-11 year old children. *Bmj.* 1995;310(6989):1225–1229.

57. Johnston NW, Sears MR. Asthma exacerbations. 1: epidemiology. *Thorax.* 2006;61(8):722–728.

58. Costa LD, Costa PS, Camargos PA. Exacerbation of asthma and airway infection: is the virus the villain? *J Pediatr (Rio J).* 2014;90(6):542–555.

59. Duenas Meza E, Jaramillo CA, Correa E, et al. Virus and Mycoplasma pneumoniae prevalence in a selected pediatric population with acute asthma exacerbation. *J Asthma.* 2016;53(3):253–260.

60. Institute of Medicine Committee on the Assessment of A. *Indoor A. Clearing the Air: Asthma and Indoor Air Exposures.* Washington (DC): National Academies Press (US) Copyright 2000 by the National Academy of Sciences; 2000. All rights reserved.

61. Kanchongkittiphon W, Mendell MJ, Gaffin JM, Wang G, Phipatanakul W. Indoor environmental exposures and exacerbation of asthma: an update to the 2000 review by the Institute of Medicine. *Environ Health Perspect.* 2015;123(1):6–20.

62. Matsui EC, Eggleston PA, Buckley TJ, et al. Household mouse allergen exposure and asthma morbidity in inner-city preschool children. *Ann Allergy Asthma Immunol.* 2006;97(4):514–520.

63. Ahluwalia SK, Peng RD, Breysse PN, et al. Mouse allergen is the major allergen of public health relevance in Baltimore City. *J Allergy Clin Immunol.* 2013;132(4):830–835.e831-832.

64. Sheehan WJ, Permaul P, Petty CR, et al. Association between allergen exposure in inner-city schools and asthma morbidity among students. *JAMA Pediatr.* 2017;171(1):31–38.

65. Reid MJ, Moss RB, Hsu YP, Kwasnicki JM, Commerford TM, Nelson BL. Seasonal asthma in northern California: allergic causes and efficacy of immunotherapy. *J Allergy Clin Immunol.* 1986;78(4 Pt 1):590–600.

66. Ito K, Weinberger KR, Robinson GS, et al. The associations between daily spring pollen counts, over-the-counter allergy medication sales, and asthma syndrome emergency department visits in New York City, 2002-2012. *Environ Health.* 2015;14:71.

67. Wark PA, Simpson J, Hensley MJ, Gibson PG. Airway inflammation in thunderstorm asthma. *Clin Exp Allergy.* 2002;32(12):1750–1756.

68. Teach SJ, Gill MA, Togias A, et al. Preseasonal treatment with either omalizumab or an inhaled corticosteroid boost to prevent fall asthma exacerbations. *J Allergy Clin Immunol.* 2015;136(6):1476–1485.

69. Guilbert TW, Morgan WJ, Zeiger RS, et al. Long-term inhaled corticosteroids in preschool children at high risk for asthma. *N Engl J Med.* 2006;354(19):1985–1997.

70. Long-term effects of budesonide or nedocromil in children with asthma. The childhood asthma management program research group. *N Engl J Med.* 2000;343(15):1054–1063.

71. Williams LK, Peterson EL, Wells K, et al. Quantifying the proportion of severe asthma exacerbations attributable to inhaled corticosteroid nonadherence. *J Allergy Clin Immunol.* 2011;128(6):1185–1191.e1182.

72. Engelkes M, Janssens HM, de Jongste JC, Sturkenboom MC, Verhamme KM. Medication adherence and the risk of severe asthma exacerbations: a systematic review. *Eur Respir J.* 2015;45(2):396–407.

73. Blaakman SW, Cohen A, Fagnano M, Halterman JS. Asthma medication adherence among urban teens: a qualitative analysis of barriers, facilitators and experiences with school-based care. *J Asthma.* 2014;51(5):522–529.

74. Burgess SW, Sly PD, Morawska A, Devadason SG. Assessing adherence and factors associated with adherence in young children with asthma. *Respirology*. 2008;13(4):559–563.

75. Pelaez S, Bacon SL, Aulls MW, Lacoste G, Lavoie KL. Similarities and differences between asthma health care professional and patient views regarding medication adherence. *Can Respir J*. 2014;21(4):221–226.

76. Foden J, Hand CH. Does use of a corticosteroid/long-acting beta-agonist combination inhaler increase adherence to inhaled corticosteroids? *Prim Care Respir J*. 2008;17(4):246–247.

77. Stoloff SW, Stempel DA, Meyer J, Stanford RH, Carranza Rosenzweig JR. Improved refill persistence with fluticasone propionate and salmeterol in a single inhaler compared with other controller therapies. *J Allergy Clin Immunol*. 2004;113(2):245–251.

78. Stanford RH, Fuhlbrigge A, Riedel A, Rey GG, Stempel DA. An observational study of fixed dose combination fluticasone propionate/salmeterol or fluticasone propionate alone on asthma-related outcomes. *Curr Med Res Opin*. 2008;24(11):3141–3148.

79. Krishnan JA, Bender BG, Wamboldt FS, et al. Adherence to inhaled corticosteroids: an ancillary study of the Childhood Asthma Management Program clinical trial. *J Allergy Clin Immunol*. 2012;129(1):112–118.

80. McNicholl DM, Stevenson M, McGarvey LP, Heaney LG. The utility of fractional exhaled nitric oxide suppression in the identification of nonadherence in difficult asthma. *Am J Respir Crit Care Med*. 2012;186(11):1102–1108.

81. Koster ES, Raaijmakers JA, Vijverberg SJ, Maitland-van der Zee AH. Inhaled corticosteroid adherence in paediatric patients: the PACMAN cohort study. *Pharmacoepidemiol Drug Saf*. 2011;20(10):1064–1072.

82. Morton RW, Everard ML, Elphick HE. Adherence in childhood asthma: the elephant in the room. *Arch Dis Child*. 2014;99(10):949–953.

83. Adams SA, Leach MC, Feudtner C, Miller VA, Kenyon CC. Automated adherence reminders for high risk children with asthma: a research protocol. *JMIR Res Protoc*. 2017;6(3):e48.

84. Grimaldi-Bensouda L, Zureik M, Aubier M, et al. Does omalizumab make a difference to the real-life treatment of asthma exacerbations?: Results from a large cohort of patients with severe uncontrolled asthma. *Chest*. 2013;143(2):398–405.

85. Busse WW, Morgan WJ, Gergen PJ, et al. Randomized trial of omalizumab (anti-IgE) for asthma in inner-city children. *N Engl J Med*. 2011;364(11):1005–1015.

86. Milgrom H, Berger W, Nayak A, et al. Treatment of childhood asthma with anti-immunoglobulin E antibody (omalizumab). *Pediatrics*. 2001;108(2):E36.

87. Custovic A, Simpson A. The role of inhalant allergens in allergic airways disease. *J Investig Allergol Clin Immunol*. 2012;22(6):393–401. qiuz follow 401.

88. Gern JE. Virus/allergen interaction in asthma exacerbation. *Ann Am Thorac Soc*. 2015;12(suppl 2):S137–S143.

89. Ortega HG, Liu MC, Pavord ID, et al. Mepolizumab treatment in patients with severe eosinophilic asthma. *N Engl J Med*. 2014;371(13):1198–1207.

90. Pavord ID, Korn S, Howarth P, et al. Mepolizumab for severe eosinophilic asthma (DREAM): a multicentre, double-blind, placebo-controlled trial. *Lancet*. 2012;380(9842):651–659.

91. Castro M, Zangrilli J, Wechsler ME, et al. Reslizumab for inadequately controlled asthma with elevated blood eosinophil counts: results from two multicentre, parallel, double-blind, randomised, placebo-controlled, phase 3 trials. *Lancet Respir Med*. 2015;3(5):355–366.

92. Ortega HG, Yancey SW, Mayer B, et al. Severe eosinophilic asthma treated with mepolizumab stratified by baseline eosinophil thresholds: a secondary analysis of the DREAM and MENSA studies. *Lancet Respir Med*. 2016;4(7):549–556.

93. Eggo RM, Scott JG, Galvani AP, Meyers LA. Respiratory virus transmission dynamics determine timing of asthma exacerbation peaks: evidence from a population-level model. *Proc Natl Acad Sci USA*. 2016;113(8):2194–2199.

94. Gerald LB, Gerald JK, Zhang B, McClure LA, Bailey WC, Harrington KF. Can a school-based hand hygiene program reduce asthma exacerbations among elementary school children? *J Allergy Clin Immunol*. 2012;130(6):1317–1324.

95. Morgan WJ, Crain EF, Gruchalla RS, et al. Results of a home-based environmental intervention among urban children with asthma. *N Engl J Med*. 2004;351(11):1068–1080.

96. Rabito FA, Carlson JC, He H, Werthmann D, Schal C. A single intervention for cockroach control reduces cockroach exposure and asthma morbidity in children. *J Allergy Clin Immunol*. 2017. http://dx.doi.org/10.1016/j.jaci.2016.10.019.

97. Woodcock A, Forster L, Matthews E, et al. Control of exposure to mite allergen and allergen-impermeable bed covers for adults with asthma. *N Engl J Med*. 2003;349(3):225–236.

98. Murray CS, Foden P, Sumner H, Shepley E, Custovic A, Simpson A. Preventing severe asthma exacerbations in children: a randomised trial of mite impermeable bedcovers. *Am J Respir Crit Care Med*. 2017;196.

99. Kercsmar CM, Dearborn DG, Schluchter M, et al. Reduction in asthma morbidity in children as a result of home remediation aimed at moisture sources. *Environ Health Perspect*. 2006;114(10):1574–1580.

100. Shirai T, Matsui T, Suzuki K, Chida K. Effect of pet removal on pet allergic asthma. *Chest*. 2005;127(5):1565–1571.

101. Dick S, Doust E, Cowie H, Ayres JG, Turner S. Associations between environmental exposures and asthma control and exacerbations in young children: a systematic review. *BMJ Open*. 2014;4(2):e003827.

102. McCarville M, Sohn MW, Oh E, Weiss K, Gupta R. Environmental tobacco smoke and asthma exacerbations and severity: the difference between measured and reported exposure. *Arch Dis Child*. 2013;98(7):510–514.

103. Baxi R, Sharma M, Roseby R, et al. Family and carer smoking control programmes for reducing children's exposure to environmental tobacco smoke. *Cochrane Database Syst Rev.* 2014;(3):CD001746. http://dx.doi.org/10.1002/14651858.

104. Ciaccio CE, Gurley-Calvez T, Shireman TI. Indoor tobacco legislation is associated with fewer emergency department visits for asthma exacerbation in children. *Ann Allergy Asthma Immunol.* 2016;117(6):641–645.

105. Tosca MA, Ruffoni S, Canonica GW, Ciprandi G. Asthma exacerbation in children: relationship among pollens, weather, and air pollution. *Allergol Immunopathol (Madr).* 2014;42(4):362–368.

106. Kim J, Kim H, Kweon J. Hourly differences in air pollution on the risk of asthma exacerbation. *Environ Pollut.* 2015;203:15–21.

107. Hasegawa K, Tsugawa Y, Chang Y, Camargo Jr CA. Risk of an asthma exacerbation after bariatric surgery in adults. *J Allergy Clin Immunol.* 2015;136(2):288–294. e288.

108. Bhogal SK, McGillivray D, Bourbeau J, Benedetti A, Bartlett S, Ducharme FM. Early administration of systemic corticosteroids reduces hospital admission rates for children with moderate and severe asthma exacerbation. *Ann Emerg Med.* 2012;60(1):84–91. e83.

109. Ganaie MB, Munavvar M, Gordon M, Lim HF, Evans DJ. Patient- and parent-initiated oral steroids for asthma exacerbations. *Cochrane Database Syst Rev.* 2016;12. http://dx.doi.org/10.1002/14651858.CD012195.pub2.

110. Johnston SL, Szigeti M, Cross M, et al. Azithromycin for acute exacerbations of asthma: the AZALEA randomized clinical trial. *JAMA Intern Med.* 2016;176(11):1630–1637.

111. Bacharier LB, Guilbert TW, Mauger DT, et al. Early administration of azithromycin and prevention of severe lower respiratory tract illnesses in preschool children with a history of such illnesses: a randomized clinical trial. *JAMA.* 2015;314(19):2034–2044.

112. Stokholm J, Chawes BL, Vissing NH, et al. Azithromycin for episodes with asthma-like symptoms in young children aged 1-3 years: a randomised, double-blind, placebo-controlled trial. *Lancet Respir Med.* 2016;4(1):19–26.

113. Beigelman A, Isaacson-Schmid M, Sajol G, et al. Randomized trial to evaluate azithromycin's effects on serum and upper airway IL-8 levels and recurrent wheezing in infants with respiratory syncytial virus bronchiolitis. *J Allergy Clin Immunol.* 2015;135(5):1171–1178. e1171.

114. Bochkov YA, Gern JE. Rhinoviruses, Their Receptors: Implications for allergic disease. *Curr Allergy Asthma Rep.* 2016;16(4):30.

115. Teran LM, Montes-Vizuet R, Li X, Franz T. Respiratory proteomics: from descriptive studies to personalized medicine. *J Proteome Res.* 2015;14(1):38–50.

116. Reisdorph N, Wechsler ME. Utilizing metabolomics to distinguish asthma phenotypes: strategies and clinical implications. *Allergy.* 2013;68(8):959–962.

117. Huang YJ, Boushey HA. The microbiome in asthma. *J Allergy Clin Immunol.* 2015;135(1):25–30.

118. Casas L, Tischer C, Taubel M. Pediatric asthma and the indoor microbial environment. *Curr Environ Health Rep.* 2016;3(3):238–249.

119. Reid M, Gunn J, Shah S, et al. Cross-disciplinary consultancy to enhance predictions of asthma exacerbation risk in Boston. *Online J Pub Health Inform.* 2016;8(3):e199.

CHAPTER 13

School-Centered Asthma Programs

LISA CICUTTO, RN, ACNP(CERT), CAE, PHD

SCHOOL AS AN IMPORTANT COMPONENT OF ASTHMA CARE

Asthma is a common chronic childhood condition associated with significant morbidity, high rates of school absenteeism, and excessive costs for the individual and society. It is estimated that billions are spent on asthma-related healthcare.[1] Every school day, 36,000 children and youth miss school because of asthma.[2] High rates of school absenteeism affect a child's ability to learn.[3] The PIAMA cohort study examined the relationships between asthma and associated school absences, family socioeconomic status, and school performance. They observed that missing more than 5 days of school because of asthma influenced school performance.[4] A healthy student with well-controlled asthma is a student ready to learn and to be a full participant in the school experience, including physical activity and sports.

Because schools provide reliable access for reaching large numbers of children with asthma, they have become a targeted setting for quality asthma care programs and initiatives that involve partnerships with schools. For low-income and ethnic minority youth, schools are often the only setting used to receive healthcare services because of limited access to traditional medical care, affordability of medical care, and, more recently for immigrant families, fear of entering the healthcare setting and becoming a target for deportation. Schools are often advocated as the ideal setting for health education, health services, and the development of supportive networks and collaborations because of their large reach. Accordingly, school settings represent an essential setting for clinicians to partner with in support of students with asthma reaching their full potential.

ASTHMA MANAGEMENT PLANS IN SCHOOLS

Two key elements to successful asthma management in school settings are beginning the school year with a completed school asthma care plan/action plan and an onsite easily accessible quick-relief inhaler that is preferably carried by the student. The purpose of the written asthma care plan or asthma action plan for the school setting is to (1) outline asthma management steps to be applied at schools, (2) serve as a medical order for schools, and (3) serve as a release of information for communication and coordination activities among schools, clinicians, students, and families. A written school asthma care plan is required so that students experiencing symptoms can use their quick-acting bronchodilator inhaler kept at school to relieve symptoms quickly, thus enabling students to return to class and avoid having to leave the school for treatment or waiting in the nurse's office while a family member brings the inhaler to school. Asthma care plans for schools differ from asthma action plans for home use in several ways and therefore home plans may not be accepted or sufficient for the school setting. Common problems of home-based asthma action plans are that they often lack a release for sharing health information among school personnel and the student's healthcare providers and lack the signed indication from a parent/guardian and healthcare provider for administering the medication, self-carrying the inhaler, or the need for assistance with medication administration. Additionally, because the action plan is seen as a medical order in schools, the inclusion of the use of maintenance asthma medication (typically an inhaled steroid) twice-daily is problematic, as it is interpreted that the school nurse is required to administer the medication daily. This later issue creates additional problems for the school in that they have insufficient personnel for daily, supervised, administration of maintenance asthma medications for all students with asthma and it requires reliance on families to supply schools with maintenance asthma medications because schools do not have funds to supply medications.

Several studies highlight that these two crucial elements to successful asthma management in schools are not being performed.[5-7] A recent study involving five Alabama school districts observed that not one student with physician-confirmed asthma had a completed school asthma care plan on file at the school. Reported rates of students with asthma having a quick-relief inhaler at school range from 14% to 39%.[6,7] This work suggests that the gap between policy and practice is dramatic and potentially life-threatening. Federal laws exist and many states and school districts have legislation and policies in place permitting students to possess quick-relief inhalers and/or to receive support from school personnel in the storage and administration of the medication.[8] However, school district policies typically require completion of a written asthma care plan for school or standard forms and authorizing signatures of students' parents/guardians and physicians/healthcare providers.

Stakeholders in San Antonio, Texas, demonstrated that a uniform, citywide asthma action care plan can be developed and implemented successfully. In addition, to providing a standardized template, annual training was provided to school nurses to support implementation that addressed: symptom recognition, response to signs and symptoms, and use of inhalers. The uniform asthma action care plan was implemented in all 16 school districts with reports of improved asthma management at schools.[9] Colorado and Minnesota have implemented similar approaches.[10-12]

SCHOOL, FAMILY, AND PROVIDER COMMUNICATION AND COORDINATION

A major obstacle to successful asthma management in schools is poor communication among students, families, healthcare providers and schools. Surveys and interviews with school nurses, school personnel, parents, and healthcare providers identified communication as the largest challenge.[11-13] Most parents of students with asthma never speak to the school nurse and too often school nurses learn of a student's diagnosis of asthma when he/she presents to the office with asthma symptoms and informs the nurse of the diagnosis.[13] Although all parties recognize that students require individualized instructions and information to support asthma management at school, this is not happening.[11] School nurses also identified the lack of parental support and involvement as a significant barrier to successful management.[11] Often there is also role confusion and unclear policies and practices for managing asthma at schools that could be addressed through clearer communication by schools of existing policies and protocols. A completed asthma care plan for the school setting is an effective tool for communicating and coordinating asthma management strategies and role expectations. If asthma management for children and youth is going to improve, it is crucial that improvements in communication occur among these parties.

Currently, communication and coordination of care that is supported by electronic health records is challenging. However, efforts are being initiated to overcome the challenges of interoperability, data access issues, and privacy regulations. A pilot study targeted children with asthma who had been hospitalized for asthma to improve coordination of care between clinicians and schools through an electronic communication system.[14] The pilot study suggested that collaborative models of care supported by electronic communication platforms can lead to reductions in hospitalizations for asthma. It is important to note that this study was a prepost design with a small sample size, but it does support feasibility of these types of initiatives. A study in Minnesota developed and implemented a secure portal designed for the electronic exchange of an asthma action care plan between providers and schools. School nurses reported that this initiative resulted in more efficient asthma management and their improved self-confidence in managing an individual student with asthma.[12] These types of interventions deserve additional investigation.

PROGRAMS AND RESOURCES TO CREATE SUPPORTIVE AND ASTHMA FRIENDLY SCHOOLS

In recognition of the important role school settings play in successful control of asthma, several stakeholders and organizations have developed dedicated websites to support effective asthma care practices in schools. Box 13.1 provides a list of websites providing guidance and resources to support best practices for asthma management in schools. One example is the School-based Asthma Management Programs (SAMPRO) supported by the American Academy of Allergy, Asthma and Immunology, which provides a framework and toolkit for clinicians to assist with the coordination and communication among schools, children and youth with asthma, and their families and clinicians.[15] The program consists of four components: establishing a circle of support around the child with asthma, facilitating bidirectional communication between clinicians and schools, comprehensive asthma education for schools, and assessment and remediation of environmental triggers.

STEPS TO BE TAKEN BY CLINICIANS TO CREATE SUPPORTIVE AND ASTHMA FRIENDLY SCHOOLS

A review by Wheeler[16] noted that the number one lesson learned from the evaluation of school asthma programs was the need to establish strong links to the asthma care providers of students. Asthma management at schools is an important consideration for all clinicians caring for children and youth with asthma, including pediatricians, family care providers, nurse practitioners, physician assistants, pediatric pulmonologists and allergists, and their clinical teams. Asthma morbidity for children and youth can be significantly reduced through the coordinated efforts of asthma care providers, families, and schools. Asthma care providers play a vital role in preparing and supporting children and youth with asthma and their families to manage asthma at school as part of the overall goal of achieving successful asthma control. Busy clinicians have limited appointment time; thus, it is important to know which actions to take that will result in the biggest benefits. These key activities are described below.

Schedule a Summer Visit for Every Child/Youth With Asthma

As part of routine care, asthma care clinicians need to ensure that they see their asthma patients during the summer months (July and August) to prepare them for a successful start to the new school year. During this visit, several activities are necessary: (1) Assess the level of asthma control and provide counsel to maintain or regain control. (2) Assess and coach for accurate inhaler technique and review indications for medications. Quick-relief inhalers are needed at school to reverse asthma symptoms; however, about half of youth with asthma over the age of 12 years report feeling uncomfortable using their inhaler at school and almost one-third report not using the inhaler despite the experience of uncomfortable symptoms.[17] Stressing the importance of teaching and discussing the use of the inhaler at school is the relationship noted between youth feeling uncomfortable using their inhalers at school and having poorly controlled asthma. [17] (3) Provide prescriptions for quick-relief inhaled bronchodilators dedicated for school use. A common issue reported by parents, children/youth, school personnel, and school health teams is the lack of access to asthma inhalers because they are not brought to the school.[5,6,18] (4) Encourage families to share with the school that a student has asthma. A major barrier reported by school personnel is that they do not know which students have asthma. Clinicians should encourage parents/guardians, and if age appropriate, children/youth to inform their teachers and other school personnel that they are in close contact with that they have asthma. (5) Complete and review the school asthma care plan with the student and family. Most students with asthma report experiencing symptoms during physical activity at school, prompting students to initiate the self-care activities of sitting out the activity, visiting the school nurse, and/or drinking water.[19] Reasons reported by children and youth for not participating in physical activity include the lack of a school asthma care plan detailing asthma management steps for physical activity such as pretreatment, lack of accessible quick-relief inhalers, poor asthma control, and stigma associated with symptoms caused by physical activity.[19] And (6) if needed, request extra support from the school healthcare team for case management and care coordination for children/youth with poorly controlled asthma. Table 13.1 summarizes key steps for clinicians that are most effective in supporting successful asthma management in schools and are complimentary to best asthma care practices.[20,21]

Consider Exposures to Triggers in the School Setting

Exposure to triggers at school, similar to home exposure, is associated with increased asthma morbidity.[22] Therefore it is important to consider and assess exposure to triggers at school, especially for those experiencing poorly controlled asthma or difficult-to-control asthma. As an example, in the Inner City Asthma Study, exposure to mouse allergen was higher in schools than in homes and lead to increased asthma symptoms and decreased lung function.[22] Of interest is that the relationship between high levels of mouse antigen exposure at school and increased morbidity was seen in all children with asthma studied, regardless of whether

they were sensitized to mouse allergen, underscoring the relevance of school-associated allergen exposure as an important contributor to asthma morbidity in children. Other important school exposures include cockroach, pet dander, dust, and mold. It can be challenging to identify levels of exposure in schools for common allergens. Often schools do not have this type of indoor air quality information, because it is not a parameter routinely monitored. Talking to teachers and the child/youth about potential exposures is a good first step and then, if indicated, speaking to environmental services at the school and district level and the principal. The U.S. Environmental Protection Agency developed resources that are easily accessible through their websites, Creating Healthy Indoor Environments in Schools: Tools for Schools and Managing Asthma in the School Environment, with the aim of improving environmental conditions in schools (see Box 13.1). Commonly, strategies used in schools to reduce exposure to triggers are the same as those used in the home. Permaul and Phipatanakul[23] in Chapter 10, Environmental Assessment and Control, provide an informative and helpful review that addresses home and school settings. Schools may be important sources of direct allergen exposure and reservoirs that could potentially contribute to allergic sensitization and asthma and allergic exacerbation in children.

Engage With Your Local Schools

Clinicians and their interdisciplinary team members can make a difference to school settings by engaging with school health teams. Several studies demonstrate that the engagement of community clinicians and their teams can lead to improvements in asthma management and asthma outcomes, such as reduced absenteeism, urgent health services use, and improved asthma control.[5,15,24-28] Strategies that community healthcare providers can use to engage and support schools include the following:

1. Provide support and assistance of clinic staff, such as asthma counselors or educators, to perform case management and communication activities among children with asthma, their families and schools and to provide self-management asthma education to children/youth with asthma.[24-26]
2. Provide asthma education workshops and consultation to school settings and school personnel to address learning gaps. Deaths from asthma in schools may be attributed to delays in school personnel providing assistance.[27] Previous studies highlight inadequate asthma management practices in schools and asthma knowledge and skill gaps of school per-

TABLE 13.1
Checklist for Summer Back to School Follow-up Visit for Asthma

Action	Helpful Hint
Assess asthma control	It is essential that children/youth start back to school with controlled asthma. During the first few weeks of school, a spike in asthma exacerbations is commonly seen in children/youth, likely related to viral infections. This sets some children/youth with asthma for a vicious cycle of exacerbations throughout the winter months. Review the importance of regular inhaled corticosteroid use.
Provide quick-relief inhaler dedicated for school use	A second and sometimes a third inhaler is necessary for use at school to relieve or prevent exercise-induced asthma symptoms. If a child/youth experiences asthma symptoms and an inhaler is unavailable, a 9-1-1 call is often required, often representing a preventable cost to schools and/or parents. Some school-aged children may need two additional inhalers, one for the school office or classroom and another for self-carrying. Some athletes require a dedicated inhaler for their sports/athletic bag, in addition to the self-carry inhaler. Inhalers need to have the prescription label attached to the inhaler that clearly delineates the name of the student and the dosing schedule.
Assess and coach for accurate inhaler technique and review indications for quick-relief inhaler use at school	Children/youth should have their inhaler technique assessed and be coached for accurate technique so the full dose is delivered. Additionally, review indications for using reliever inhalers, such as in response to asthma symptoms, the prevention of exercise-induced asthma symptoms, and for control of trigger exposure. Schools represent a setting where many children/youth are initiating asthma self-care activities; therefore understanding the use of reliever inhalers is essential.
Encourage family to share with the school community that the student has asthma	If schools do not know the student has asthma, school personnel are unable to meet the student's needs. Explain the necessity and importance to the family in the case of an asthma emergency for recognizing and responding appropriately to the situation.
Complete and review with the family the school asthma care plan/action plan for use during school	The school asthma care plan/action plan serves as the order for the use of an inhaled reliever at school. Most school districts have their own form. However, in some jurisdictions there are standard forms that cross districts, and the SAMPRO website (see Box 13.1) provides forms for use at school and home. However, you will need to check with the school district to see what forms are permissible. School district forms can be found off of their websites. Some districts may not have a specific asthma form and the completion of a medication administration form will be necessary. Completion of this form should involve the child/youth and parent/guardian as it dictates how the inhaled reliever is to be used during school hours and activities. The form outlines when and how much of the inhaled reliever is to be used in response to symptoms for relief and to prevent symptoms (pretreat) in response to exposure to physical activity, cold weather, or other triggers. Typically, this form also permits communication about the child's health and asthma in school settings and among the healthcare provider, child/youth, and parents/guardians. Because the form serves as a medication order and release of information, signatures of both the physician/prescriber and parent/guardian are required.
If needed, request extra support for case management and care coordination for children/youth with poorly controlled asthma	If extra support is needed to assist a child/youth with poorly controlled or difficult to control asthma, a call to the school nurse should be made for consultation and to determine what additional services can be provided. For instance, for a student with chronically poorly controlled asthma, directly observed therapy of an inhaled corticosteroids may be considered.

sonnel.[5,28–32] School teachers report low levels of confidence, knowledge, and skills for recognizing and responding to worsening asthma, managing an asthma exacerbation, and the proper use of asthma medications.[5,17] Training school staff (administrators, secretaries, teachers, etc.) in the recognition of and appropriate response to worsening asthma and asthma medications led to improvements in asthma knowledge and practice.[28–32] School personnel are enthusiastic about receiving training about asthma in schools. Contact the school health nurse and offer to provide a 10-min overview of asthma for a school staff meeting or professional development day.

3. Serve as an asthma consultant to school nurses and school health teams. Although not evaluated through controlled studies, the availability of a consulting physician one half-day per week to work with school nurses noted improvements in the administration of quick-relief inhalers at school instead of home, which lead to reductions in the number of students leaving school or requiring a 9-1-1 call for urgent care thus keeping students engaged in school activities.[33,34]

SUMMARY

Second to their home, children and youth spend the largest portions of their day at school. The Centers for Disease Control,[35,36] professional organizations,[15,20,21] advocacy groups,[36] and multiple studies highlight the need for schools, youth with asthma and their families, and asthma care providers to work together to control asthma.[15,24–26,37,38] Schools absolutely need the involvement and cooperation of asthma clinicians to help students successfully manage their asthma. Efforts of asthma care clinicians and schools, individually and collectively, should address the medical, psychosocial, and educational needs of the child/youth. The synergy created by each party playing an active role in asthma management assists students and their families to achieve asthma control and to reduce associated morbidity. If asthma is well controlled, students will experience fewer school absences, be more productive, and be engaged in school.

REFERENCES

1. Hasegawa K, Tsugawa Y, Brown DF, Camargo CA Jr. Childhood asthma hospitalizations in the United States, 2000-2009. *J Pediatr.* 2013;163:1127–1133.e3.
2. Asthma and Allergy Foundation of America. Asthma Facts and Figures. http://www.aafa.org/display.cfm?id=9&sub=42.
3. Basch CE. Healthier students are better learners: a missing link in school reforms to close the achievement gap. *J Sch Health.* 2011;81:593–598.
4. Ruijsbroek A, Wijga AH, Gehring U, Kerkhof M, Droomers M. School performance: a matter of health or socioeconomic background? Findings from the PIAMA Birth Cohort Study. *PLoS One.* 2015;6:e0134780.
5. Cicutto L, Conti E, Evans H, et al. Creating asthma-friendly schools: a public health approach. *J Sch Health.* 2006;76:255–258.
6. Gerald JK, Stroupe N, McClure LA, et al. Availability of asthma quick relief medication in five Alabama School Systems. *Pediar Allergy Immunol Pulmonol.* 2012;25:11–16.
7. Taras H, Wright S, Brennan J, et al. Impact of school nurse case management on students with asthma. *J Sch Health.* 2004;74:213–219.
8. Jones SE, Wheeler L. Asthma inhalers in schools: rights of students with asthma to a free appropriate education. *Am J Public Health.* 2004;94:1102–1108.
9. Staudt AM, Alamgir H, Long DL, et al. Developing and implementing a citywide asthma action plan: a community collaborative partnership. *South Med J.* 2015;108:710–714.
10. Cicutto L, Shocks D, Gleason M, et al. Creating district readiness for implementing evidence-based school-centered asthma management programs: Denver Public Schools as a case study. *NASN Sch Nurse.* 2016;31:112–118.
11. Egginton JS, Textor L, Knoebel E, et al. Enhancing school asthma action plans: qualitative results from southeast Minnesota Beacon stakeholder groups. *J Sch Health.* 2013;83:885–895.
12. Hanson TK, Aleman M, Hart L, Yawn B. Increasing availability to and ascertaining value of asthma action plans in schools through use of technology and community collaboration. *J Sch Health.* 2013;83:915–920.
13. Liberatos P, Leone J, Craig AM, et al. Challenges of asthma management for school districts with high asthma hospitalization rates. *J Sch Health.* 2013;8:867–875.
14. Reeves KW, Taylor Y, Tapp H, et al. Evaluation of a pilot asthma care program for electronic communication between school health and healthcare system's electronic medical record. *Appl Clin Inform.* 2016;7:969–982.
15. Lemanske RF, Kakumanu S, Shanovich K, et al. Creation and implementation of SAMPRO™: a school-based asthma program. *J Allergy Clin Immunol.* 2016;138:711–723.
16. Wheeler L, Buckley R, Gerald L, et al. Working with school to improve pediatric asthma management. *Pediatr Asthma Allergy Immunol.* 2009;22:197–207.
17. Harris K, Mosler G, Williams SA, et al. Asthma control in London secondary school children. *J Asthma.* 2017;23:1–8.
18. Cain A, Reznik M. Asthma management in New York schools: a classroom teacher perspective. *J Asthma.* 2016;53:744–750.
19. Walker TJ, Reznik M. In-school asthma management and physical activity: children's perspectives. *J Asthma.* 2014;14:1–6.

20. *Global Initiative for Asthma Report. 2107 Global Strategy for Asthma Management and Prevention. 2017.* at http://ginasthma.org/2017-gina-report-global-strategy-for-asthma-management-and-prevention/.

21. National Institutes of Health. National Heart, Lung, Blood Institute. *National Asthma Education and Prevention Program. Expert Panel Report 3: Guidelines for the Diagnosis and Management of Asthma.* NIH Publication; August 2007. No. 07-4051 http://www.nhlbi.nih.gov/guidelines/asthma/index.htm.

22. Sheehan WJ, Permaul P, Petty CR, et al. Association between allergen exposure in inner-city schools and asthma morbidity among students. *JAMA Pediatr.* 2017;17:31–38.

23. Permaul P. and Phipatanakul W. [Chapter X]. Environmental Assessment and Control.

24. Liptzin DR, Gleason MC, Cicutto L, et al. Developing, implementing and evaluating a school-centered asthma program: step-Up Asthma Program. *J Allergy Clin Immunol Pract.* 2016;4:972–979.

25. Cicutto L, Gleason M, White M, et al. Building Bridges for Better Asthma Care: a program connecting schools, students with asthma and their health care providers for optimizing outcomes. *Am J Respir Crit Care Med.* 2014;189:A2453.

26. Cicutto L, Murphy S, Coutts D, et al. Breaking the access barrier: evaluating and asthma center's efforts to provide education to children with asthma in schools. *Chest.* 2005;128:1928–1935.

27. Greiling AK, Boss LP, Wheeler LS. A preliminary investigation of asthma mortality in schools. *J Sch Health.* 2005;75:286–290.

28. Cicutto L, To T, Murphy S. A randomized controlled trial of a public health nurse delivered asthma program to elementary schools. *J Sch Health.* 2013;83:876–884.

29. Eisenberg JD, Moe EL, Stillger CF. Educating school personnel about asthma. *J Asthma.* 1993;30:351–358.

30. Neuharth-Pritchett S, Getch YQ. Asthma and the school teacher: the status of teacher preparedness and training. *J Sch Nurse.* 2001;17:323–328.

31. Goei R, Boyson AR, Lyon-Callo SK, et al. Developing an asthma tool for schools: the formative evaluation of Michigan's asthma school packet. *J Sch Health.* 2006;76:259–263.

32. Keysser J, Splett PL, Ross S, et al. Statewide asthma training for Minnesota school personnel. *J Sch Health.* 2006;76:264–268.

33. Richmond CM, Sterling D, Huang X, et al. Asthma 411-addition of a consulting physician to enhance school health. *J Sch Health.* 2006;76:333–335.

34. Wilson KD, Moonie S, Sterling DA, et al. Examining the consulting physician model to enhance school nurse role for children with asthma. *J Sch Health.* 2009;79:1–7.

35. Centers for Disease Control. School and Childcare Providers. http://www.cdc.gov/asthma/schools.html.

36. Centers for Disease Control. Initiating Change: Creating an Asthma Friendly School. http://www.cdc.gov/HealthyYouth/asthma/creatingafs/. Accessed on April, 1 2017.

37. Coffman JM, Cabana MD, Yelin EH. Do school-based asthma education programs improve self-management and health outcomes? *Pediatrics.* 2009;124:729–742.

38. Al Aloola NA, Naik-Panvelkar P, Nissen L, et al. Asthma interventions in primary schools- a review. *J Asthma.* 2014;19:1–20.

CHAPTER 14

Systems Biology Approaches to Asthma Management

YASMEEN NKRUMAH-ELIE, PHD • MARC ELIE, PHD •
NICHOLE REISDORPH, PHD, MS

ABBREVIATIONS

BALF   Bronchoalveolar lavage fluid
CAAPA   Consortium on Asthma among African-ancestry Populations in the Americas
DNA   Deoxyribonucleic acid
EBC   Exhaled breath condensate
ELF   Epithelial lining fluid
FENO   Fractional exhaled nitric oxide
GWAS   Genome-wide association studies
HAT   Histone acetyl transferase
IgE   Immunoglobulin E
MeDALL   Mechanisms of the Development of ALLergy
mRNA   Messenger ribonucleic acid
MS   Mass spectrometry
NGS   Next-generation sequencing
NMR   Nuclear magnetic resonance
RANTES   Regulated on activation, normal T cell expressed and secreted
RNA   Ribonucleic acid
RNA-seq   RNA sequencing
Th2   Helper-inducer T-lymphocytes type 2
VOC   Volatile organic compounds

WHAT IS SYSTEMS BIOLOGY?

Systems biology is a scientific discipline that aims to elucidate the complex interactions of multiple components within a biologic system using various technologies and computational tools. This approach integrates information from a molecular level to a pathway level, from multiple organs to an organism, and eventually from individuals to entire populations.[1] Different components, which are themselves dynamic and/or temporal, contribute to the whole; hence, a holistic approach is required to elucidate the complexity of an entire biologic system. Each of these components may require a different approach to measure its contribution to a system; therefore, systems biology requires multiple

'omics technologies including genomics, epigenomics, transcriptomics, proteomics, and metabolomics. Additional disciplines including microbiome analysis, nutritional research, and pharmacogenomics may also be included. To provide a fully comprehensive analysis of health and disease, systems biology also takes into account clinical outcomes and measurements. Finally, bioinformatics and computational approaches are used to analyze individual datasets and to combine information from multiple sources.

In addition to understanding how a healthy system functions, this relatively new scientific discipline integrates information from advanced technologies with traditional clinical measures with the goal of more effectively treating disease. End goals include establishing molecular fingerprints and/or biomarkers to improve all aspects of clinical care; these include assessing disease susceptibility, developing prognostic indicators, predicting optimal treatments, and developing strategies for disease prevention.

SYSTEMS BIOLOGY APPROACHES ARE NECESSARY TO FULLY UNDERSTAND ASTHMA

One example of a complex system is the respiratory system, which includes multiple organs, cell types, and individual molecules that are influenced by both endogenous interactions and exogenous stimuli. The complexity of the respiratory system is emphasized when considering asthma, a multifaceted disease that can manifest with a variety of clinical symptoms or phenotypes. Several asthma phenotypes, which can be defined as the observable characteristics, exist. These include early-onset allergic, late-onset eosinophilic, obesity-related, exercised-induced, and neutrophilic asthma.[2] Understanding the biologic pathways and pathophysiologic mechanisms that result in phenotypic characteristics can be termed "endotyping." Several biomarkers attempting to distinguish between phenotypes and endotypes, and asthma in general, have been shown to be nonspecific, and new biomarkers and clinical indicators are needed. This highlights the multifactorial nature and overall complexity of asthma and emphasizes the need for a systems approach in developing new clinical tools. For example, diagnostic tools that can be used to classify asthma phenotypes or predict responsiveness to asthma therapy are sorely needed. However, to date, no single technology or approach has been successful in this regard. This review describes the various technologies available to conduct systems biology, offers examples where these technologies have been successful in understanding asthma, and addresses some future directions for applications of systems biology approaches to asthma diagnostic, mechanistic, and therapeutic research.

TOOLS THAT ARE AVAILABLE TO ASSIST RESEARCHERS IN APPLYING A SYSTEMS BIOLOGY APPROACH

The complexity and heterogeneity of asthma make both its clinical management and investigation challenging; therefore, a systems biology approach has the potential to model the myriad connections and interdependencies that ultimately lead to diverse disease phenotypes and treatment responses across individuals.[3] The increasing availability of high-throughput technologies has enabled global profiling of the genome, transcriptome, proteome, microbiome, and metabolome; these provide means for systems biology approaches to examine asthma at a more holistic level. The following paragraphs focus on 'omics tools that are currently being used to assist researchers in developing better diagnosis, monitoring, prevention, and treatment strategies for asthma. Furthermore, the huge potential of 'omics data integration strategies within the clinical context is described, as is its key role for the clinical actionability of 'omics-based biomarkers.

High-Throughput Sequencing Technologies

High-throughput sequencing, also known as next-generation sequencing (NGS), is the comprehensive term used to describe technologies that sequence DNA and RNA in a rapid and cost-effective manner. Sequencing methods differ primarily by how the DNA or RNA samples are obtained; for example, the methods will depend on the organism, tissue type, disease state, and experimental conditions. Methods for data analysis will also vary, allowing researchers to ask virtually any question related to the genome, transcriptome, or epigenome. The particular applications of this technology are described below.

Genomics

From the sequencing of the first human genome in 2001 to the completion of the Human Genome Project, genomic studies have reported the association of large numbers of candidate biomarkers to multiple diseases, including asthma. For example, several genes have been found to be significantly induced in asthmatics, including chemokine ligands (CCL8, CCL5, CCL11, and CCL24), SERPINs (SERPINB2, SERPINB4, and SERPINA1), and carboxypeptidaseA3. Genome-wide association studies (GWAS), which determine if associations exist between genotype and phenotype, enable the unbiased identification of genetic loci for asthma. GWAS has been used to discover several chromosomal regions that are linked to asthma phenotype; for example, a nucleotide substitution in the promoter region of IL-4 receptor; IL-13; HLA-II alleles; regulated on activation, normal T cell expressed and Secreted (RANTES); and CC-chemokine ligands were found to be strongly associated with asthma.[4,5] Although more work is needed, genomics is poised to become the first NGS-based technology to be introduced into the clinic.

Epigenomics

Epigenomics is addressing the gaps in our understanding of the complex interaction between genes and the environment and how they contribute to asthma pathogenesis. Chemical modifications, including methylation and acetylation, of DNA, histones, nonhistone chromatin proteins, and nuclear RNA define the epigenome. Modifications can be due to environmental exposures, such as pollution or cigarette smoke, and affect gene expression without altering the base sequence.[6] For example, it has been found that reduced histone deacetylase activity and increased histone acetyl transferase (HAT) activity jointly promote the expression of multiple inflammatory genes associated with asthma; however, inhaled steroids reduce HAT activity to the normal level.[7] External stimuli such as allergen exposure, cigarette smoke, traffic exhaust, and folate-rich diet cause methylation-mediated silencing of genes such as IFNγ, Fox-P3, IL-2, iNOS; conversely, these cause hypomethylation-mediated activation of genes including IL-6, IL-4, IL-8, and acylCoA. The latter causes an overall increase in the so-called helper-inducer T-lymphocytes type 2 (Th2) phenotype.[8] The study of such epigenetic changes complements genome-wide and transcriptomic approaches for studying disease, because it can characterize DNA sequence–independent modification contributing to transcriptomic variation and downstream phenotype. Overall, epigenomic studies provide a potential mechanistic bridge between environmental exposures and the development of asthma.

Transcriptomics

Transcriptomics comprises the quantitation of RNA species such as messenger RNAs (mRNA), noncoding RNAs, and small RNAs. Using one type of this technology, namely microarrays, it is possible to detect variations in expression of many, but not all, transcribed genes under both normal and perturbed conditions. For example, transcriptomics has confirmed the presence of distinct subsets of mild/moderate asthmatic patients on the basis of their expression of Th2 cytokines; it has further shown that gene expression profiles in airway epithelial cells can be used to predict drug responsiveness.[9] As an alternative to microarray technologies, RNA sequencing (RNA-seq) is considered unbiased, because it does not rely on a set of predefined probes selected for the array chip and covers the whole transcriptome, enabling the discovery of novel exons, isoforms, and even previously undetected transcripts.[10] In asthma, RNA-seq profiles of lower and upper airway biospecimens distinguish subjects with the disease from those without asthma. A comparison of RNA-seq profiles of endobronchial biopsies from steroid-free atopic asthma patients and healthy nonatopic controls demonstrated 46 differentially expressed genes, including SLC26A4, POSTN, and BCL2.[10] RNA-seq profiles of nasal brushings from 10 asthma and 10 control subjects showed that nasal airway gene expression profiles can identify subjects with asthma driven by IL-33, which was previously implicated in GWAS of asthma.[3]

Regardless of the platform used, genetic-based studies have shown that the 17q21 gene locus, which encompasses *ORMDL3*, *GSDMB*, *ZPBP2*, and *IKZF3*, is associated with asthma,[3] although it does not explain the full genetic risk for asthma. Single nucleotide polymorphisms to 17q12-21 IKZF3-ZPBP2-GSDMB-ORMDL3 region have been identified and validated in several studies as strong genetic markers for childhood-onset asthma, particularly in Caucasian children.[11] It seems that the contribution of genotype to effectiveness of drug response is more prominent in children than in adults.[12] ADRB2, the gene that encodes the β2-adrenergic receptor is one of the most studied genes in drug response.[12] Adverse events, including hospital admissions, during long-acting β-agonist therapy in African Americans, non-Hispanic whites, and Puerto Ricans, have been associated with Ile164 and Ile376 rare variants of ADRB2.[13]

Mass Spectrometry-Based 'Omics

Mass spectrometry (MS) measures the mass-to-charge ratios (m/z) of molecules, including proteins, peptides, and several classes of small molecules. MS analysis can be semiquantitative in an untargeted fashion using high-resolution MS instruments or quantitative through targeted analysis using tandem MS. MS-based 'omics include proteomics and metabolomics, both of which have been applied to the study of asthma.[14,15]

Proteomics

The proteome consists of all the proteins expressed by a biologic system; these include both modified and unmodified proteins. Proteomics biomarker discovery has been applied to a variety of clinical sample types that contain protein, including induced sputum, exhaled breath condensate (EBC), epithelial lining fluid (ELF), bronchoalveolar lavage fluid (BALF), plasma, and serum. Proteomic approaches have been widely used to identify the expression level and modification of proteins toward improved understanding of the pathophysiology of asthma. For example, S100A8 and S100A9 (singularly and as a ratio), albumin, cytokeratins, actin, complement C, hemoglobin, and α2-macroglobulin are protein biomarkers associated with asthma that have been identified in multiple studies and/or multiple biofluids.[15] Overall, clinical proteomics for the purpose of biomarker discovery faces several challenges, including depth of coverage, cost, and standardized sampling techniques. However, given that proteins are the functional units of genes, understanding the role of proteins in asthma is an essential component to a systems biology approach.

Metabolomics

Metabolomics has been shown to be a valuable tool for the discovery of biomarkers and for the elucidation of complex mechanisms in several complex diseases, including asthma.[14,16] Metabolomics is a growing field that includes lipidomics, metabolic measurements, nutritional markers, metabolite profiling, and targeted analyses. Metabolomics can be conducted using both MS-based and nuclear magnetic resonance (NMR)-based platforms; however, because of the relatively lower sensitivity of NMR, MS-based platforms have become increasingly adopted by clinical and research laboratories. Several disease biomarkers have been discovered using this important systems biology tool. For example, amino acid metabolism, hypoxia response pathways, immune and inflammatory pathways, lipid metabolism, oxidative stress, and tricarboxylic acid cycle have been found to be significantly changed in more than one clinical asthma metabolomics study.[17] Finally, individual small molecules, such as leukotrienes, have been found in various associations with disease, including severity and ability to predict response to medication.[18]

Other Technologies

Other technologies that are being applied to studying asthma include microbiome research, MS-based imaging of tissues and biofilms, analysis of breath volatiles, and exposomics.[16,19] For example, in young children, a change in the intestinal microbial flora may precede the symptomatic development of allergic disease.[20] Furthermore, the diversity of the airway microbiome of asthmatics is increased and more heavily populated by *Proteobacteria* when compared with nonasthmatics.[20] Additional information on the impact of the microbiome on asthma phenotypes and diagnostics is presented in Chapter 16, Preventing the Development of Asthma: Early Intervention Strategies in Children. Breath-based diagnostics are based on the noninvasive measurement and profile of EBC, which contains a complex gas mixture of volatile organic compounds and a composite of nonvolatile compounds; these may be easily perturbed by inflammatory lung diseases such as asthma.[21] Imaging MS is an invaluable tool for visualizing the cellular and subcellular distribution and metabolism of asthma drug and drug metabolites, as well as the localization of endogenous protein, peptide, and lipid biomarkers.[22] Together, these data can aid in identifying the tissue compartments involved in drug uptake, transfer, and metabolism. Finally, recent efforts have focused on measuring the contribution of various environmental and diet-related effects on lung health; this is termed the "exposome." Although still nascent fields, the benefits of these approaches to an overall clinical understanding of asthma are readily apparent.

Bioinformatics

One defining feature of the systems biology approach is the plethora of data resulting from the different sources of technologies and clinical metadata. Such complexity arises from the diversity of biological components (genes, proteins, mRNA, and metabolites), the high selectivity of molecular interactions, and a nonlinear nature of these interactions. Therefore, it is not surprising that the need for mathematical and computational models for effective integration of quantitative omics measurements and the demand to handle increasingly large amounts of biologic data have prompted the use of bioinformatics. Bioinformatics comprises the storage, retrieval, and analysis of biomedical information and omics datasets; furthermore, it suggests optimal strategies for deciphering this information through statistics and visualization.[23] Bioinformatics is essential to understand the complexity of biologic systems; however, the development and application of such tools for systems biology is a significant challenge. Examples of such difficulties include the sophisticated data processing and analysis required for omics data, the slow development and population of data repositories, and challenges in developing simulation software to aid in visualization of biochemical networks. In spite of challenges, large-scale system biology studies, such as MeDALL (Mechanisms of the Development of ALLergy), are making significant strides in establishing the bioinformatics infrastructure necessary to integrate and understand multidimensional datasets to better understand the mechanisms of asthma.[9]

HOW CAN SYSTEMS BIOLOGY HELP US UNDERSTAND TREATMENT OPTIONS AND EFFICACY?

While progress has been made in effectively diagnosing and treating asthma using clinical measurements, more remains to be done. To date, no clear clinical biomarkers have been found that effectively distinguish between asthma subtypes; furthermore, the use of such markers in the clinic has proven difficult. For example, high serum immunoglobulin E (IgE) is effective in diagnosing only atopic asthma. Sputum eosinophil levels, although effective in identifying airway inflammation, can be difficult to collect from children in a clinical setting. Serum periostin, a protein involved in subepithelial fibrosis, has potential as a clinical biomarker for asthma; however, it may have low diagnostic value for some asthma phenotypes.[24] All told, these examples emphasize the need for integrative 'omic studies, i.e., systems biology, that provide panels of biomarkers that tell a more complete story of an individual's condition.

Systems biology research explores high-dimensional interactions to obtain a comprehensive understanding of complex molecular interactions[3]; this in turn gives rise to the development of systems medicine, the application of systems biology discoveries in the clinical setting.[25] Although several translational research discoveries have resulted from individual and integrative 'omics studies, application in the clinical setting has not yet been employed. For example, metabolomics research has identified leukotriene E4 levels as a possible urinary biomarker of childhood asthma[26]; when combined with levels of impulse oscillometry reactance area, this marker can distinguish treatment responses in children with uncontrolled asthma.[18] McGeachie and colleagues utilized a systems biology approach by combining plasma lipidomics, genotyping, gene expression, and methylation data as analyzed by a Conditional Gaussian Bayesian Network to identify four single-nucleotide polymorphisms (rs9522789, rs7147228, rs2701423, rs759582) and two metabolites (monoHETE_0863 and sphingosine-1-phosphate) that predicted asthma control by short-acting β-agonists with 95% accuracy (n = 20).[27] However, neither of these have been translated into a clinical test.

This gap between discovery and clinical translation is due to a variety of factors; challenges include studies lacking the necessary statistical power to adequately demonstrate their results, replicating results in different cohorts, and funding limitations preventing validation in multiple cohorts. For example, it has become apparent that the genetic factors that result in adult-onset asthma differ from those of childhood-onset asthma.[2] There are also likely genetic contributions to asthma that differ in various racial groups, and thus many of the discoveries of genetic markers of asthma in those with primarily European ancestry often do not translate to individuals of other races. This is especially highlighted in the Consortium on Asthma among African-ancestry Populations in the Americas (CAAPA) project, which found extensive ancestry-related biases in precision genomic medicine when applied to asthmatic populations.[28] This is a huge disservice, because globally, whites only represent about 16% of the global population, and asthma burden is now more prominent in low- to middle-income countries, which are often dominated by people of color.[29]

In spite of challenges, several significant discoveries have been validated in multiple cohorts and different biofluids, and have helped propel asthma research forward (Table 14.1). Although many studies have utilized a single or even dual 'omics approach, very few asthma studies have employed a complete systems biology approach. The resources required to complete such high dimensionality studies make them unfeasible for single laboratories; however, through multiple collaborations, such studies have become possible. The US-based National Heart, Lung, and Blood Institute's AsthmaNet is a clinical consortium developed to execute clinical asthma studies aimed to improve asthma management and develop effective asthma treatments.[30] Within the AsthmaNet network, clinical sites are collecting samples from both child and adult asthmatics with one possible goal of performing longitudinal, 'omics-based studies.

Although many of the studies are still in progress, one study has demonstrated that in young children requiring Step 2 asthma therapy, the best response to daily inhaled corticosteroid therapy was observed in children with aeroallergen sensitization and high blood eosinophil counts.[31]

The MeDALL study provided a true systems biology approach to studying asthma and allergies in a European population.[25] This longitudinal study included 44,000 participants from 14 cohorts throughout Europe; participants were evaluated from birth to age 20 years. Blood samples provided longitudinal data for GWAS, epigenomics, transcriptomics, proteomics, IgE, and microarray data; estimates of ambient air pollution exposure in 10,000 of the participants were also included. Results of the study identified exposure to nitrogen dioxide and fine particulate matter early in life as risk factors for developing asthma. Low levels of club cell secretory protein16 was found to be a predictor of poor forced expiratory volume 1 (FEV1). Finally, consistent and substantial impacts of maternal smoking on offspring's DNA methylome was discovered. One deliverable was the development of the "MeDALL allergen-chip," a combination of 170 allergen molecules noted to have higher sensitivity than the traditional Immuno-CAP, for use in allergic asthma diagnosis. The study was effective in the application of systems biology for biomarker discovery and development of models that ruled out asthma development, although the goal of developing models to predict asthma was not successful.[25]

CURRENT LIMITATIONS AND FUTURE PROJECTIONS FOR USING A SYSTEMS BIOLOGY APPROACH IN ASTHMA RESEARCH AND CLINICAL CARE

To date, no tool exists that can distinguish between the myriad of asthmatic phenotypes and endotypes, highlighting the multifactorial nature and overall complexity of asthma and emphasizing the need for not only multiplex tests but also multiple platforms of discovery. In spite of a large number of studies, in fact, very few biomarkers from any of the 'omics technologies have moved from discovery to clinical applications.[32] Limitations of the various technologies include a need for optimization and standardization of methods for clinical sample collection, storage, and preparation of samples including unique respiratory fluids such as BALF, EBC, ELF, and induced sputum. Analytical standardization will also help to increase biomarker discovery reproducibility and robustness; this will push the movement toward systems medicine into clinical

TABLE 14.1

Summary of Recent Significant Discoveries Validated in Multiple Cohorts or Different Biofluids Using Systems Biology Approaches for Clinical Asthma

Author and Year	Study Purpose	Study Population	Omics Platform Used	Sample Source	Results and Knowledge Gained
Moffat[5]	Genome-wide association study by genotyping persons with physician-diagnosed asthma and unaffected persons, all of whom were matched for ancestry	Asthma patients (n = 10,365) vs. healthy control individuals (n = 16,110) (patients were European or of European descent and were recruited from 23 different studies)	Genome-wide association studies (GWAS)	Whole blood DNA	Associations were observed between asthma and six SNPs, implicating IL1RL1/IL18R1, HLA-DQ, IL-33, SMAD3, IL2RB in the entire population and ORMDL3/GSDMB only in those with childhood onset of asthma. Elevation of total serum IgE levels has a minor role in the development of asthma
Mc-Geachie[27]	Identify novel predictors of asthma control	Stable asthmatics (n = 20)	Metabolomics	Plasma	Altered sphingolipid metabolism represents an underlying feature of both asthma control and cellular response to albuterol (bronchodilator). Lipid mediators play an important role in airway inflammation and asthma
Woodruff[9]	Determine whether the heterogeneity of asthma reflects heterogeneity in underlying molecular mechanisms related to Th2 inflammation	Patients with mild-to-moderate asthma (n = 42) vs. healthy control subjects (n = 28)	Transcriptomics (microarray)	Basal cells (airway epithelial brushings)	Asthma can be divided into at least two distinct molecular phenotypes defined by degree of Th2 inflammation. Therapies targeting Th2 cytokines may be effective in only a subset of patients with asthma. Non–Th2-driven asthma represents a significant proportion of patients and responds poorly to current therapies
Breton[6]	Examine the epigenome as a potential mechanistic bridge between environmental exposures and the development of asthma	Children aged 5–12 years with asthma (n = 527)	Epigenomics	Whole blood DNA	Screening loci for differential methylation related to prenatal smoke exposure, adjusting for gender, age, and clinical site. Prenatal smoke exposure was associated with methylation at 19 CpG loci, demonstrating that prenatal tobacco exposure may be associated with epigenetic changes that persist into childhood

TABLE 14.1
Summary of Recent Significant Discoveries Validated in Multiple Cohorts or Different Biofluids Using Systems Biology Approaches for Clinical Asthma—cont'd

Author and Year	Study Purpose	Study Population	Omics Platform Used	Sample Source	Results and Knowledge Gained
Smolinska[16]	Metabolomic profile of asthma vs. transient wheeze	Asthma (n = 343) vs. healthy (185) and transient wheezers (n = 546)	Breath-based diagnostics	Exhaled breath condensate	PLS-DA model based on 17 volatile organic compounds (VOCs) distinguished asthmatic children from transient wheezers with a prediction rate of 80%. VOCs in the exhaled breath predict the subsequent development of asthma that might guide early treatment
Bousquet[25]	Assess antiinflammatory club cell secretory protein (CC16) levels in airways between asthma and healthy patients	Control patients without asthma (n = 19), patients with nonrefractory asthma (n = 28), and patients with refractory asthma (n = 52)	Proteomics	Bronchoalveolar lavage (BAL)	Low serum levels of CC16 have been previously associated with an accelerated FEV1 decline. Significant CC16 deficits are present in the airways of patients with asthma and suggest that reduced lung CC16 expression or decreased CC16-producing epithelial cells may be responsible
Marri[19]	Differences in microbial composition of asthmatic vs. nonasthmatic subjects	Nonasthmatic subject (n = 10) vs. patients with mild active asthma (n = 10) not using inhaled corticosteroids	Microbiome	Sputum	Samples from asthmatic patients had greater bacterial diversity compared with samples from nonasthmatic subjects. Proteobacteria were present in higher proportions in asthmatic patients

FEV1, forced expiratory volume 1; *IgE*, immunoglobulin E; *SNP*, single-nucleotide polymorphism.

trials and application. Additional challenges include limited sample sizes and lack of validation cohorts. Exploratory 'omics studies are often ancillary to larger clinical trials that focus on specific phenotypic or mechanistic questions or on response to medication. This necessarily biases an after-the-fact study toward the original question being asked and, because sample numbers are often limited, does not enable the exploration of broader questions. Conservative standardized approaches in bioinformatics and statistics are also necessary as there is extensive variability into what is scientifically and clinically significant. This will propel the next step in the development and validation of networks that can combine all of the 'omics and microbiome data into true systems biology models.

One of the major limitations in existing systems biology and clinical asthma research is the lack of repeated measures to address the potential circadian and longitudinal manifestations of asthma and its associated biomarkers. Dopico et al. demonstrated the seasonal and geographic variation in the immune system gene expression and blood cellular composition[33] The Airways Disease Endotyping for Personalized Therapeutics study conducted on adults with mild, moderate, and severe asthma discovered significant individual longitudinal variation in bronchodilator reversibility, responses to the asthma control questionnaire, fractional exhaled nitric oxide (FENO) in the FENO-high (≥35 ppb) phenotype, and sputum phenotype markers over 12 months.[34] These variations may have resulted from seasonal allergen exposure, resulting in an increase in Th2 inflammation, viral infections and other illnesses, diet, medication changes, treatment compliance, and other environmental factors. Even within 24 h, significant nondiurnal variation in blood eosinophil counts has been seen in mild and moderate asthmatics,[35] whereas diurnal FeNO variation is significantly more extensive in uncontrolled asthmatics versus controlled asthmatics.[36] It will be valuable for future studies to employ intraday and longitudinal sampling points to address intraindividual variation, seasonal and environmental influences, diurnal differences, medication influences, and comorbidities of the measurable levels of existing and novel asthma biomarkers. Additionally, standardization will be required to determine normality of within-subject and population variability as these biomarkers are validated.

Another challenge in systems biology research is the predominance of European/white-based data in clinical databases from genetic analysis to metabolomics. European genetics are more homogenous than that of African genetics, for example, and thus do not provide an ample model for all people because they are biased toward European ancestry.[28] Future 'omics studies and movements toward personalized medicine will need to take into account these Eurocentric database limitations and move toward global sampling to improve the implementation of systems biology analysis for all asthmatics, regardless of ancestry and geography.

A challenge that will need to be addressed, as new biomarkers and clinical methods are developed and validated, is that of the need for clinics to have specialized instruments and training of its personnel, because this is already proving to be a challenge for some diagnostic tests in clinics. For example, the diagnostic utilization of sputum induction, to decipher some asthma endotypes, is only conducted at specialized medical centers, because it is considered technically complex and variable.[37] Similarly, urinary leukotriene E4 has been shown to be higher in asthmatics and may predict tobacco smoke and environmentally induced exacerbations,[38] although it is speculated that its lack of widespread applications in clinical settings may be due to analysis instrument costs and technical requirements. As developments are made, effective strategies to improve costs, ease of applicability, and standardization for Good Laboratory Practice requirements will need to be addressed.

The movement toward improved systems biology studies for applications of systems medicine can potentially be modeled after the AsthmaNet, CAAPA, and MeDALL strategies. These studies serve as a platform for the future of asthma research, clinical diagnosis, and treatment. These and similar strategies have higher probabilities of success because of several factors: they focus on broad and specific populations, they use technology to answer specific questions, they are working to discover specific biomarker signatures of various phenotypes and endotypes, and they have strong informatics components. Overall, technologic advances in every area from data collection and analysis to communication and project management is helping to move asthma from a disease of unknowns to a curable or preventable condition. They will also help to identify poor responders and reveal complex pathways in the various endotypes. As technologies mature and research progresses, systems approaches promise to provide truly personalized medicine to asthmatics. An example of this is illustrated in Fig. 14.1, where a variety of sample types are interrogated using several technologic platforms. In one fictitious example, blood is used to perform genomics, which results in information regarding phenotype and adverse responses to medication. Small molecules are measured in plasma and EBC to further narrow down a phenotype and to determine disease severity. Other plasma protein and metabolite markers, in combination with microbiome analysis, are used to predict an individual's response to medication. Overall, a personalized approach to medicine will first require a systems approach to research.

SUMMARY AND FUTURE DIRECTIONS

As illustrated below, future diagnostics may include a combination of tests to create the final diagnosis and treatment plan. Additionally, personally collected data such as activity levels, dietary intake, sleep patterns, and other personalized health monitoring on smart phones and other mobile devices will contribute to diagnosis and monitoring of disease status. Hospital and doctor visits only provide single data points on the temporal pathology of asthma. Phenotypes may become apparent when clinical data are combined with personalized monitoring and environmental assessments. Asthma diagnosis and treatment will no longer be based on averages, but rather on true personalized medicine.

Through the extensive data collected, bioinformatics will reveal networks that combine genomic, proteomic, metabolomic, and microbiome discoveries. These systems biology networks will not only provide models for understanding mechanisms of asthma phenotypes but can also be used to improve diagnosis and develop new therapeutic targets. They will propel the development of improved diagnostic testing and help scientists

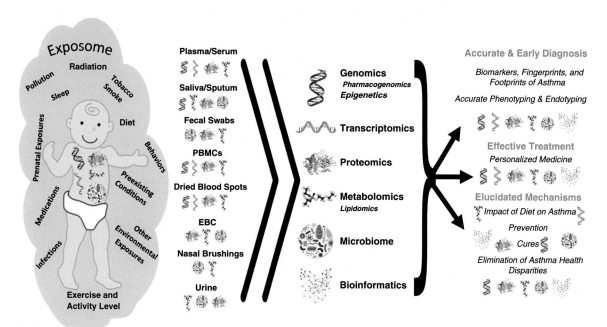

FIG. 14.1 How a systems biology approach to asthma research can result in improved diagnostics, treatments, and mechanistic elucidation. An individual is exposed to many external stimuli (i.e., exposome) that can have direct and indirect effects on health. A variety of biospecimens can reflect, for example pollutant exposure, through changes in DNA methylation or in levels of small molecules. These changes can be measured through a variety of technologies, including genomics, proteomics, metabolomics, and microbiome analysis. Information from each of these areas can be combined using bioinformatics to determine an overall effect of external stimuli on molecular pathways and networks; this in turn can be used to understand the pathogenesis of disease and how individuals respond to treatment. The end result is improved and personalized diagnostics and treatment strategies for individuals suffering from asthma.

to figure out which questions we need to ask to best treat each patient, and how can we improve our technology to employ efficient systems biology analysis at the individual patient level. These discoveries will also aid in prevention and ultimately in curing asthma. With the advancement of technologies, including instrumentation, software, and computational strategies, there is high potential for success, and in the near future, we expect to see several novel diagnostic approaches for asthma.

REFERENCES

1. Thamrin C, Frey U, Kaminsky DA, et al. Systems biology and clinical practice in respiratory medicine. The Twain Shall meet. *Am J Respir Crit Care Med.* 2016;194(9):1053–1061.
2. Wenzel SE. Asthma phenotypes: the evolution from clinical to molecular approaches. *Nat Med.* 2012;18(5):716–725.
3. Bunyavanich S, Schadt EE. Systems biology of asthma and allergic diseases: a multiscale approach. *J Allergy Clin Immunol.* 2015;135(1):31–42.
4. Toda M, Ono SJ. Genomics and proteomics of allergic disease. *Immunology.* 2002;106(1):1–10.
5. Moffatt MF, Gut IG, Demenais F, et al. A large-scale, consortium-based genomewide association study of asthma. *N Engl J Med.* 2010;363(13):1211–1221.
6. Breton CV, Siegmund KD, Joubert BR, et al. Prenatal tobacco smoke exposure is associated with childhood DNA CpG methylation. *PLoS One.* 2014;9(6):e99716.
7. Ito K, Caramori G, Lim S, et al. Expression and activity of histone deacetylases in human asthmatic airways. *Am J Respir Crit Care Med.* 2002;166(3):392–396.
8. Durham AL, Wiegman C, Adcock IM. Epigenetics of asthma. *Biochim Biophys Acta.* 2011;1810(11):1103–1109.
9. Woodruff PG, Modrek B, Choy DF, et al. T-helper type 2-driven inflammation defines major subphenotypes of asthma. *Am J Respir Crit Care Med.* 2009;180(5):388–395.
10. Wang Z, Gerstein M, Snyder M. RNA-Seq: a revolutionary tool for transcriptomics. *Nat Rev Genet.* 2009;10(1): 57–63.
11. Dijk FN, de Jongste JC, Postma DS, Koppelman GH. Genetics of onset of asthma. *Curr Opin Allergy Clin Immunol.* 2013;13(2):193–202.

12. Davis JS, Weiss ST, Tantisira KG. Asthma pharmacogenomics: 2015 update. *Curr Allergy Asthma Rep.* 2015;15(7):42.

13. Ortega VE. Pharmacogenetics of beta2 adrenergic receptor agonists in asthma management. *Clin Genet.* 2014;86(1):12–20.

14. Reisdorph N, Wechsler ME. Utilizing metabolomics to distinguish asthma phenotypes: strategies and clinical implications. *Allergy.* 2013;68(8):959–962.

15. Terracciano R, Pelaia G, Preiano M, Savino R. Asthma and COPD proteomics: current approaches and future directions. *Proteomics Clin Appl.* 2015;9(1–2):203–220.

16. Smolinska A, Klaassen EM, Dallinga JW, et al. Profiling of volatile organic compounds in exhaled breath as a strategy to find early predictive signatures of asthma in children. *PLoS One.* 2014;9(4):e95668.

17. Kelly RS, Dahlin A, McGeachie MJ, et al. Asthma metabolomics and the potential for integrative omics in research and the clinic. *Chest.* 2017;151(2):262–277.

18. Rabinovitch N, Mauger DT, Reisdorph N, et al. Predictors of asthma control and lung function responsiveness to step 3 therapy in children with uncontrolled asthma. *J Allergy Clin Immunol.* 2014;133(2):350–356.

19. Marri PR, Stern DA, Wright AL, Billheimer D, Martinez FD. Asthma-associated differences in microbial composition of induced sputum. *J Allergy Clin Immunol.* 2013;131(2):346–352. e341–e343.

20. Noval Rivas M, Crother TR, Arditi M. The microbiome in asthma. *Curr Opin Pediatr.* 2016;28(6):764–771.

21. Horvath I, Hunt J, Barnes PJ, et al. Exhaled breath condensate: methodological recommendations and unresolved questions. *Eur Respir J.* 2005;26(3):523–548.

22. Nilsson A, Fehniger TE, Gustavsson L, et al. Fine mapping the spatial distribution and concentration of unlabeled drugs within tissue micro-compartments using imaging mass spectrometry. *PLoS One.* 2010;5(7):e11411.

23. Bernstam EV, Smith JW, Johnson TR. What is biomedical informatics? *J Biomed Inf.* 2010;43(1):104–110.

24. Wagener AH, de Nijs SB, Lutter R, et al. External validation of blood eosinophils, FENO and serum periostin as surrogates for sputum eosinophils in asthma. *Thorax.* 2015;70(2):115–120.

25. Bousquet J, Anto JM, Akdis M, et al. Paving the way of systems biology and precision medicine in allergic diseases: the MeDALL success story: mechanisms of the development of allergy; EU FP7-CP-IP; Project No: 261357; 2010-2015. *Allergy.* 2016;71(11):1513–1525.

26. Armstrong M, Liu AH, Harbeck R, Reisdorph R, Rabinovitch N, Reisdorph N. Leukotriene-E4 in human urine: comparison of on-line purification and liquid chromatography-tandem mass spectrometry to affinity purification followed by enzyme immunoassay. *J Chromatogr B Anal Technol Biomed Life Sci.* 2009;877(27):3169–3174.

27. McGeachie MJ, Dahlin A, Qiu W, et al. The metabolomics of asthma control: a promising link between genetics and disease. *Immun Inflamm Dis.* 2015;3(3):224–238.

28. Kessler MD, Yerges-Armstrong L, Taub MA, et al. Challenges and disparities in the application of personalized genomic medicine to populations with African ancestry. *Nat Commun.* 2016;7:12521.

29. Network GA. *Global asthma report 2014* Global burden of disease due to asthma. 2016.

30. Sutherland ER, Busse WW, National Heart L, Blood Institute's A. Designing clinical trials to address the needs of childhood and adult asthma: the National Heart, Lung, and Blood Institute's AsthmaNet. *J Allergy Clin Immunol.* 2014;133(1):34–38.e31.

31. Fitzpatrick AM, Jackson DJ, Mauger DT, et al. Individualized therapy for persistent asthma in young children. *J Allergy Clin Immunol.* 2016;138(6):1608–1618.e1612.

32. Teran LM, Montes-Vizuet R, Li X, Franz T. Respiratory proteomics: from descriptive studies to personalized medicine. *J Proteome Res.* 2014;14(1):38–50.

33. Dopico XC, Evangelou M, Ferreira RC, et al. Widespread seasonal gene expression reveals annual differences in human immunity and physiology. *Nat Commun.* 2015;6:7000.

34. Silkoff PE, Laviolette M, Singh D, et al. Longitudinal stability of asthma characteristics and biomarkers from the airways disease endotyping for personalized therapeutics (ADEPT) study. *Respir Res.* 2016;17:43.

35. Spector SL, Tan RA. Is a single blood eosinophil count a reliable marker for "eosinophilic asthma?". *J Asthma.* 2012;49(8):807–810.

36. Saito J, Gibeon D, Macedo P, Menzies-Gow A, Bhavsar PK, Chung KF. Domiciliary diurnal variation of exhaled nitric oxide fraction for asthma control. *Eur Respir J.* 2014;43(2):474–484.

37. Vijverberg SJ, Hilvering B, Raaijmakers JA, Lammers JW, Maitland-van der Zee AH, Koenderman L. Clinical utility of asthma biomarkers: from bench to bedside. *Biologics.* 2013;7:199–210.

38. Rabinovitch N, Reisdorph N, Silveira L, Gelfand EW. Urinary leukotriene E(4) levels identify children with tobacco smoke exposure at risk for asthma exacerbation. *J Allergy Clin Immunol.* 2011;128(2):323–327.

The Microbiome in Asthma: Potential Impact on Phenotype and Medication Response

YVONNE J. HUANG, MD

ABBREVIATIONS

CF   Cystic fibrosis
COPD   Chronic obstructive pulmonary disease
FEV1   Forced expiratory volume in 1 s
ICS   Inhaled corticosteroid
IL-13   Interleukin-13
rRNA   Ribosomal RNA
SCFA   Short-chain fatty acids
Th2   T-helper type 2

WHAT IS THE MICROBIOME?

Human-associated microbes exist as consortia of mixed-species communities—inclusive of bacteria, archaea, fungi, and viruses—that colonize mucosal surfaces and the skin.[1] Patterns of microbial colonization are niche-specific, and thus the microbial burden and types of *microbiota* found in different organ systems and anatomic locations vary greatly.[1] Collectively, however, the genomic content and therefore functional potential of our microbiota are many orders of magnitude greater than that encoded by human genes. Thus microbiota confer a vast array of functions to human hosts, many of which are important for human survival and defense.[2,3] Mutualistic interactions between microbiota and hosts have coevolved over millennia, resulting in effects that can be beneficial or detrimental to the host. The human body therefore can be viewed as a complex ecosystem, wherein microbes and their functional interactions within a given niche ("microbiome") represent distinct anatomic habitats.[4]

Tremendous knowledge about microbial ecologic interactions within humans has been gleaned from studies of the intestinal microbiome. Insights into microbial properties and mechanisms by which innate and adaptive immune responses are molded or become dysregulated within the gut have significantly advanced the understanding of the pathogenesis of inflammatory bowel disease and other conditions.[3,5] This knowledge includes a new extensive understanding of how microbial-host interactions within the gut, especially in early life, shape maturation of the immune system and the consequence of particular immune phenotypes impacting susceptibility to allergic diseases. Investigations of the gut microbiome in this context represent the mechanistic arm of research related to the "hygiene hypothesis," which originated in epidemiologic findings of birth order and Westernized lifestyles, both associated with reduced environmental microbial exposures, as contributing to the current high prevalence of allergic diseases.[6] Furthermore, findings from gut microbiome studies have since spurred research on characteristics of microbiota present in other body habitats such as the respiratory system, which was not included in the NIH Human Microbiome Project.[1] Although undoubtedly lower in microbial biomass compared with the intestine, thus challenging its investigation, both the upper and lower respiratory tracts are now recognized to harbor ecosystems that differ in compositional complexity.[7] Furthermore, characteristics of respiratory microbiomes differ in the presence of airway disease versus health.[8,9] However, our understanding of longitudinal variations in respiratory microbiota composition, their ecologic interactions, and local influences on respiratory mucosal immune responses and ultimately lung disease features remains nascent.

It is important to highlight in this introduction that, like all habitats, myriad extrinsic and intrinsic factors shape the composition of respiratory microbiota, the functions they express, and in turn their influence on immune responses and respiratory disease. Moreover, it is inevitable that host-microbial interactions are bidirectional. It is well recognized that microenvironmental and physiologic conditions dictate the composition and ecology of microbial consortia. This is true of observed topographical differences along skin surfaces and also along extensive mucosal surfaces such as those found in the gastrointestinal and respiratory tracts.[10-12] Microbial composition and functional activities in any environment are influenced by factors such as temperature, pH, salinity, oxygen availability, and many other factors. The presence of host-derived nutrients, such as mucins and lipids (as found in sebum and surfactant) and, of course, immune cells, further shape microbial activities.[7] Finally, interactions among microbes themselves influence the behaviors of respective species such as through the production of microbial signaling molecules (quorum-sensing) that influence biofilm production and expression of microbe-specific pathogenic traits.

HOW DOES THE MICROBIAL ENVIRONMENT AFFECT ASTHMA DEVELOPMENT?

Numerous studies, and accordingly many reviews, have been dedicated to discussions of the many ways by which microbiota and specific microbial products can shape immune responses and counterregulatory processes that impact the development of allergic inflammation. The reader is referred to several recent papers that provide a concise overview of primary evidence supporting the role of microbial exposures, establishment of gut microbiota patterns in early life, and mechanisms of immune stimulation that shape allergic immune responses in the gut as well as in the lungs.[9,13,14] The following aspects are highlighted.

Animal models, supplementing epidemiologic studies, have demonstrated the direct impact of microbiota on the development of allergic responses and allergic airway inflammation.

Seminal epidemiologic investigations from cohort studies in Europe and the United States brought to the fore recognition that differences in microbial exposures, related to lifestyle practices, are an important factor in the prevalence of allergic diseases.[15-17] Recent reports have corroborated the longitudinal impact of these early life exposure differences on continued differences in the prevalence of atopic diseases and asthma in later life.[18] From animal models, the importance of microbiota to immune system maturation is most prominently highlighted by the fact that germ-free mice at baseline have exaggerated susceptibility to allergic responses, which can be modified by exposure to microbes before allergen exposure to sensitize the animals.[19] Additional

studies in animal models have elucidated the effects that microbial components have on targets in specific immune cells (e.g., dendritic cells, epithelial cells) and regulation of allergic inflammation downstream.[20-23]

In addition to the antigenic properties of bacteria that stimulate local innate and adaptive immune responses, studies have also examined the role of bacterial metabolic products such as short-chain fatty acids (SCFAs). SCFAs in the gut are generated from fermentation of dietary fiber and exert a range of effects including maintenance of gut epithelial health, energy homeostasis,[24] and regulation of inflammatory processes outside of the gut.[23,25] Recent studies in mice have demonstrated that circulating SCFAs influence the maturation of dendritic cell progenitors in the bone marrow, resulting in attenuation of their ability to initiate type 2 immune responses in the lungs.[23] Other microbiota products of interest include the essential amino acid tryptophan, which is biotransformed by mammalian enzyme systems into other effectors with immunoregulatory properties.[26] The mechanisms by which SCFAs, tryptophan, and other microbial metabolites, including potentially from fungi,[27] ultimately shape respiratory immune responses are active areas of research interest.

Studies of the human gut microbiome, and more recently of the nasopharyngeal microbiome, have identified patterns of microbiota composition associated with asthma risk in children.

Much evidence from human studies now exists linking alterations in the gut microbiome to risk of allergic disease in childhood, including asthma. Recent studies, coupling clinical findings with in vivo or ex vivo experiments, have forged new ground toward elucidating underlying mechanisms for the associations.[28,29] Additionally, other omic methods such as metabolomics have been leveraged to identify metabolites that may mediate microbial-host interactions leading to observed associations with atopy or allergic inflammation.[28,29] The focus in such studies has predominantly been on childhood-onset asthma rather than adult-onset disease.

Emerging evidence also suggests the nasopharyngeal microbiome may play a role in childhood asthma development. Because studying the lower airways invasively in children poses a significant challenge for research, studies have pursued analysis of upper airway samples collected by different methods and accessing different niches. These methods include use of swabs, aspirates, or lavage to sample the deep throat, nasal, or nasopharyngeal passages. Interpreting findings from disparate methods remains a topic of debate.[30] Nonetheless, findings from these studies, largely based on bacterial 16S rRNA gene sequencing, have been broadly concordant in that a relative increase in particular bacterial genera (e.g., *Moraxella, Haemophilus, Streptococcus*) is associated with asthma or exacerbations related to more severe viral respiratory infections in children.[31-33]

It is noteworthy that differences in microbiota composition associated with asthma risk in the larger studies, both in the intestinal and upper respiratory tracts, were detected in very early infancy (<3 months of age).[28,33] This highlights the dynamic development of the human microbiome perinatally, possibly even in utero.[34,35] Such clinical findings also coincide with data from many mouse model studies demonstrating the plasticity of immune system responses when modulated by interventions, including microbial transfer, in very early life but not at older ages.[21,28,36]

POTENTIAL IMPACT OF THE MICROBIOME ON ASTHMA PHENOTYPE AND MEDICATION RESPONSE

The clinical heterogeneity of asthma is defined by the significant variability observed in disease severity and control and, accordingly, differences in asthma-related impairment and risk for adverse outcomes.[37] Underscoring these are differences between patients in their responses to therapeutic approaches to minimize impairment and risk. The efficacy of current standard therapies for asthma is now known to be associated with differences in genotype (e.g., β-agonists) and molecular inflammatory phenotype (e.g., inhaled corticosteroids).[38,39] Thus the biologic mechanisms driving particular asthma phenotypes will determine to a large extent therapeutic strategies and their effectiveness. The hypothesis that responses to inhaled medications may be influenced by respiratory microbiota is drawn from recent translational clinical studies, discussed next, on differences in the lower airway microbiome associated with differences in asthma features, including response to inhaled corticosteroids.[40-44]

Phenotypic Features of Asthma and the Airway Microbiome

Many asthma phenotypes have been described typically incorporating demographic, clinical, and/or inflammatory features.[45,46] To incorporate known biology and more precisely define phenotypes based on distinct molecular underpinnings, identifying asthma "endotypes"[47] has been proposed as a goal to better tailor treatments.[48] However, many features overlap between observed phenotypes, and it seems likely that

overlapping mechanisms would also contribute to different endotypes.

Most relevant to this chapter's focus on the microbiome is the dichotomy in asthma inflammatory phenotypes defined by the presence or absence of significant airway inflammation due to T-helper (Th) type 2 immune responses. Based on assessments of airway cellular inflammation, eosinophil- or noneosinophil-predominant inflammation has long been recognized in asthma,[49,50] and recent molecular studies of airway gene expression patterns identified concordant patterns of high or low expression of genes related to type 2 inflammation.[39,51,52] Initial work focused on identifying signature bronchial epithelial cell genes responsiveness to IL-13.[39,51] Asthmatic subjects with a Th2-high epithelial gene expression pattern demonstrated significant improvements in FEV1 after a course of inhaled corticosteroids (ICSs) compared with those without a Th2-high pattern.[39] Studies of sputum cell expression of genes for type 2 cytokines, IL-13 responsive epithelial genes, and non–type 2 cytokines also led to identification of asthmatic subgroups with type 2-"high" versus type 2-"low" asthma.[52] It is estimated that up to 50% of asthmatic adult patients may not have significant underlying type 2 airway inflammation. However, it must be noted that type 2 cytokines derive also from other sources besides classic Th2 lymphocytes (e.g., innate lymphoid cells). Alternate sources of type 2 inflammation or etiologies of steroid insensitivity likely are important in severe asthma patients who display persistent eosinophilia despite high-dose steroid treatment.

In contrast, subjects with a type 2-"low" inflammatory profile of asthma are unified by generally poor response to steroids and few treatment options. This large subgroup encompasses several subtypes with likely different underlying mechanisms that are incompletely understood.[53] One long-standing postulate has been the potential role of chronic airway infection or colonization by particular bacterial species (e.g., *Mycoplasma pneumoniae*) in adults with stable asthma.[54,55] Recent studies of the respiratory microbiome have expanded on this postulate, leveraging advances in molecular high-throughput approaches to profile bacterial communities based on conserved but phylogenetically discriminatory gene sequences (e.g., 16S rRNA gene). This has led to an increasing number of studies examining characteristics of the lower airway microbiome in asthmatic, mostly adult, subjects.[40-43,56-58] Beyond simply identifying differences in airway microbiota composition associated with asthma versus health, some of these studies have further identified relationships between the airway microbiome and phenotypic features of asthma, including airway inflammation patterns related to type 2 and non–type 2 responses.[40-43] Highlights of these studies in adult subjects, which have been recently reviewed,[14,59] are presented here as they inform the hypothesis that the airway microbiome has the potential to influence responses to medications, in particular to inhaled corticosteroids.

First, a consistent finding across several studies of the respiratory microbiome in adults, as well as children, with asthma is a relative increase in the abundance of particular members of the Proteobacteria, a large phylum that represents many potential respiratory pathogens. This includes reports of airway enrichment in members of the following bacterial genera or family (since 16S rRNA-based analyses do not reliably resolve species-level identities): *Haemophilus* (Pasteurellaceae family), *Moraxella, Neisseria,* and *Streptococcus.*[31,33,41,43,56,57,60] An issue to be aware of is that differences exist across studies in reported asthma-associated bacteria because of variability in subject's age, asthma severity, and sampling and analysis protocols (e.g., nasopharyngeal vs. oral swab or bronchial epithelial brushing; platforms used for analyses). Although these issues are not trivial but are also difficult to resolve, it is important to recognize these data provide information only on bacterial identities based on phylogenetic similarity of their 16S rRNA gene sequences. Analytic methods that expand on these findings to determine functional capacities of bacterial microbiota of interest are available and have been applied.[61]

Secondly, recent studies of asthmatic adult patients have uncovered significant relationships between characteristics of the lower airway microbiome and clinical features of interest in asthma.[40-44] These include differences in bronchial airway bacterial composition related to the severity of airway hyperresponsiveness[43] and airflow obstruction.[40] In severe asthma, differences in the bronchial microbiome associated with obesity and stability of asthma control also were identified.[42] Interestingly, obese severe asthma patients demonstrated significant bronchial enrichment in members of the Bacteroidetes or Firmicutes phylum rather than Proteobacteria; Bacteroidetes and Firmicutes represent the most prevalent bacteria found in the gastrointestinal system. In severe asthma patients whose Asthma Control Questionnaire (ACQ) scores indicated interim worsening of asthma control, over 90% of the bronchial bacterial communities whose relative abundance correlated positively with the change in ACQ were members of the Proteobacteria, in particular

Gammaproteobacteria/Enterobacteriaceae. This contrasted with the predominance of Actinobacteria correlating with a change in ACQ indicative of stable or improved asthma control in severe asthma subjects.

Thirdly, significant associations between bronchial epithelial gene expression signatures and members of the bronchial bacterial microbiota have been found. Such findings were initially detected among severe asthma subjects in whom epithelial gene expression for type 2–related inflammation, Th17-related inflammation, and molecular response to steroids were determined.[42] Somewhat surprisingly, no positive relationships between type 2–related gene expression and airway bacterial composition were identified. Further analyses confirmed that severe asthma subjects with higher numbers of airway eosinophils harbored significantly lower airway bacterial burden. However, significant positive associations were seen between the Th17-related gene expression patterns and several members of the bacterial microbiota including *Klebsiella* spp. This initial observation of a difference in the airway bacterial microbiome related to level of type 2 airway inflammation has since been corroborated in a multicenter study of mild asthma subjects not using inhaled steroids at baseline.[41] Applying the same approach for epithelial gene expression analysis to define type 2-"high" versus type 2-"low" asthma, a striking difference in bronchial bacterial burden was observed (Fig. 15.1). Fig. 15.1 also presents a summary of three major bronchoscopy-based studies of the bronchial bacterial microbiome performed to date, two of which were performed by NIH asthma clinical research networks. In further support of the finding that molecular-based assessments of *low* type 2 airway inflammation were associated with higher airway bacterial burden, a significant proportion of the subjects in each study in whom the bacterial community could be profiled had sputum eosinophils of <2%. Similar findings of a relationship between higher bacterial burden and fewer airway eosinophils were recently reported in another cohort.[44]

Influence of the Airway Microbiome on Medication Responses in Asthma

It is clear from studies to date that the composition of the airway microbiome differs across asthma severity. Escalation of steroid therapy is common and guideline-driven for more severe asthma but often insufficient to control asthma and minimize risks. Although biologics targeting type 2 inflammation are now available as adjunctive therapies, treatment options for those with predominantly type 2-low asthma remain limited. A

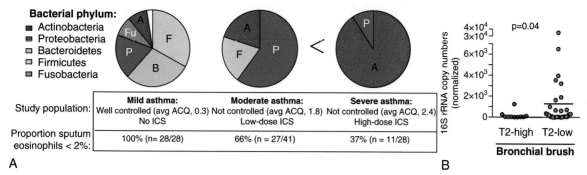

FIG. 15.1 **(A)** The composition of bronchial bacterial microbiota differs by asthma severity and asthma control. Pie charts generated from studies in which same bronchial sampling method (protected epithelial brushings) was used for 16S rRNA-based analyses. Direct comparison of severe versus moderate asthma subjects was performed since the same molecular platform was used to generate bacterial profiles in those two studies. **(B)** Data from mild asthma subjects not on corticosteroid therapy showing differences in bacterial burden by level of type 2 airway inflammation. (Data from Durack J, Lynch SV, Nariya S, et al. Features of the bronchial bacterial microbiome associated with atopy, asthma, and responsiveness to inhaled corticosteroid treatment. *J Allergy Clin Immunol.* 2016;140(1); Huang YJ, Nariya S, Harris JM, et al. The airway microbiome in patients with severe asthma: associations with disease features and severity. *J Allergy Clin Immunol.* 2015;136(4):874–884; Huang YJ, Nelson CE, Brodie EL, et al. Airway microbiota and bronchial hyperresponsiveness in patients with suboptimally controlled asthma. *J Allergy Clin Immunol.* 2011;127(2):372–381.e371–373.)

role for chronic treatment of asthma with macrolides has been extensively studied without clear findings of overall benefit.[62] However, previous studies may not have targeted asthma subgroups most likely to benefit from chronic intervention with macrolides. In the AZISAST study,[63] a randomized placebo-controlled trial in which subjects with exacerbation-prone severe asthma took azithromycin for 6 months, a prespecified analysis found that azithromycin was associated with a significantly lower rate of respiratory events only in subjects with noneosinophilic inflammation, a difference not seen in the study cohort as a whole.

An increased interest in the microbiome and its role in asthma and also chronic obstructive pulmonary disease (COPD) has led to exploration of the effects that therapies have on the airway microbiome or, conversely, the potential influence of the microbiome on treatment response. The use of antibiotics to acutely treat respiratory exacerbations in COPD or bronchiectasis (cystic fibrosis and non-CF-related) is common. Although broad-spectrum antibiotics have more variable effects on the sputum microbiome of CF patients,[64] likely due to more fixed characteristics of the CF airway microbiome typically dominated by *Pseudomonas aeruginosa*, two recent investigations of the sputum microbiome in COPD patients treated for exacerbations identified significant changes in airway bacterial diversity.[65,66] A detailed analysis of bacterial

community dynamics in this setting found a significant reduction in many members of the Proteobacteria phylum in COPD subjects treated with antibiotics alone or in combination with steroids, the latter suggesting an antibiotic-dominant effect.[65] The effect of macrolide antibiotics on the microbiome, when utilized as a chronic suppressive and antiinflammatory approach, is less well studied. When impacts on the airway microbiome of non-CF bronchiectasis or COPD patients have been examined, the actual effects reported on airway bacterial composition have been unclear or inconsistent,[67,68] potentially due to limited power related to heterogeneity in the baseline bacterial microbiota of subjects. In an analysis[43] of whether the efficacy of clarithromycin treatment for 16 weeks in subjects with moderate asthma differed by baseline (pretreatment) bronchial microbiota characteristics, the investigators found that airway bacterial diversity was higher in those whose bronchial hyperresponsiveness improved. Overall, such findings highlight the importance of ecologic interactions within a microbial community, which shape community resilience and its response to perturbations that can impact the detected outcome of an intervention. This concept is well recognized in the gut microbiome field.[69,70]

Corticosteroids have been a cornerstone of asthma treatment for decades. Although unquestionably effective for many patients, variability in treatment responses does exist, which, as discussed earlier, relates at least in part to differences in underlying disease mechanisms. Because steroids have immunosuppressive properties that could increase host susceptibility to microbial colonization, a question in the field has been whether observed airway microbiome differences by airway disease severity are influenced by concurrent ICS treatment. To address this and other questions, the NIH AsthmaNet consortium designed a study to examine characteristics of the bronchial microbiome in mild asthma subjects with well-controlled disease who were not on ICS at baseline.[41] These asthmatic subjects were randomized to inhaled fluticasone or placebo inhaler treatment for 6 weeks, after which bronchoscopy was repeated to collect airway samples for analysis. Significant changes in the relative abundance of several bacterial groups were observed and, importantly, the patterns of change differed between the fluticasone and placebo-treated groups. This suggests specific consequences of ICS treatment on the bronchial microbiome that are not simply reflective of usual variation that might be expected and seen in the placebo group. The investigators further analyzed if differences in predicted functional features of the bacterial microbiome were associated with clinical response to ICS, defined by a significant improvement in bronchial hyperresponsiveness. Predicted microbial genes linked to pathways for metabolism of xenobiotics were the most overrepresented functional group in the baseline microbiome of asthmatic subjects who did not respond to ICS.

FUTURE DIRECTIONS

Collectively, recent studies have elucidated the complexity of the upper and lower respiratory microbiota and features of these communities that are differentially associated with asthma and specific phenotypic features. Despite the unique challenges to studying the lower airway microbiome, current evidence drawn from studies of different asthma cohorts supports the possibility that microbiomes specific to each patient may not only influence the phenotype but also modulate responses to medications. These represent novel hypotheses for the respiratory microbiome field but are not entirely new concepts. For example, differences in gut microbiome features affect susceptibility to *Clostridium difficile* infection and responses to treatment including fecal transplantation.[69,71] Moreover, gut microbiota are known to biotransform therapeutic compounds, impacting their efficacy or toxicity, such

as for chemotherapeutic agents and digoxin.[72,73] The list of xenobiotics and other chemicals that could be modulated by microbiota or that impact microbiota functions is likely much more extensive than currently appreciated.[74–76] Naturally, the focus of such studies has been in the gut microbiome where microbial activities are greatest.

Because of its much lower microbial biomass compared with the intestine, the possibility that the respiratory tract could harbor microbiota whose functions are directly modulated by xenobiotic compounds, or even the possibility of respiratory microbes biotransforming them, may at first seem implausible. However, recent data coupled with evidence from other research fields collectively support these as plausible possibilities. First, antibiotics and host-targeted drugs clearly affect the functional activities of gut microbiota, as was recently shown in an elegant study using a combination of techniques.[74] Thus, it is certainly conceivable that drugs, including host-targeted medications, could impact the functional activities of respiratory microbiota even if smaller in scale.

Further evidence in support of the above arguments is gleaned from recent studies exploring functional effects of steroidal compounds, including glucocorticoids, on specific bacteria or bacterial-steroid interactions on host responses. In one study *Haemophilus parainfluenzae* was reported as being more prevalent in a group of steroid-resistant asthma patients.[77] The investigators then tested whether coculture of this species with macrophages altered responses of the macrophages to dexamethasone. Significant differences in dexamethasone-induced macrophage responses were seen with *H. parainfluenzae* coculture, in contrast to coculture with *Prevotella melaninogenica*. Another study examined the effect of beclomethasone on *Haemophilus influenzae* demonstrating through RNA-seq and biofilm studies changes in the transcription of several bacterial genes involved in stress responses, iron acquisition, and biofilm formation.[78] Moreover, beclomethasone-exposed *H. influenzae* induced a more sustained level of lung inflammation in mice infected in an immunosuppressed pneumonia model, compared with nonsteroid-exposed bacteria. Finally, a number of studies from the environmental microbiology or microbial ecology field have reported on the capabilities of both specific Proteobacteria and Actinobacteria members to biotransform steroidal compounds.[79–81] Thus, the emerging paradigm that inhaled medications could directly shape the respiratory microbiome or, conversely, that microbiota could modulate xenobiotic activities is supported

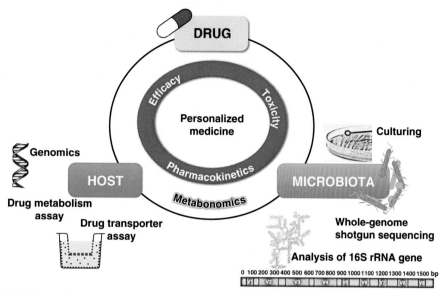

FIG. 15.2 Integrative approach to study host-respiratory microbiota interactions in pharmaceutical-related research. (From Yip LY, Chan EC. Investigation of host-gut microbiota modulation of therapeutic outcome. *Drug Metab Dispos.* 2015;43(10):1619–1631; with permission.)

by combined evidence from several different lines of investigation including insights from human-based studies.[41]

Dissecting the microbial players and mechanisms by which medications and other xenobiotics interact with the respiratory microbiome is an immensely daunting task (Fig. 15.2). This is compounded by (1) the challenges of performing large-scale studies of the lower airway microbiome in diverse human populations and (2) determining in vivo the relative contribution of involved microbial versus host metabolic pathways and ultimately the impact on respiratory disease phenotype. Related to this, a committee recently established by the National Academy of Science, Engineering and Medicine was charged with developing a research strategy to assess the effect of chemical exposures on human microbiomes and the role of chemical-microbiota interactions on related health effects.[82] Finally, a variety of investigative approaches will need to be deployed to understand how medications interact with the respiratory microbiome. These range from focused studies of particular compounds and respiratory microbes to broader studies examining systems-level metabolic readouts of the microbiome and host in particular compartments which has been coined "metabonomics."[83] As with all new horizons, the challenge is daunting but also an exciting new frontier for asthma research and pulmonary medicine.

REFERENCES

1. Consortium HMP. Structure, function and diversity of the healthy human microbiome. *Nature.* 2012;486(7402): 207–214.
2. Lynch SV, Pedersen O. The human intestinal microbiome in health and disease. *N Engl J Med.* 2016;375(24):2369–2379.
3. Round JL, Mazmanian SK. The gut microbiota shapes intestinal immune responses during health and disease. *Nat Rev Immunol.* 2009;9(5):313–323.
4. Marchesi JR, Ravel J. The vocabulary of microbiome research: a proposal. *Microbiome.* 2015;3:31.
5. Levy M, Kolodziejczyk AA, Thaiss CA, Elinav E. Dysbiosis and the immune system. *Nat Rev Immunol.* 2017;17(4).
6. Okada H, Kuhn C, Feillet H, Bach JF. The "hygiene hypothesis" for autoimmune and allergic diseases: an update. *Clin Exp Immunol.* 2010;160(1):1–9.
7. Huffnagle GB, Dickson RP, Lukacs NW. The respiratory tract microbiome and lung inflammation: a two-way street. *Mucosal Immunol.* 2017;10(2):299–306.
8. Huang YJ, Lynch SV. The emerging relationship between the airway microbiota and chronic respiratory disease: clinical implications. *Expert Rev Respir Med.* 2011;5(6):809–821.
9. Marsland BJ, Gollwitzer ES. Host-microorganism interactions in lung diseases. *Nat Rev Immunol.* 2014;14(12): 827–835.
10. Bassis CM, Erb-Downward JR, Dickson RP, et al. Analysis of the upper respiratory tract microbiotas as the source of the lung and gastric microbiotas in healthy individuals. *mBio.* 2015;6(2):e00037.

11. Dickson RP, Erb-Downward JR, Freeman CM, et al. Bacterial topography of the healthy human lower respiratory tract. *mBio.* 2017;8(1).

12. Grice EA, Kong HH, Conlan S, et al. Topographical and temporal diversity of the human skin microbiome. *Science.* 2009;324(5931):1190–1192.

13. Fujimura KE, Lynch SV. Microbiota in allergy and asthma and the emerging relationship with the gut microbiome. *Cell Host Microbe.* 2015;17(5):592–602.

14. Huang YJ, Marsland BJ, Bunyavanich S, et al. The microbiome in allergic disease: current understanding and future opportunities – 2017 PRACTALL document of the American Academy of Allergy, Asthma & Immunology and the European Academy of Allergy and Clinical Immunology. *J Allergy Clin Immunol.* 2017;139(4).

15. Braun-Fahrlander C, Riedler J, Herz U, et al. Environmental exposure to endotoxin and its relation to asthma in school-age children. *N Engl J Med.* 2002;347(12):869–877.

16. Haahtela T, Laatikainen T, Alenius H, et al. Hunt for the origin of allergy – comparing the Finnish and Russian Karelia. *Clin Exp Allergy.* 2015;45(5):891–901.

17. Ownby DR, Johnson CC, Peterson EL. Exposure to dogs and cats in the first year of life and risk of allergic sensitization at 6 to 7 years of age. *JAMA.* 2002;288(8):963–972.

18. Ruokolainen L, Paalanen L, Karkman A, et al. Significant disparities in allergy prevalence and microbiota between the young people in Finnish and Russian Karelia. *Clin Exp Allergy.* 2017;47(5).

19. Herbst T, Sichelstiel A, Schar C, et al. Dysregulation of allergic airway inflammation in the absence of microbial colonization. *Am J Respir Crit Care Med.* 2011;184(2):198–205.

20. Nembrini C, Sichelstiel A, Kisielow J, Kurrer M, Kopf M, Marsland BJ. Bacterial-induced protection against allergic inflammation through a multicomponent immunoregulatory mechanism. *Thorax.* 2011;66(9):755–763.

21. Olszak T, An D, Zeissig S, et al. Microbial exposure during early life has persistent effects on natural killer T cell function. *Science.* 2012;336(6080):489–493.

22. Schuijs MJ, Willart MA, Vergote K, et al. Farm dust and endotoxin protect against allergy through A20 induction in lung epithelial cells. *Science.* 2015;349(6252):1106–1110.

23. Trompette A, Gollwitzer ES, Yadava K, et al. Gut microbiota metabolism of dietary fiber influences allergic airway disease and hematopoiesis. *Nat Med.* 2014;20(2):159–166.

24. Canfora EE, Jocken JW, Blaak EE. Short-chain fatty acids in control of body weight and insulin sensitivity. *Nat Rev Endocrinol.* 2015;11(10):577–591.

25. Thorburn AN, McKenzie CI, Shen S, et al. Evidence that asthma is a developmental origin disease influenced by maternal diet and bacterial metabolites. *Nat Commun.* 2015;6:7320.

26. Steinmeyer S, Lee K, Jayaraman A, Alaniz RC. Microbiota metabolite regulation of host immune homeostasis: a mechanistic missing link. *Curr Allergy Asthma Rep.* 2015;15(5):24.

27. Wheeler ML, Limon JJ, Bar AS, et al. Immunological consequences of intestinal fungal dysbiosis. *Cell Host Microbe.* 2016;19(6):865–873.

28. Arrieta MC, Stiemsma LT, Dimitriu PA, et al. Early infancy microbial and metabolic alterations affect risk of childhood asthma. *Sci Transl Med.* 2015;7(307):307ra152.

29. Fujimura KE, Sitarik AR, Havstad S, et al. Neonatal gut microbiota associates with childhood multisensitized atopy and T cell differentiation. *Nat Med.* 2016;22(10):1187–1191.

30. Perez-Losada M, Crandall KA, Freishtat RJ. Two sampling methods yield distinct microbial signatures in the nasopharynges of asthmatic children. *Microbiome.* 2016;4(1):25.

31. Kloepfer KM, Lee WM, Pappas TE, et al. Detection of pathogenic bacteria during rhinovirus infection is associated with increased respiratory symptoms and asthma exacerbations. *J Allergy Clin Immunol.* 2014;133(5):1301–1307. 1307.e1301–e1303.

32. Perez-Losada M, Alamri L, Crandall KA, Freishtat RJ. Nasopharyngeal microbiome diversity changes over time in children with asthma. *PloS One.* 2017;12(1):e0170543.

33. Teo SM, Mok D, Pham K, et al. The infant nasopharyngeal microbiome impacts severity of lower respiratory infection and risk of asthma development. *Cell Host Microbe.* 2015;17(5):704–715.

34. Aagaard K, Ma J, Antony KM, Ganu R, Petrosino J, Versalovic J. The placenta harbors a unique microbiome. *Sci Transl Med.* 2014;6(237):237ra265.

35. Chu DM, Ma J, Prince AL, Antony KM, Seferovic MD, Aagaard KM. Maturation of the infant microbiome community structure and function across multiple body sites and in relation to mode of delivery. *Nat Med.* 2017;23(3):314–326.

36. Gollwitzer ES, Saglani S, Trompette A, et al. Lung microbiota promotes tolerance to allergens in neonates via PD-L1. *Nat Med.* 2014;20(6):642–647.

37. Global Initiative for Asthma. *Global Strategy for Asthma Management and Prevention;* 2016. Available from: http://www.ginasthma.org.

38. Wechsler ME, Kunselman SJ, Chinchilli VM, et al. Effect of beta2-adrenergic receptor polymorphism on response to longacting beta2 agonist in asthma (LARGE trial): a genotype-stratified, randomised, placebo-controlled, crossover trial. *Lancet.* 2009;374(9703):1754–1764.

39. Woodruff PG, Modrek B, Choy DF, et al. T-helper type 2-driven inflammation defines major subphenotypes of asthma. *Am J Respir Crit Care Med.* 2009;180(5):388–395.

40. Denner DR, Sangwan N, Becker JB, et al. Corticosteroid therapy and airflow obstruction influence the bronchial microbiome, which is distinct from that of bronchoalveolar lavage in asthmatic airways. *J Allergy Clin Immunol.* 2016;137(5):1398–1405.e1393.

41. Durack J, Lynch SV, Nariya S, et al. Features of the bronchial bacterial microbiome associated with atopy, asthma, and responsiveness to inhaled corticosteroid treatment. *J Allergy Clin Immunol.* 2016;140(1).

42. Huang YJ, Nariya S, Harris JM, et al. The airway microbiome in patients with severe asthma: associations with disease features and severity. *J Allergy Clin Immunol.* 2015;136(4):874–884.

43. Huang YJ, Nelson CE, Brodie EL, et al. Airway microbiota and bronchial hyperresponsiveness in patients with suboptimally controlled asthma. *J Allergy Clin Immunol.* 2011;127(2):372–381.e371–e373.

44. Sverrild A, Kiilerich P, Brejnrod A, et al. Eosinophilic airway inflammation in asthmatic patients is associated with an altered airway microbiome. *J Allergy Clin Immunol.* 2016. http://dx.doi.org/10.1016/j.jaci.2016.10.046.

45. Moore WC, Meyers DA, Wenzel SE, et al. Identification of asthma phenotypes using cluster analysis in the Severe Asthma Research Program. *Am J Respir Crit Care Med.* 2010;181(4):315–323.

46. Wenzel SE. Asthma phenotypes: the evolution from clinical to molecular approaches. *Nat Med.* 2012;18(5):716–725.

47. Lotvall J, Akdis CA, Bacharier LB, et al. Asthma endotypes: a new approach to classification of disease entities within the asthma syndrome. *J Allergy Clin Immunol.* 2011;127(2):355–360.

48. Chung KF. Asthma phenotyping: a necessity for improved therapeutic precision and new targeted therapies. *J Intern Med.* 2016;279(2):192–204.

49. Douwes J, Gibson P, Pekkanen J, Pearce N. Non-eosinophilic asthma: importance and possible mechanisms. *Thorax.* 2002;57(7):643–648.

50. McGrath KW, Icitovic N, Boushey HA, et al. A large subgroup of mild-to-moderate asthma is persistently noneosinophilic. *Am J Respir Crit Care Med.* 2012;185(6):612–619.

51. Woodruff PG, Boushey HA, Dolganov GM, et al. Genome-wide profiling identifies epithelial cell genes associated with asthma and with treatment response to corticosteroids. *Proc Natl Acad Sci USA.* 2007;104(40):15858–15863.

52. Peters MC, Mekonnen ZK, Yuan S, Bhakta NR, Woodruff PG, Fahy JV. Measures of gene expression in sputum cells can identify TH2-high and TH2-low subtypes of asthma. *J Allergy Clin Immunol.* 2014;133(2):388–394.

53. Fahy JV. Type 2 inflammation in asthma–present in most, absent in many. *Nat Rev Immunol.* 2015;15(1):57–65.

54. Kraft M, Cassell GH, Pak J, Martin RJ. Mycoplasma pneumoniae and Chlamydia pneumoniae in asthma: effect of clarithromycin. *Chest.* 2002;121(6):1782–1788.

55. Sutherland ER, Martin RJ. Asthma and atypical bacterial infection. *Chest.* 2007;132(6):1962–1966.

56. Green BJ, Wiriyachaiporn S, Grainge C, et al. Potentially pathogenic airway bacteria and neutrophilic inflammation in treatment resistant severe asthma. *PloS One.* 2014;9(6):e100645.

57. Hilty M, Burke C, Pedro H, et al. Disordered microbial communities in asthmatic airways. *PloS One.* 2010;5(1):e8578.

58. Marri PR, Stern DA, Wright AL, Billheimer D, Martinez FD. Asthma-associated differences in microbial composition of induced sputum. *J Allergy Clin Immunol.* 2013;131(2):346–352.e341–e343.

59. Ndum O, Huang YJ. Asthma phenotypes and the microbiome. *Eur Med J Allergy Immunol.* 2016;1(1):82–90.

60. Bisgaard H, Hermansen MN, Buchvald F, et al. Childhood asthma after bacterial colonization of the airway in neonates. *N Engl J Med.* 2007;357(15):1487–1495.

61. Langille MG, Zaneveld J, Caporaso JG, et al. Predictive functional profiling of microbial communities using 16S rRNA marker gene sequences. *Nat Biotechnol.* 2013;31(9):814–821.

62. Kew KM, Undela K, Kotortsi I, Ferrara G. Macrolides for chronic asthma. *Cochrane Database Syst Rev.* 2015;(9):Cd002997.

63. Brusselle GG, Vanderstichele C, Jordens P, et al. Azithromycin for prevention of exacerbations in severe asthma (AZISAST): a multicentre randomised double-blind placebo-controlled trial. *Thorax.* April 2013;68(4):322–329.

64. Huang YJ, LiPuma JJ. The microbiome in cystic fibrosis. *Clin Chest Med.* 2016;37(1):59–67.

65. Huang YJ, Sethi S, Murphy T, Nariya S, Boushey HA, Lynch SV. Airway microbiome dynamics in exacerbations of chronic obstructive pulmonary disease. *J Clin Microbiol.* 2014;52(8):2813–2823.

66. Wang Z, Bafadhel M, Haldar K, et al. Lung microbiome dynamics in COPD exacerbations. *Eur Respir J.* 2016;47(4):1082–1092.

67. Rogers GB, Bruce KD, Martin ML, Burr LD, Serisier DJ. The effect of long-term macrolide treatment on respiratory microbiota composition in non-cystic fibrosis bronchiectasis: an analysis from the randomised, double-blind, placebo-controlled BLESS trial. *Lancet Respir Med.* 2014;2(12):988–996.

68. Segal LN, Clemente JC, Wu BG, et al. Randomised, double-blind, placebo-controlled trial with azithromycin selects for anti-inflammatory microbial metabolites in the emphysematous lung. *Thorax.* 2017;72(1):13–22.

69. Buffie CG, Pamer EG. Microbiota-mediated colonization resistance against intestinal pathogens. *Nat Rev Immunol.* 2013;13(11):790–801.

70. Byrd AL, Segre JA. Infectious disease. Adapting Koch's postulates. *Science.* 2016;351(6270):224–226.

71. Rao K, Young VB. Fecal microbiota transplantation for the management of Clostridium difficile infection. *Infect Dis Clin North Am.* 2015;29(1):109–122.

72. Alexander JL, Wilson ID, Teare J, Marchesi JR, Nicholson JK, Kinross JM. Gut microbiota modulation of chemotherapy efficacy and toxicity. *Nat Rev Gastroenterol Hepatol.* 2017;14(6).

73. Haiser HJ, Gootenberg DB, Chatman K, Sirasani G, Balskus EP, Turnbaugh PJ. Predicting and manipulating cardiac drug inactivation by the human gut bacterium Eggerthella lenta. *Science.* 2013;341(6143):295–298.

74. Maurice CF, Haiser HJ, Turnbaugh PJ. Xenobiotics shape the physiology and gene expression of the active human gut microbiome. *Cell.* 2013;152(1–2):39–50.

75. Spanogiannopoulos P, Bess EN, Carmody RN, Turnbaugh PJ. The microbial pharmacists within us: a metagenomic view of xenobiotic metabolism. *Nat Rev Microbiol.* 2016;14(5):273–287.

76. Yip LY, Chan EC. Investigation of host-gut microbiota modulation of therapeutic outcome. *Drug Metab Dispos.* 2015;43(10):1619–1631.

77. Goleva E, Jackson LP, Harris JK, et al. The effects of airway microbiome on corticosteroid responsiveness in asthma. *Am J Respir Crit Care Med.* 2013;188(10):1193–1201.

78. Earl CS, Keong TW, An SQ, et al. Haemophilus influenzae responds to glucocorticoids used in asthma therapy by modulation of biofilm formation and antibiotic resistance. *EMBO Mol Med.* 2015;7(8):1018–1033.

79. Bergstrand LH, Cardenas E, Holert J, Van Hamme JD, Mohn WW. Delineation of steroid-degrading microorganisms through comparative genomic analysis. *mBio.* 2016;7(2):e00166.

80. Donova MV, Egorova OV. Microbial steroid transformations: current state and prospects. *Appl Microbiol Biotechnol.* 2012;94(6):1423–1447.

81. Li Z, Nandakumar R, Madayiputhiya N, Li X. Proteomic analysis of 17beta-estradiol degradation by Stenotrophomonas maltophilia. *Environ Sci Technol.* 2012;46(11):5947–5955.

82. http://www8.nationalacademies.org/cp/projectview.aspx?key=49795.

83. Nicholson JK, Lindon JC. Systems biology: metabonomics. *Nature.* 2008;455(7216):1054–1056.

CHAPTER 16

Preventing the Development of Asthma: Early Intervention Strategies in Children

JEFFREY R. STOKES, MD • LEONARD B. BACHARIER, MD

Asthma represents the source of substantial health burden among children. In 2015, the prevalence of asthma among US children was 8.4% or 6.2 million affected individuals.[1] In 2014, 3 million children experienced one or more asthma attacks, 136,000 were hospitalized for their asthma, and 187 died from asthma.[2] Recurrent wheezing in early life, a typical antecedent to a diagnosis of asthma, is common in preschool children, with 50% of children having at least one wheezing episode during their first 6 years of life. Fortunately, 60% of children who wheeze by 3 years of age experience resolution of their symptoms by 6 years of age.[3] The onset of asthmalike symptoms occurs before 6 years of age in 80%–90% of cases.[4] These findings highlight the early life onset of asthma and present a potential window for intervention for the primary prevention of childhood asthma.

Environmental and host factors influence the progression from wheezing illnesses to subsequent asthma, with respiratory viral infections and aeroallergen sensitization being dominant risk factors.[5] Other important and potentially modifiable environmental contributors are early life microbial exposures, environmental tobacco smoke, air pollution, dietary factors (vitamin D, long-chain polyunsaturated fatty acids), and stress. In addition, host factors include genetic predisposition (often reflected by a parental history of asthma), race, gender, and weight gain/obesity (Fig. 16.1).

Several trials have examined the potential effect of treatment of asthma in early childhood on the natural course of the disease, and while showing that inhaled corticosteroids, the gold standard for asthma therapy, lead to symptomatic improvement during therapy, there is no evidence that this therapy alters the overall course of disease once treatment is stopped.[6,7] These studies suggest that interventions may need to be applied prior to the emergence of asthma symptoms

(i.e., primary prevention) in early life to effectively prevent early life asthma. The prevention of asthma hinges on defining children at greatest risk for asthma and targeting interventions aimed at altering these key environmental factors. In 2015, Beasley et al. reviewed numerous risk factors for the development of asthma, including both effective and ineffective primary prevention strategies.[8] Although not the focus of this chapter, the effect of early life pet exposure has yielded conflicting results on allergic disease depending on age of exposure, and no clinical trials evaluating the effect of pet exposure on asthma prevention have been undertaken. Although exclusive breastfeeding has been associated with reduced allergic disease, there is no evidence for breastfeeding in the prevention of asthma.[8] This chapter will discuss recent interventions aimed at several key environmental factors that augment asthma risk, in efforts to prevent the development of asthma.

VITAMIN D SUPPLEMENTATION

Vitamin D deficiency has been identified as a potential explanation for the rising prevalence of allergic diseases, including asthma, for over a decade. Blood levels of 25-hydroxyvitamin D_3 (25OHD), which define vitamin D deficiency (<20 ng/mL) and insufficiency (20–30 ng/mL), are based on the effect of vitamin D on bone metabolism; slightly higher levels of 30–40 ng/mL have been suggested as the lower level for the immune effects of vitamin D.[9] In the United States, the prevalence of vitamin D insufficiency almost doubled from the late 1980s through the early 2000s. This rise in prevalence has paralleled a worldwide increase in asthma prevalence, leading to a multitude of investigations into the relationships between these two concurrent epidemics. The potential link between these two conditions is supported by the multiple key roles

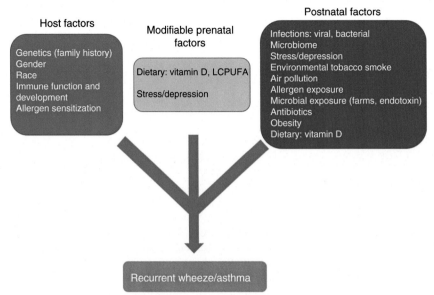

Host factors

Genetics (family history)
Gender
Race
Immune function and
development
Allergen sensitization

Modifiable prenatal
factors

Dietary: vitamin D, LCPUFA

Stress/depression

Postnatal factors

Infections: viral, bacterial
Microbiome
Stress/depression
Environmental tobacco smoke
Air pollution
Allergen exposure
Microbial exposure (farms, endotoxin)
Antibiotics
Obesity
Dietary: vitamin D

Recurrent wheeze/asthma

FIG. 16.1 Contributing factors for the development of asthma in children. *LCPUFA*, long-chain polyun-saturated fatty acids.

identified for vitamin D in intrauterine and postnatal lung development, along with modulation of the immune system and antimicrobial mechanisms.[9]

The relationship between maternal vitamin D intake during pregnancy and the development of allergic disease in their offspring was initially identified from studies using food-frequency questionnaires. In a population cohort study from Finland, 1669 children were evaluated for the development of asthma, allergic rhinitis, and atopic dermatitis at the age of 5 years.[10] Maternal dietary intake of vitamin D, as reported by questionnaire, was inversely related to the risk asthma and allergic rhinitis. A prospective prebirth cohort in Massachusetts assessed maternal intake of vitamin D during the entire pregnancy, based on questionnaires, and recurrent wheeze in children by the age of 3 years.[11] Mothers who were in the highest quartile of intake of vitamin D during pregnancy experienced a significantly lower risk of having a child with recurrent wheeze than those in the lowest quartile of intake.

A birth cohort study from France investigated the relationship of a direct assessment of vitamin D status, cord blood vitamin D levels, and the development of asthma, allergic rhinitis, atopic dermatitis, or wheezing in early life.[12] No association was noted for asthma, but cord serum vitamin D levels were inversely associated with transient early wheezing at 5 years of age.

Of note, both the mean and median cord vitamin D levels were 17.8 ng/mL, indicating that at least half the study population would be classified as vitamin D deficient. The Childhood Asthma Study from Australia enrolled children at high risk for allergy and asthma and followed them from birth to 10 years of age.[13] Multiple measurements (8 follow ups) of serum vitamin D levels were examined for associations with asthma. Overall, vitamin D levels were lowest at birth (median 26.2 nmol/L [equal to 10.4 ng/mL]) and highest at 5 years of age (89 nmol/L [35.6 ng/mL]). Multivariate analysis showed that the number of visits where vitamin D levels were deficient was positively associated with risk for asthma/wheeze, eczema, and allergen sensitization at 10 years of age. The authors suggested that low vitamin D levels may contribute to asthma development by modulating early allergen sensitization by 2 years of age and/or lower respiratory infection with fever (e.g., bacterial colonization).

A metaanalysis including data from the French birth cohort and three additional studies found no association between maternal vitamin D levels and childhood asthma or wheezing.[12,14] However, these findings are limited by important differences in the assessments of maternal vitamin D status (cord blood vitamin D levels, maternal serum vitamin D levels, and reported oral intake). In contrast, a metaanalysis of 16 birth cohort studies suggested an inverse relationship of in utero exposure to vitamin D and asthma or wheezing,[15] although this association only became significant for wheeze when cord blood vitamin D level was the assessment measure.

To determine if vitamin D deficiency was causally related to the risk of recurrent wheezing in early life, two recent trials have examined the effect of vitamin D supplementation during pregnancy on early life respiratory and allergic outcomes.[16,17] In a Danish study, 623 pregnant women were randomized to receive either the standard recommended dose of vitamin D during pregnancy (400 IU/day) or an additional 2400 IU/day (total of 2800 IU/day) starting at week 24 of gestation and continuing through 1 week postpartum.[16] The primary outcome of this trial was persistent wheeze in the children during the first 3 years of life. Of the 581 children examined, persistent wheeze was diagnosed in 16% of the vitamin D group and 20% in the control group, a nonsignificant difference of 4%. Although the high-dose vitamin D group experienced fewer episodes of troublesome lung symptoms, the two groups did not differ in asthma prevalence at 3 years of age, rates of respiratory tract infections, allergic sensitization, or eczema. A multicenter trial from the United States by Litonjua and colleagues enrolled 881 pregnant women at risk of having a child with asthma based on a parental history of asthma, allergic rhinitis, or eczema and evaluated the effect of vitamin D supplementation on recurrent wheezing or asthma in their offspring by the age of 3 years.[17] This double-blind, placebo-controlled study also provided 400 IU/day of vitamin D3 in the control group, but the supplementation group received an additional 4000 IU/day (total of 4400 IU/day). Women were randomized earlier in gestation than the previous study, this time at 10–18 weeks' gestation compared with 24 weeks. The primary outcome was either physician-diagnosed asthma or recurrent wheezing through 3 years of age in the 806 children. Of those women in the 4400 IU/day treatment group, 75% had vitamin D levels of 30 ng/mL or higher by the third trimester, compared with only 34% in the control group. Asthma or recurrent wheeze was present in 24.3% of children in the treatment group and 30.4% in the control group. This 6.1% lower absolute difference in the prevalence of asthma or recurrent wheeze at 3 years of age was not statistically significant (hazard ratio 0.8; 95% CI, 0.6–1.0; $P = .051$). The difference between the two groups of children decreased with age with an 8.9% difference at 1 year of age, 7.4% at 2 years, and 6.1% difference at 3 years of age. Fewer children born to mothers in the 4400 IU/day group had evidence of allergic sensitization, but there were no between group differences in the development of eczema, lower respiratory tract infections, or total IgE levels.

There are several potential explanations as to why neither of these trials of prenatal vitamin D supplementation demonstrated significant reduction in wheezing or asthma diagnosis in early life. Each of these studies may have been underpowered to detect a significance difference in the primary outcome, particularly the study by Litonjua and colleagues, where the P-value for the primary outcome was .051.[17] The initiation of supplementation, even by 10–18 weeks, may have been too late in gestation and missed a critical period of time for lung development. Neither study enrolled mothers based on their vitamin D levels at the time of entry into the study. Further analysis of the study by Litonjua and colleagues found that mothers with initial vitamin D level ≥30 ng/mL who were randomized to the 4400 IU/day vitamin D group had a significant reduction in asthma/recurrent wheezing in their children compared with women with a baseline level <20 ng/mL and randomized to the standard 400 IU/day of vitamin D (OR 0.42, 95% CI, 0.19–0.91),[18] suggesting that sufficient levels in the first trimester (and potentially in the preconception period), combined with ongoing supplementation throughout pregnancy, may be necessary to maximize the effect of vitamin D supplementation on asthma prevention. Finally, neither trial included vitamin D supplementation for the infants, and it is possible that maintenance of vitamin D sufficiency during early postnatal life may also be necessary.

Overall, maternal vitamin D status during pregnancy seems to be related to the risk of recurrent wheeze in early life. Although the mechanisms through which vitamin D influences these outcomes remain uncertain, these may include effects on lung development, immune regulation, microbiome composition, and/or genomic effects.[19] Supplementation with vitamin D during pregnancy, and potentially preconception, potentially even for mothers who are vitamin D sufficient, along with maintenance of normal levels during early childhood, may be necessary for the prevention of asthma and wheezing illnesses.

FISH OIL SUPPLEMENTATION

N-6 polyunsaturated fatty acids (e.g., arachidonic acid) have been recognized as having proinflammatory properties, and increased levels have been associated with both elevated exhaled nitric oxide and asthma symptoms.[20] Early observational studies suggested that a diet deficient in the antiinflammatory n-3 long-chain polyunsaturated fatty acids (LCPUFAs), eicosapentaenoic acid (EPA), and docosahexaenoic acid (DHA) during pregnancy may increase the risk of asthma or wheezing in children.[20] This may be due to their protective ability to displace arachidonic acid in membrane phospholipids, thus reducing potential leukotriene synthesis. Fish oil contains both EPA and DHA in varying amounts and thus is a good vehicle for LCPUFA supplementation.

A Cochrane review involving 3300 women and their children included six trials studying the administration of at least 1 g of fish oil supplement daily during pregnancy in a high-risk population resulting in reduced risks of atopic eczema in children 1–3 years of age and allergen sensitization at 1 year compared with children whose mothers did not receive fish oil.[21] No effect was noted on asthma or wheezing. Since that review, two recent large placebo-controlled studies (reviewed below) have demonstrated beneficial effect of high-dose fish oil supplementation during pregnancy on subsequent respiratory outcomes.[22,23]

In a single-center, double-blind, placebo-controlled, parallel-group trial, 736 pregnant women were randomized at 24 weeks gestation to treatment with either 2.4 g/day of LCPUFAs (fish oil) or placebo (olive oil).[22] A total of 695 children were followed for 5 years. Those children whose mothers had LCPUFA supplementation had a 30.7% reduction in the risk of persistent wheeze or asthma at the 3- to 5-year follow-up relative to the placebo group. In contrast to the effect of vitamin D supplementation, children born to women with the lowest baseline LCPUFA levels before the intervention and who received LCPUFA supplementation experienced the greatest reduction in risk (54.1%).[18,22] In addition, fish oil supplementation reduced the risk of lower respiratory tract infections. Beneficial effects were most noticeable in the children of mothers with a variant in the *FADS* gene that has been associated with low levels of EPA and DHA. The number of women needed to treat to prevent one case of persistent wheeze or asthma was 15 overall, but only 6 among women with baseline EPA and DHA levels in the lowest tertile.[22]

These findings were supported by a randomized control trial of 533 women who were assigned to receive fish oil, olive oil, or no oil starting at 30 weeks' gestation.[23] At 24 years of age, the children born to mothers in the fish oil group had a significantly lower risk of hospital discharge diagnosis of asthma (3%) compared with the olive oil group (10%). In addition, the use of asthma medication was significantly less likely among the fish oil group compared with the olive oil group. The dose of LCPUFA used in these two studies is estimated to be 10 times the normal daily intake in Denmark and 20 times in the United States.[22] Thus, supplementation with fish oil, presumably through improvements in levels of n-3 LCPUFAs, is associated with reduced risks of persistent wheeze and asthma, with one study suggesting long-standing protection for at least 24 years.

MICROBIOME MODIFICATION

There is strong evidence that the composition of the enteral and respiratory microbiomes plays a key role in the development of asthma[24–29] and multiple other conditions. Exposure to environmental microbes, including bacterial and fungal components such as endotoxins, influences the development of the human microbiome. Environmental microbial exposures have been identified as an explanation for the lower rates of atopic disease among children from farming communities compared with those from rural and urban areas.[30] Among children growing up in urban areas, exposure to high levels of indoor allergens, along with high levels of microbial richness in house dust, was associated with the lowest likelihood of atopic wheezing during the first 3 years of life, further supporting the influence of environmental exposures on asthma risk.[31]

Once thought to be sterile, it has become clear that a lung microbiome indeed exists, and the composition of the lung microbiome differs between adults with asthma, who have greater amounts of proteobacteria, relative to healthy adults.[29] In addition, there seems to be an interplay between viruses (respiratory syncytial virus [RSV], rhinovirus) and bacteria (*Haemophilus influenzae, Streptococcus pneumoniae, Staphylococcus aureus,* and *Moraxella catarrhalis*) that predispose children to wheeze in early life.[32] The gut microbiome composition is affected by race, mode of delivery, breastfeeding, antibiotic use, and vitamin D level.[33] In fact, infants at risk for asthma exhibit transient gut microbial dysbiosis during their first 3 months of life.[34] The gastrointestinal tract microbiome may also affect airway inflammation via the induction and migration of regulatory T cells.[32]

Given the emerging evidence of the importance of the enteral microbiome on subsequent disease development, research has begun to explore strategies aimed at modification of the microbiome. Potential strategies include enhancing the presence of organisms that exert protective effects and/or reduction of organisms with disease-promoting effects. Primary asthma prevention through microbiome targeting may focus on the microbiome of gastrointestinal system early in life, or even in utero, which may exert prenatal priming or epigenetic effects.[32] Secondary prevention, aimed at children who have shown a history of wheezing, may occur through altering the microbiome of the respiratory and/or gastrointestinal tracts with antibiotics, prevention of RSV infection with anti-RSV antibodies, or with immunostimulants acting on the gastrointestinal tract microbiome.[32]

The administration of probiotics (live microorganisms that provide health benefits) has been proposed as a method of primary prevention via Th1 stimulation, leading to a potential decrease in the development of allergic disease such as allergic asthma. Numerous trials have examined the effects of probiotics on these outcomes, using many different study designs, timing of probiotic use, multiple different probiotic products, dosing regimens, and varying durations of follow-up. A metaanalysis of 29 studies evaluated the use of probiotics for the prevention of allergic diseases.[35] The only benefit noted was a reduction in eczema in children when probiotics were used in the following scenarios: use in the third trimester, during breastfeeding, or when directly given directly to the infant. Another metaanalysis of 20 studies encompassing nearly 5000 children evaluated probiotic use during pregnancy or when given to infants in the first year of life.[36] These authors also found no evidence to support a preventative effect of probiotics on wheezing or asthma. Future trials examining other strategies, including prebiotics, combinations of probiotics, and other approaches to microbiome manipulation, are needed to fully understand if this approach can lessen the risk of allergic diseases, including asthma.

RESPIRATORY TRACT INFECTIONS

Respiratory tract infections are a key factor in the expression of asthma, both in terms of conferring asthma risk and contributing to asthma episodes. The viruses most strongly linked with the development of recurrent wheezing or asthma are RSV and rhinovirus.[37] The mechanisms through which these viruses participate in asthma pathogenesis remain uncertain.

Recent research has begun to explore strategies to lessen the impact of viral infections in early life and reduce the risk of subsequent asthma. Two potential avenues of primary prevention have included the primary prevention of viral infections and the use of substances to stimulate the immune system.

Given the strong association between severe RSV infection and subsequent asthma, primary prevention of RSV infection could reduce the risk of subsequent recurrent wheeze and asthma.[38] An effective vaccine

against RSV has not yet been developed. However, palivizumab, a humanized monoclonal antibody against the RSV fusion protein, reduces serious lower respiratory tract infections because of RSV in high-risk infants.[39] The double-blind, placebo-controlled MAKI trial evaluated the effectiveness of palivizumab in preventing wheezing lower respiratory tract infections during the first year of life in otherwise healthy late preterm (33–36 weeks gestation) infants.[40] Palivizumab reduced the total number of wheezing days by 61% and the proportion of infants with recurrent wheeze by 10 percentage points, suggesting that primary prevention of RSV infection reduced the risk of subsequent wheeze from all causes, and this effect persisted even after conclusion of the RSV season. A multicenter, prospective, matched, double-cohort observational study in 27 centers in both Europe and Canada examined the effect of palivizumab administration on preventing recurrent wheeze in over 400 premature (<36 weeks) infants.[41] By the age of 5 years, physician-diagnosed recurrent wheeze was reduced by 68% in those children with no family history of asthma and by 80% with no family history of atopy or food allergy. In those children with a family history of atopy or food allergy, palivizumab had no effect on subsequent recurrent wheezing. A recent report from a case-control study of 444 infants born at 33–35 weeks gestational age, receipt of palivizumab during the first year of life was associated with significantly lower rates of recurrent wheezing among treated children, but there was no difference in the incidence of atopic asthma at age 6 years between treated and untreated children.[42] Thus, while prevention of RSV infection with palivizumab seems to reduce wheezing illnesses early in life, its effect on subsequent allergic asthma development has not yet been demonstrated, and its efficacy may differ based on underlying atopy risk factors.

Acute severe RSV bronchiolitis is associated with neutrophilic airway inflammation and a heightened risk of asthma by age 7 years.[43]. Macrolide antibiotics, such as azithromycin, have been demonstrated to have antiinflammatory properties as well as antibacterial effects.[37] Given the high risk of asthma following severe RSV bronchiolitis, a proof-of-concept trial in 40 healthy infants hospitalized with RSV bronchiolitis randomized participants to receive either azithromycin or placebo for 14 days.[44] Azithromycin treatment resulted in a longer time to a third wheezing episode, fewer days with respiratory symptoms, and a lower risk of recurrent wheezing in the 12 months following bronchiolitis. The mechanisms of these effects are not fully understood but may be related to changes in the inflammatory response reflected by lower levels of IL-8 in nasal secretions[44] and/or alterations in the upper airway microbiome composition. These results have prompted an ongoing trial to evaluate if the addition of azithromycin to routine bronchiolitis care, among infants hospitalized with RSV bronchiolitis, reduces the occurrence of recurrent wheeze during the preschool years (ClinicalTrials.gov NCT02911935).

Another potential approach toward the prevention of asthma is through the nonspecific prevention of viral respiratory tract infections. OM-85 BV is an immunostimulatory agent composed of lyophilized bacterial lysates of *Haemophilus influenzae, Diplococcus pneumoniae, Klebsiella pneumoniae* and *ozaenae, Staphylococcus aureus, Streptococcus pyogenes* and *viridans,* and *Neisseria catarrhalis.*[45] OM-85 BV has been used in Europe for the prevention of respiratory illness for over 25 years. Although its mechanisms of action remain uncertain, in a randomized, double-blind, placebo-controlled study in 75 children with a history of recurrent wheezing, treatment with OM-85 BV during viral season was associated with a 38% reduction in wheezing lower respiratory tract infections and a shorter duration of illness by 2 days.[45] A Cochrane metaanalysis of 61 placebo-controlled clinical trials involving over 4000 children 6 months to 18 years of age evaluated the use of immune stimulants, such as OM-85 BV, on acute respiratory infections.[46] Of these studies, 40 used bacterial products, with 12 studies using OM-85 BV. Overall, the administration of immune stimulants reduced the incidence of acute respiratory tract infections by 40%. The effect of OM-85 BV was a 36% reduction in respiratory infections compared with placebo.[46] Based on these findings, there is a multicenter, randomized, placebo-controlled study under way (ClinicalTrials.gov NCT02148796) to evaluate if OM-85 BV given regularly for 2 years to high-risk infants 6–18 months of age, potentially by reducing the frequency of viral respiratory infections, also reduces the likelihood of developing wheezing lower respiratory tract illnesses during a third observation year while off therapy.

CONCLUSIONS

The era of primary asthma prevention is under way. Driven by findings from epidemiologic studies, clinical trials have been undertaken to determine if therapeutic efforts targeting these epidemiologic findings result in clinically relevant asthma prevention. To date, positive effects have been demonstrated for supplementation during pregnancy with fish oil and potentially with high-dose vitamin D. Strategies targeting viral infections and the microbiome remain in their relative infancies, with more research required to determine if such interventions can exert protective effects. Further research will hopefully include multiple simultaneous interventions, such as supplementation with vitamin D and/or fish oil along with microbiome and immune stimulation, to minimize the risk of subsequent asthma. More precise identification of children at risk for asthma, along with improved insights into the mechanisms underlying the multiple endotypes and phenotypes of asthma, will enable more specific and targeted interventions in the highest-risk populations. In addition to efforts aimed at primary asthma prevention, several strategies for the secondary prevention of asthma, along with modification of the course and severity, are being developed. The coming decade will hopefully begin to bring the totality of these approaches to bear and may finally allow clinicians to act early in life to reduce the overall burden of childhood asthma.

DISCLOSURE

Dr. Bacharier reported receiving grant support from NIH; serving as a consultant to Aerocrine, GlaxoSmithKline, Genentech/Novartis, Cephalon, Teva, Circassia, and Boehringer Ingelheim; serving on advisory boards for Merck, Sanofi, and Vectura; serving on data and safety monitoring boards for DBV Technologies; and receiving honoraria for lectures or continuing medical education development from Aerocrine, GlaxoSmithKline, Genentech/Novartis, Merck, Cephalon, Teva, AstraZeneca, WebMD/Medscape, and Boehringer Ingelheim.

REFERENCES

1. CDC/NCHS. *National Health Interview Survey;* 2015. https://www.cdc.gov/asthma/nhis/2015/table3-1.htm.
2. CDC/NCHS. *National Health Interview Survey;* 2014. http://www.cdc.gov/nchs/nhis/SHS/tables.htm.
3. Martinez FD, Wright AL, Taussig LM, et al. Asthma and wheezing in the first six years of life. *N Engl J Med.* 1995;1995(332):133–138. http://dx.doi.org/10.1056/NEJM199501193320301.
4. Yunginger JW, Reed CE, O'Connell EJ, et al. A community-based study of the epidemiology of asthma. Incidence rates, 1964-1983. *Am Rev Respir Dis.* 1992;146(4):888–894.
5. Jackson DJ, Hartert TV, Martinez FD, et al. Asthma: NHLBI workshop on the primary prevention of chronic lung diseases. *Ann Am Thorac Soc.* 2014;11(suppl 3):S139–S145. http://dx.doi.org/10.1513/AnnalsATS.201312-448LD. Review. PMID: 24754822.

6. Guilbert TW, Morgan WJ, Zeiger RS, et al. Long-term inhaled corticosteroids in preschool children at high risk for asthma. *N Engl J Med.* 2006;354(19):1985–1997. PMID: 16687711.

7. Bisgaard H, Hermansen MN, Loland L, et al. Intermittent inhaled corticosteroids in infants with episodic wheezing. *N Engl J Med.* 2006;354(19):1998–2005. PMID: 16687712.

8. Beasley R, Semprini A, Mitchell EA. Risk factors for asthma: is prevention possible? *Lancet.* 2015;386(9998):1075–1085. http://dx.doi.org/10.1016/S0140-6736(15)00156-7.

9. Mirzakhani H, Al-Garawi A, Weiss ST, et al. Vitamin D and the development of allergic disease: how important is it?. *Clin Exp Allergy.* 2015;45(1):114–125. http://dx.doi.org/10.1111/cea.12430. Review. PMID: 25307157.

10. Erkkola M, Kaila M, Nwaru BI, et al. Maternal vitamin D intake during pregnancy is inversely associated with asthma and allergic rhinitis in 5-year-old children. *Clin Exp Allergy.* 2009;39(6):875–882. http://dx.doi.org/10.1111/j.1365-2222.2009.03234.x.

11. Camargo Jr CA, Rifas-Shiman SL, Litonjua AA, et al. Maternal intake of vitamin D during pregnancy and risk of recurrent wheeze in children at 3 y of age. *Am J Clin Nutr.* 2007;85(3):788–795.

12. Baïz N, Dargent-Molina P, Wark JD, et al. Cord serum 25-hydroxyvitamin D and risk of early childhood transient wheezing and atopic dermatitis. *J Allergy Clin Immunol.* 2014;133(1):147–153. http://dx.doi.org/10.1016/j.jaci.2013.05.017. PMID: 23810764.

13. Hollams EM, Teo SM, Kusel M, et al. Vitamin D over the first decade and susceptibility to childhood allergy and asthma. *J Allergy Clin Immunol.* 2017;139(2):472–481: e9. http://dx.doi.org/10.1016/j.jaci.2016.07.032.

14. Wei Z, Zhang J, Yu X. Maternal vitamin D status and childhood asthma, wheeze, and eczema: a systematic review and meta-analysis. *Pediatr Allergy Immunol.* 2016;27(6):612–619. http://dx.doi.org/10.1111/pai.12593. [Epub July 20, 2016] PMID: 27726947.

15. Feng H, Xun P, Pike K, et al. In utero exposure to 25-hydroxyvitamin D and risk of childhood asthma, wheeze, and respiratory tract infections: a meta-analysis of birth cohort studies. *J Allergy Clin Immunol.* 2016. http://dx.doi.org/10.1016/j.jaci.2016.06.065. pii:S0091-6749(16)30962-9. [Epub ahead of print].

16. Chawes BL, Bønnelykke K, Stokholm J, et al. Effect of vitamin D3 supplementation during pregnancy on risk of persistent wheeze in the offspring: a randomized clinical trial. *JAMA.* 2016;315(4):353–361. http://dx.doi.org/10.1001/jama.2015.18318.

17. Litonjua AA, Carey VJ, Laranjo N, et al. Effect of prenatal supplementation with vitamin D on asthma or recurrent wheezing in offspring by age 3 years: the VDAART randomized clinical trial. *JAMA.* 2016;315(4):362–370. http://dx.doi.org/10.1001/jama.2015.18589. PMID: 26813209.

18. Wolsk HM, Harshfield BJ, Laranjo N, et al. In utero exposure to 25-hydroxyvitamin D and risk of childhood asthma, wheeze, and respiratory tract infections: a meta-analysis of birth cohort studies. *J Allergy Clin Immunol.* 2017;139(5). Published online 2017.

19. Litonjua AA, Weiss ST. Vitamin D status through the first 10 years of life: a vital piece of the puzzle in asthma inception. *J Allergy Clin Immunol.* 2016;139(2):459–461.

20. Willers SM, Devereux G, Craig LC, et al. Maternal food consumption during pregnancy and asthma, respiratory and atopic symptoms in 5-year-old children. *Thorax.* 2007;62(9):773–779. [Epub March 27, 2007].

21. Best KP, Gold M, Kennedy D, et al. Omega-3 long-chain PUFA intake during pregnancy and allergic disease outcomes in the offspring: a systematic review and meta-analysis of observational studies and randomized controlled trials. *Am J Clin Nutr.* 2016;103(1):128–143. http://dx.doi.org/10.3945/ajcn.115.111104. Review. PMID: 26675770.

22. Bisgaard H, Stokholm J, Chawes BL, et al. Fish oil-derived fatty acids in pregnancy and wheeze and asthma in offspring. *N Engl J Med.* 2016;375(26):2530–2539. http://dx.doi.org/10.1056/NEJMoa1503734.

23. Hansen S, Strøm M, Maslova E, et al. Fish oil supplementation during pregnancy and allergic respiratory disease in the adult offspring. *J Allergy Clin Immunol.* 2017;139(1):104–111.e4. http://dx.doi.org/10.1016/j.jaci.2016.02.042. PMID: 27246522.

24. Bisgaard H, Li N, Bonnelykke K, et al. Reduced diversity of the intestinal microbiota during infancy is associated with increased risk of allergic disease at school age. *J Allergy Clin Immunol.* 2011;128(3):646–652.e1-5. http://dx.doi.org/10.1016/j.jaci.2011.04.060. [Epub July 22, 2011].

25. Arrieta MC, Stiemsma LT, Dimitriu PA, et al. Early infancy microbial and metabolic alterations affect risk of childhood asthma. *Sci Transl Med.* 2015;7(307):307ra152. http://dx.doi.org/10.1126/scitranslmed.aab2271.

26. Simonyte Sjödin K, Vidman L, Rydén P, et al. Emerging evidence of the role of gut microbiota in the development of allergic diseases. *Curr Opin Allergy Clin Immunol.* 2016;16(4):390–395. http://dx.doi.org/10.1097/ACI.0000000000000277.

27. Bridgman SL, Kozyrskyj AL, Scott JA, et al. Gut microbiota and allergic disease in children. *Ann Allergy Asthma Immunol.* 2016;116(2):99–105. http://dx.doi.org/10.1016/j.anai.2015.10.001.

28. Teo SM, Mok D, Pham K, et al. The infant nasopharyngeal microbiome impacts severity of lower respiratory infection and risk of asthma development. *Cell Host Microbe.* 2015;17(5):704–715. http://dx.doi.org/10.1016/j.chom.2015.03.008. [Epub April 9, 2015].

29. von Mutius E. The microbial environment and its influence on asthma prevention in early life. *J Allergy Clin Immunol.* 2016;137(3):680–689. http://dx.doi.org/10.1016/j.jaci.2015.12.1301. Review. PMID: 26806048.

30. Ege MJ, Mayer M, Normand AC, et al. Exposure to environmental microorganisms and childhood asthma. *N Engl J Med.* 2011;364(8):701–709. http://dx.doi.org/10.1056/NEJMoa1007302. PMID: 21345099.

31. Lynch SV, Wood RA, Boushey H, et al. Effects of early-life exposure to allergens and bacteria on recurrent wheeze and atopy in urban children. *J Allergy Clin Immunol.* 2014;134(3)593–601.e12. http://dx.doi.org/10.1016/j.jaci.2014.04.018. [Epub June 4, 2014].

32. Smits HH, Hiemstra PS, Prazeres da Costa C, et al. Microbes and asthma: opportunities for intervention. *J Allergy Clin Immunol.* 2016;137(3):690–697. http://dx.doi.org/10.1016/j.jaci.2016.01.004. Review. PMID: 26947981.

33. McLoughlin RM, Mills KH. Influence of gastrointestinal commensal bacteria on the immune responses that mediate allergy and asthma. *J Allergy Clin Immunol.* 2011;127(5): 1097–1107:quiz 1108-9. http://dx.doi.org/10.1016/j.jaci.2011.02.012. [Epub March 21, 2011].

34. Sordillo JE, Zhou Y, McGeachie MJ, et al. Factors influencing the infant gut microbiome at age 3-6 months: findings from the ethnically diverse Vitamin D Antenatal Asthma Reduction Trial (VDAART). *J Allergy Clin Immunol.* 2017;139(2):482–491.e14. http://dx.doi.org/10.1016/j.jaci.2016.08.045.

35. Cuello-Garcia CA, Brożek JL, Fiocchi A, et al. Probiotics for the prevention of allergy: a systematic review and meta-analysis of randomized controlled trials. *J Allergy Clin Immunol.* 2015;136(4):952–961. http://dx.doi.org/10.1016/j.jaci.2015.04.031. [Epub June 2, 2015].

36. Azad MB, Coneys JG, Kozyrskyj AL, et al. Probiotic supplementation during pregnancy or infancy for the prevention of asthma and wheeze: systematic review and meta-analysis. *BMJ.* 2013;347. http://dx.doi.org/10.1136/bmj.f6471. Review. PMID: 24304677.

37. Beigelman A, Bacharier LB. Early-life respiratory infections and asthma development: role in disease pathogenesis and potential targets for disease prevention. *Curr Opin Allergy Clin Immunol.* 2016;16(2):172–178. http://dx.doi.org/10.1097/ACI.0000000000000244.

38. Beigelman A, Bacharier LB. Infection-induced wheezing in young children. *J Allergy Clin Immunol.* 2014;133(2):603–604. http://dx.doi.org/10.1016/j.jaci.2013.12.001.

39. American Academy of Pediatrics Committee on Infectious Diseases. American Academy of Pediatrics Bronchiolitis Guidelines Committee. Updated guidance for palivizumab prophylaxis among infants and young children at increased risk of hospitalization for respiratory syncytial virus infection. *Pediatrics.* 2014;134(2):e620–e638. http://dx.doi.org/10.1542/peds.2014-1666. PMID: 25070304.

40. Blanken MO, Rovers MM, Molenaar JM, et al. Respiratory syncytial virus and recurrent wheeze in healthy preterm infants. *N Engl J Med.* 2013;368(19):1791–1799. http://dx.doi.org/10.1056/NEJMoa1211917. Erratum in: N Engl J Med. 2016 Jun 16;374(24):2406. PMID: 2365664.

41. Simões EA, Carbonell-Estrany X, Rieger CH, et al. The effect of respiratory syncytial virus on subsequent recurrent wheezing in atopic and nonatopic children. *J Allergy Clin Immunol.* 2010;126(2):256–262. http://dx.doi.org/10.1016/j.jaci.2010.05.026. PMID: 20624638.

42. Mochizuki H, Kusuda S, Okada K, et al. Palivizumab prophylaxis in preterm infants and subsequent recurrent wheezing: 6 Year follow up study. *Am J Respir Crit Care Med.* 2017. http://dx.doi.org/10.1164/rccm.201609-1812OC. [Epub ahead of print].

43. Bacharier LB, Cohen R, Schweiger T, et al. Determinants of asthma after severe respiratory syncytial virus bronchiolitis. *J Allergy Clin Immunol.* 2012;130(1):91–100.e3. http://dx.doi.org/10.1016/j.jaci.2012.02.010. PMID: 22444510; PMCID: PMC3612548.

44. Beigelman A, Isaacson-Schmid M, Sajol G, et al. Randomized trial to evaluate azithromycin's effects on serum and upper airway IL-8 levels and recurrent wheezing in infants with respiratory syncytial virus bronchiolitis. *J Allergy Clin Immunol.* 2015;135(5):1171–1178.e1. http://dx.doi.org/10.1016/j.jaci.2014.10.001. [Epub November 18, 2014].

45. Razi CH, Harmancı K, Abacı A, et al. The immunostimulant OM-85 BV prevents wheezing attacks in preschool children. *J Allergy Clin Immunol.* 2010;126(4):763–769. http://dx.doi.org/10.1016/j.jaci.2010.07.038.

46. Del-Rio-Navarro BE, Espinosa Rosales F, Flenady V, et al. Immunostimulants for preventing respiratory tract infection in children. *Cochrane Database Syst Rev.* 2006;(4). http://dx.doi.org/10.1002/14651858.CD004974.pub2.

CHAPTER 17

Identifying and Preventing the Progression of Asthma to Chronic Obstructive Pulmonary Disease

PADMAJA SUBBARAO, MD, MSC • MALCOLM R. SEARS, MB

Asthma is the most common chronic disease of childhood and yet its causes, and factors related to its remission or persistence, remain to be fully understood. Asthma refers to a group of disorders that are characterized by the common symptoms of wheezing, cough, and shortness of breath and manifested physiologically by variable airflow obstruction. In many children, these effects are transient, but in a substantial minority, symptoms and airflow obstruction persist and may become more severe and even permanent in adolescence and adulthood. Persistent asthma can be associated with a degree of fixed airflow obstruction similar to that generally associated with chronic obstructive pulmonary disease (COPD).

NATURAL HISTORY OF CHILDHOOD WHEEZING

Wheezing, a sentinel symptom of asthma, was documented in almost 50% of all children enrolled in the Tucson longitudinal study.[1] In another longitudinal study, recurrent wheeze, the primary risk factor for persistent asthma, occurred in 40% of preschool children.[2,3] Typically, many children with these early wheezing disorders experience remission by school age, but some 15% continue to suffer persistent symptoms into the school-age years and into adult life.[4] An understanding of the difference in risk factors for wheezing episodes that persist or remit in childhood and for asthma in older children and adults may shed light on underlying biologic mechanisms related to persistence and concomitant airflow obstruction.

Viral infections underlie the majority of episodes of early life wheezing in preschool children; these viral infections cause narrowing in these structurally smaller airways. The type of viral infection associated with wheezing may be relevant in predicting the persistence of asthma. In a high-risk cohort of children with known parental atopy, up to 90% of children with wheezing associated with infection by rhinovirus had persistent school age asthma.[5] Severe respiratory syncytial virus (RSV) infection has been associated with persistent wheezing in non–high-risk cohorts.[6,7]

In early childhood, viral infections are more frequent triggers of wheezing episodes than is sensitization to inhalant allergens, but by adulthood, many asthmatics have evidence of aeroallergen sensitization and experience exacerbations of symptoms when exposed either to allergens or to viral infections. Several lines of evidence suggest that early life atopic sensitization with a second "hit" of an early severe respiratory viral infection will significantly increase the risk of persistent asthma.[8] Birth cohort studies following the development of aeroallergen sensitization have consistently supported the importance of atopy in the persistence and severity of asthma. Early sensitization, especially to multiple allergens, is strongly associated with the development of both persistent asthma[9,10] and more severe asthma symptoms.

LUNG FUNCTION AND WHEEZING SYNDROMES

Low lung function is consistently associated with persistent asthma. Longitudinal general population cohort studies serially measuring lung function suggest that subjects destined to have persistent adult asthma demonstrate a stable and persistent loss of lung function from early childhood (Fig. 17.1).[4] However, whether low lung function is present at birth and is a primary risk factor for the development of asthma is less certain. This may be dependent on the population under study. Data from two general population cohorts with infant pulmonary function from 1 month of age suggest that low lung function at 1 month is not associated with

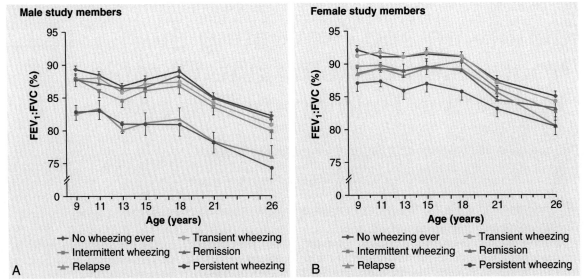

Male study members

Female study members

FIG. 17.1 Tracking of lung function with age in males **(A)** and females **(B)** participating in the Dunedin Multidisciplinary Research and Development study, demonstrating the loss of function already evident at age 9 years in study members found to have persistent or relapsing asthma at age 26 years. (From Sears MR, Greene JM, Willan AR, et al. A longitudinal, population-based, cohort study of childhood asthma followed to adulthood. *N Engl J Med.* 2003;349:1414–1422; with permission.)

persistent asthma at school age but rather is associated with transient wheeze that resolves by school age.[1,11] On the other hand, data from the high-risk cohort in Copenhagen suggest that low lung function at 1 month is indeed a risk factor for the development of asthma.[12] What has been consistently shown is that asthma and atopy are associated with a sustained decrease in lung function from an early age, as illustrated in Fig. 17.2. The trajectory of low lung function and the critical period for damage seems to occur very early in life for those with persistent early wheeze and seems to be related to parental history of asthma as well as early onset of atopy.[13] The combination of early life insults on a backdrop of an immune system primed toward allergy likely leads to airway inflammation and the structural changes associated with persistent asthma.

Further complicating this issue is that lung function, like height, is normally distributed in the general population. Therefore, "low" lung function is normal in a small proportion of the population. However, lung function toward the lower end of the normal range does seem to be of physiologic relevance to the development of asthma and is known to be related to factors such as cigarette smoke exposure in utero,[14] low birth weight, and early gestational age. Additionally, in two cohorts, maternal asthma was a risk factor for low lung function.[13,14] Low lung function in infancy, whether present at birth

or developing shortly after, provides a template for the adverse effect of severe viral infections,[15] which may cause further airway injury and impaired or low lung function.

Genetic studies suggest that the heritability characteristics of low lung function may be independent of asthma but rather are related to lung growth and morphogenesis.[16] General population birth cohort studies have indicated that for children with transient wheezing, genes associated with COPD are a more important risk factor for low lung function than are genes associated with asthma.[16] Two general population birth cohorts that incorporated lung function measurements suggest that although low lung function from infancy is associated with transient wheeze, low lung function may persist into adulthood in the absence of symptoms.[17,18] The role of low lung function as a risk factor for the development of symptoms may be modified by lifestyle characteristics such as cigarette smoking.

GENETIC, GENE-ENVIRONMENT, AND EPIGENETIC EFFECTS ON LUNG FUNCTION

In the Dunedin general population birth cohort followed into midadulthood, there was a clear impact of genetic risk on the likelihood of childhood asthma persisting to adulthood and for development of chronic airflow obstruction.[19] A genetic risk score (GRS) was determined

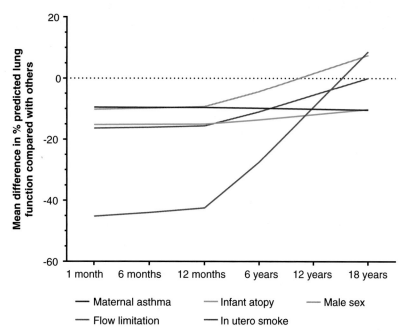

FIG. 17.2 The mean difference in percent predicted lung function at ages 1 month to 18 years for those exposed to identified risk factors compared with individuals without those factors, representing trajectories of altered lung growth from infancy due to risk factors. (Adapted from Turner S, Fielding S, Mullane D, et al. A longitudinal study of lung function from 1 month to 18 years of age. *Thorax*. 2014;69:1015–1020; with permission.)

in each of 880 Caucasian study members, based on the actual number of alleles of 15 asthma-associated single nucleotide polymorphisms (SNPs) as reported in previous genome wide association studies, including SNPs located in or near the genes *IL18R1, IL13, HLA-DQ, IL33, SMAD3, ORMDL3, GSDMB, GSDMA,* and *IL2RB.* The population distribution of the 15 examined SNPs (30 alleles) was bell-shaped, with a median GRS of 13.7 alleles and SD 4.4. Individuals with a low asthma GRS (defined as GRS 2.0 SD below median) had a 13% risk of developing irreversible airflow obstruction by age 38 years, compared with a 37% risk for those with a high asthma GRS (2.0 SD above median) (Fig. 17.3).

Yamada et al.[20] demonstrated that a multi-SNP GRS for lower FEV_1/FVC (forced exhaled volume in 1 s/ forced vital capacity) was consistently associated with the onset of asthma in two independent populations as well as with the onset of COPD defined by lung function parameters. An increased GRS score may be responsible for the development of a particular phenotype of asthma characterized by early onset, atopy, and more severe airflow obstruction. In the Childhood Asthma Management Program (CAMP) study[21] an intergenic SNP rs4445257 on chromosome 8 was strongly associated with the pattern of normal lung function growth followed by early decline compared

with all other pattern groups. Intriguingly, this variant also appeared to protect against early decline in lung function in groups with reduced lung growth. Associations were determined in nonsmokers in the LifeLines cohort[22] between the FEV_1/FVC ratio and the genes *HHIP* and *FAM13A*, indicating a genetic risk for airway obstruction not driven by cigarette smoking.

Gene-environment interactions likewise have an impact on lung function. In a Latino population,[23] a genetic variant of *Plasminogen activator inhibitor-1 (PAI-1)*, in association with early life viral bronchiolitis, increased the risk of asthma and reduced the lung function. Further evidence of gene-environment interactions impacting lung function was provided by Forno et al.[24] who demonstrated in a Puerto Rican population that house-dust mite allergen exposure modified the effect of the SNP rs117902240 on lung function, being positively associated with FEV_1 in children exposed to low levels of mite allergen, but negatively associated with FEV_1 in children exposed to high levels, suggesting this SNP may have transcription factor regulatory functions.

Data from the Isle of Wight cohort[25] indicated the importance of epigenetics in impacting lung function in asthma. DNA methylation at a specific site was influenced by the interaction of maternal smoking during pregnancy and the functional SNP *rs20541* of the *IL-13*

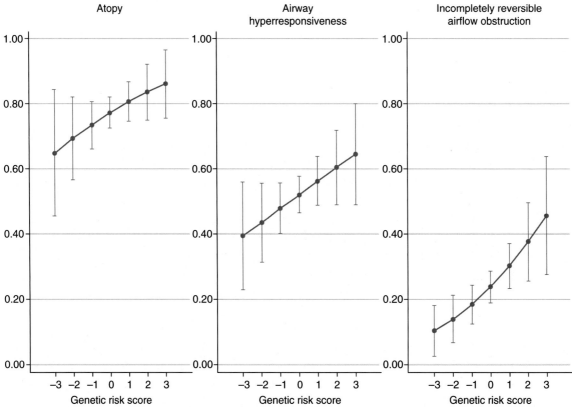

FIG. 17.3 Relationship between genetic risk score (X-axis, shown as median and standard deviations [z-scores] for number of asthma-related alleles) and prevalence of characteristics of asthma (atopy, airway hyperresponsiveness, and incompletely reversible airflow obstruction) in Caucasian participants in the Dunedin Multidisciplinary Research and Development study, demonstrating increased likelihood of persistent airflow obstruction in those at greater genetic risk. (From Belsky DW, Sears MR, Hancox RJ, et al. Polygenic risk and the development and course of asthma: An analysis of data from a four-decade longitudinal study. *Lancet Respir Med*. 2013;1:453–461; with permission.)

gene, while another *IL-13* SNP rs1800925 interacted with that methylation site to significantly affect airflow limitation and airway responsiveness. A later report from the same study[26] linked other methylation sites to airway obstruction and asthma, with replication of the direction of effect in the Barn Allergi Miljo Stockholm Epidemiologi (BAMSE) cohort in Sweden. A recent randomized controlled trial suggested administration of vitamin C may normalize DNA methylation related to maternal smoking, offering a possible therapeutic option for mitigating this epigenetic effect.[27]

PROGRESSION OF ASTHMA TO CHRONIC OBSTRUCTIVE PULMONARY DISEASE

COPD is a heterogeneous disease, classically encompassing both primarily airway pathology (chronic bronchitis)

and destructive alveolar disease (emphysema), and is often associated with a neutrophilic inflammatory response of the lungs in response to noxious agents.[28] The diagnosis is usually considered in patients with a history of exposure to known risk factors, especially cigarette smoking. Like asthma, COPD is classically defined as a lung disease characterized by symptoms of wheezing, cough, sputum production, and/or dyspnea, but unlike asthma, it is generally associated with smoking and is characterized by chronic airflow obstruction that is not fully reversible spontaneously or with bronchodilators. These symptoms may precede the development of airflow limitation, and vice versa.

The severity of COPD is measured not only by symptoms but now primarily by lung function, namely FEV_1 and its relation to FVC as the ratio, FEV_1/FVC. These measurements have been shown to correlate with pathologic findings[29] and to predict mortality.[30] These functional criteria for assessment of COPD have led to a greater awareness of airflow obstruction developing in the absence of identifiable noxious inhalants (particularly cigarette smoking) in up to 20%–25% of individuals.[31] Recently, the definition of COPD has tended to be based solely on spirometric measurements, namely FEV_1 <70% predicted or FEV_1/FVC ratio <0.7. This definition has resulted in the recognition of, or at least suggested, a somewhat controversial new phenotype of lung disease, the asthma-COPD overlap syndrome (ACOS), encompassing individuals who have features of both asthma and COPD; this may include asthma that has developed progressive and partly irreversible airflow obstruction, with or without exposure to known risk factors for COPD.

HISTORICAL CONCEPTS OF DEVELOPMENT OF CHRONIC OBSTRUCTIVE PULMONARY DISEASE

Fletcher and Peto[32] described the development of COPD in a prospective cohort study of respiratory symptoms in a large group of working men and theorized that smoking caused an accelerated irreversible loss of lung function in susceptible individuals leading to COPD and symptoms. A key feature of the Fletcher and Peto theory was that adults attain maximal lung function before experiencing accelerated decline. However, they concluded their paper with several key questions including the role of childhood infections in impairing lung function.

In the same year, Burrows et al.[33] examined the relationship between a retrospectively recalled history of childhood respiratory problems and chronic obstructive symptoms in a population-based cohort of adults. They described a relationship between a history of childhood respiratory problems and lower maximally attained adult lung function. Furthermore, they theorized that acute respiratory infections of childhood not only lead to a decrease in maximal adult lung function but also increased the individual's susceptibility to a more rapid decline in adulthood. Notably the childhood respiratory problems were due to asthma in a third of cases in this data set.

Advocates of the Dutch hypotheses[34,35] posit that there is a wide variation in adult lung function and that susceptibility to COPD is partly determined by early life factors. Furthermore, there are likely multiple distinct heterogeneous pathways to the development of COPD in adulthood, including failure to attain normal adult peak lung function followed by a normal decline, as well as accelerated adult decline in lung function regardless of the peak adult lung function.

ASTHMA EVOLUTION INTO FUNCTIONALLY DEFINED CHRONIC OBSTRUCTIVE PULMONARY DISEASE

Multiple large cohort studies have confirmed that the risk of COPD in adulthood, as defined by lung function, is increased among those with a history of childhood asthma.[35-37] This relationship is sustained in the absence of smoking and is not related to social status. The pathway to COPD, however, differs across studies and asthma definitions.

Several studies suggest that chronic or severe childhood asthma is associated with lower peak adult lung function but not necessarily an accelerated decline in adulthood.[36-38] A longitudinal study of lung function in a cohort of children with mild to moderate asthma enrolled at a mean age of 9 years and followed through the first three decades of life (CAMP) shed light on four different possible patterns of lung function growth[39] (Fig. 17.4). Normal lung growth is characterized by a steep increase in adolescence, a plateau in early adulthood, and a gradual decline with aging. Abnormal lung growth patterns included normal childhood growth and an early and accelerated decline; reduced childhood growth with suboptimal peak in adult lung function but usual rate of decline; and, finally, reduced childhood growth with an early and accelerated decline. Only 25% of the CAMP study children with asthma were classified as having a normal pattern of growth of lung function; 26% had normal childhood growth but early decline; 23% had reduced childhood growth in lung function; and 26% showed reduced childhood lung function growth and early decline. Participants with reduced lung growth patterns met spirometric criteria for COPD as early as their third decade of life. Risk factors for reduced growth patterns included lower lung function at enrollment, lower bronchodilator responsiveness, increased airway hyperresponsiveness, longer duration of asthma, male sex, and greater number of atopic skin prick tests. Of these, the strongest risk factors appeared to be impaired lung function at an early age and male sex.

Berry and colleagues reported similar findings in the Tucson general population cohort, which was followed up to the fourth decade of life, with serial measurements of lung function.[40] Latent class analysis was used to cluster participants based on lung function patterns. Persistent low lung function was observed in 9%; these individuals were more likely to have asthma, to

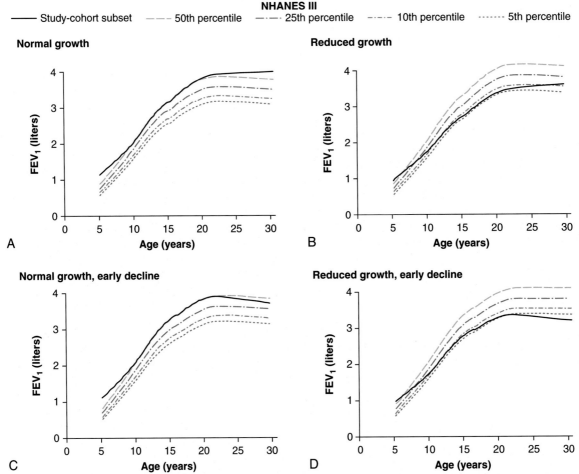

FIG. 17.4 Trajectories of lung function growth and decline in the Childhood Asthma Management Program (CAMP) study, demonstrating **(A)** normal growth, **(B)** reduced growth without decline, **(C)** normal growth with early decline, and **(D)** reduced growth with early decline. (From McGeachie MJ, Yates KP, Zhou X, et al. Patterns of Growth and Decline in Lung Function in Persistent Childhood Asthma. *N Engl J Med*. 2016;374:1842–1852; with permission.)

have a maternal history of asthma, and to have had an increased risk of lower respiratory tract illness due to RSV in their first 3 years of life.

NEONATAL CONTRIBUTION TO FUNCTIONALLY DEFINED CHRONIC OBSTRUCTIVE PULMONARY DISEASE

The Barker hypothesis, now generally referred to as the Developmental Origins of Health and Disease (DOHaD), posits that long-term programming occurs through intrauterine and early childhood exposures, setting an individual's trajectory toward the

development of adult health and disease.[41] This theory challenged the prior view that degenerative diseases resulted primarily from an interaction between genes and adverse adult environment exposures. Specifically, longitudinal studies of birth records of some 5000 individuals in England during the 1900s suggest that birth weight and lower respiratory infection during infancy were strong predictors of adult lung function independent of smoking status and social class.[42] Later studies and metaanalyses have confirmed the positive association between increasing birth weight and FEV_1.[43] Other cohorts examining in utero factors underlying the association suggest that maternal undernutrition may play an important role.[44,45] Studies during the Dutch famine suggest that the period of greatest risk is early- to mid-estation,[45] whereas other studies suggest the early critical window may extend from in utero through the first year of life. In a cohort comprising both small for gestational age and appropriate for gestational age infants, impairment in lung function in early life related not only to birth weight but also to a complex causal relationship with postnatal social disadvantage.[46–48] Furthermore, early life tracking of these initial decrements in lung function[48] proved that they persisted through infancy. In turn, low lung function acts during early childhood as a risk factor for severe lower respiratory illnesses causing further lung injury and subsequent further progression of a worsening trajectory of lung function growth[49] and asthma.[50]

THE ASTHMA-CHRONIC OBSTRUCTIVE PULMONARY DISEASE OVERLAP SYNDROME

In recent years, the term asthma-COPD overlap syndrome has been used to describe patients with airway disease with characteristics of both asthma and COPD.[51,52] In the majority of studies examining characteristics of ACOS, the detection of COPD was predicated by an impairment of lung function with a postbronchodilator FEV_1 below 70% predicted or FEV_1/FVC ratio below 0.7. Longitudinal follow-up in the Dunedin study provided evidence of airway remodeling and progression of functional loss leading to a degree of fixed or less reversible airflow obstruction as early as age 18 years.[53] It seems probable that the majority of individuals with ACOS have asthma with remodeling and a component of irreversible airflow obstruction that meets the spirometric criteria for COPD, without having the usual clinical features of COPD. Not surprisingly, given this definition, many of these "ACOS" patients do not have any of the usual risk factors for classic COPD such as smoking or other noxious substance exposure. Detailed analyses of characteristics of these "ACOS" patients show that the majority of features are consistent with asthma, with greater eosinophilia, greater airway hyperresponsiveness, greater response to corticosteroids, and greater bronchodilator responses than seen in studies of patients with classic COPD.[54–58] These patients should be recognized as having chronic persistent asthma with airway remodeling, which has progressed to less reversible airflow obstruction, rather than being considered to have two diseases as implied in the "ACOS" designation.

Bui et al.[59] recently described adult outcomes of the Tasmanian longitudinal health study and showed that being in the lowest quartile for lung function at age 7 years had long-term consequences for the development of COPD and ACOS by middle age. In this study, COPD, and therefore ACOS, was defined solely on the basis of spirometric measurements showing airflow obstruction. Among those with a history of asthma and meeting criteria for ACOS, 93% were using inhaled medications, whereas among those without a history of asthma but who met the same physiologic criteria for COPD, none was using medication, indicating essentially asymptomatic airflow obstruction and not the classic disease known as COPD. This underscores the point that ACOS most often represents progression of chronic asthma causing airflow obstruction rather than a combination of two separate diseases. Several authors have suggested that the term ACOS should be abandoned.[60,61]

EARLY DETECTION OF ASTHMA AND PREVENTION OF PROGRESSION

The ultimate goal of primary prevention of asthma remains elusive, as discussed by Stokes and Bacharier elsewhere in this volume, but recent cohort findings related to the gut microbiome certainly suggest this may not be an impossible target.[62] Secondary and tertiary prevention measures have been invoked for many decades, focusing on lifestyle, avoidance of exposures, and optimal pharmacotherapy, but little is known about how these strategies impact the trajectory of asthma through the life-course and whether they reduce the progression of disease toward chronic and irreversible airflow obstruction.

Early Detection of Loss of Function in Children With Asthma

Early recognition of the development of asthma manifested by a history of recurrent episodes of wheezing in early childhood, especially if accompanied by allergen sensitization, should prompt regular and routine lung function monitoring, which is strongly encouraged for all children with asthma. Those with early and persistent loss of function indicating obstruction should be even more closely monitored. It is important to recognize that the "normal values" for lung function parameters are substantially different in young children, e.g., the normal FEV_1/FVC ratio in a 5-year-old is not >75% but in fact >90%.[63] Physical growth also changes lung function parameters so that simply following serial absolute numbers for spirometric variables may obscure functional abnormalities. The FEV_1/FVC ratio gradually declines from >90% to 82%–85% in adolescence and is appropriate to monitor. Younger children (preschoolers) may be able to perform spirometry with good coaching, but very young children may require other measures such as lung clearance index based on inert gas washout techniques in a specialized laboratory.[64]

Lifestyle Factors

Lung protection strategies such as avoidance of noxious inhalants including cigarette and other inhaled smoke (passive and active) should be implemented, together with awareness and avoidance of relevant deleterious occupational exposures. The recent decrease in the prevalence of childhood recurrent wheezing and asthma in many developed countries may reflect the substantial decrease in maternal smoking during pregnancy. In the ongoing Canadian Healthy Infant Longitudinal Development study,[65] less than 4% of mothers admitted to smoking during pregnancy. Although 13% of fathers or visitors to the home smoked, almost all indicated they smoked outdoors or away from the pregnant mother or young child.

Reduction of Allergen Sensitization

A recent analysis from the Dunedin longitudinal birth cohort study showed that adults with asthma and persistent airflow obstruction were almost all atopic (Fig. 17.5).[19] If sensitization can be reduced, asthma may be reduced, and persistence and severity particularly favorably impacted.

Measures to reduce the likelihood of allergen sensitization have been widely studied, with conflicting and often disappointing results. Allergen avoidance, such as banning pets in the home, using dust-impermeable bedding to reduce house dust mite allergen exposure, have had limited success, in part because interventions such as these likely need to be multiple[66,67] and secondly because avoidance may, in fact, be the wrong strategy as now recognized with peanut allergy.[68] Many cohort studies now clearly indicate that exposure to a farming environment, farm animals, and domestic pets (especially dogs) confers substantial protection against development of inhalant sensitization.[69,70] Early rather than delayed introduction of "allergenic" foods appears to induce tolerance and reduce the risk of food sensitization,[68,71] which may reduce the risk of initiation of the "atopic march" from atopic dermatitis in infancy to childhood asthma.

Pharmacologic Management

It is unclear at this time whether pharmacologic treatments or other strategies can prevent the loss of lung

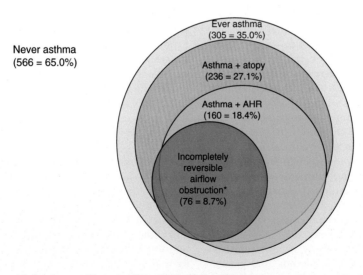

*defined as post-bronchodilator FEV$_1$/FVC >2SD below mean for normal subjects

FIG. 17.5 Prevalence of characteristics of asthma (atopy, airway hyperresponsiveness, and incompletely reversible airflow obstruction) in 871 Caucasian participants in the Dunedin Multidisciplinary Research and Development study, demonstrating that 90% of adult study members with persisting airflow obstruction are atopic with airway hyperresponsiveness (AHR). (From Belsky DW, Sears MR, Hancox RJ, et al. Polygenic risk and the development and course of asthma: an analysis of data from a four-decade longitudinal study. *Lancet Respir Med*. 2013;1:453–461; with permission.)

function or restore lost function. The CAMP study[39] failed to show any protection against lung function decline among children given inhaled corticosteroid treatment. These data are consistent with several other studies that have shown that, despite improved symptoms, no currently available therapies improve lung growth or return impaired lung function to normal.[72,73]

There have been some intriguing insights into the use of antioxidants in improving lung function. One randomized controlled trial of vitamin C supplementation in pregnant smoking women showed an improvement in lung function of their infants.[74] In this study 179 women were randomized to receive vitamin C supplementation or placebo during pregnancy. Infant lung function along with wheeze phenotypes were assessed up to 1 year of age. Newborn pulmonary function was improved slightly in those treated with antioxidants, with almost 50% reduction in wheeze. However, the effects on lung function were not sustained through the first year of life. Finally, there was a gene-environment interaction in that mothers with polymorphisms in the nicotinic acetylcholine receptor, which have been associated with COPD, showed the greatest impact of maternal smoking on lung function.[74]

There is increasing evidence that low levels of vitamin D in early childhood have an impact on childhood lung function. In the Perth birth cohort, vitamin D deficiency was associated with impaired lung function in children of both sexes at age 6 years ($P<.02$ for both) and threefold increased risk of asthma in boys ($P=.04$).[75] Similarly, in the Generation R study, in which vitamin D levels were measured in maternal blood in midgestation maternal blood and again in cord blood, children in the lowest tertile of vitamin D levels at birth had a higher airway resistance compared with those in the highest tertile.[76] Adjustment for current vitamin D levels at age 6 years reduced the effect size of the association, suggesting the loss of function could be improved by improving childhood vitamin D intake. Among full-term infants in Taiwan, low cord blood levels were significantly associated with poorer lung function and a higher likelihood of respiratory infection before 6 months of age ($P<.01$ for both outcomes).[77]

Other pertinent risk factors include severe lower respiratory tract infections, both viral and bacterial in early life. The advent of novel approaches of examining the microbiome have shed new light on colonization of the lower airways in infants destined to develop asthma and may indicate a group with altered host-immune responses and therefore increased susceptibility to severe lower airway infection. This may provide a mechanism for immune alteration using probiotics and potential prevention of chronic airway disease.

SUMMARY

Chronic airway disease manifested as asthma is influenced by exposures during critical periods of prenatal and postnatal lung growth and development, as well as by genetic risk. Further studies must focus on discerning more precisely the effects of putative risk factors, which in some instances may be dependent on the timing of exposure during critical developmental windows. Strategies to reduce the early development of allergy and asthma, through a combination of lifestyle factors in pregnancy and early infancy, together with novel immunologic and pharmacologic interventions throughout childhood, may provide tools to limit the progression of airway pathology and the development of persistent airflow obstruction.

Despite the availability of therapies effective in controlling symptoms in asthma, there are currently no proven therapeutic options to improve or halt the loss of lung function in subjects with asthma. Therefore, current strategies must be aimed at secondary prevention of progression which may be achieved by the following:

1. **Early identification of at-risk individuals using pulmonary function assessments**
   Use of standardized pulmonary function tests should be implemented as early as possible to identify those individuals whose function is falling below the limits of normality after race correction. It is important to consider the population studied to develop reference equations for lung function. If the population used to generate normative date include subjects who are exposed to known lung-damaging agents such as secondary smoke exposure, the broader limits of normality due to the inclusion of subjects with early subtle lung damage may result in underestimation of disease. Additionally, studies of healthy populations must further define normal longitudinal growth trajectories in healthy children, which will allow clinicians to identify children with abnormal growth patterns earlier.
2. **Targeted lung health promotion strategies** such as directed counseling to avoid cigarette smoke exposure and harmful occupational inhalant exposures should be aimed at individuals identified as at higher risk based on impaired pulmonary function.

REFERENCES

1. Martinez FD, Wright AL, Taussig LM, Holberg CJ, Halonen M, Morgan WJ, Asthma and wheezing in the first six years of life. The Group Health Medical Associates. *N Engl J Med*. 1995;332:133–138.
2. Henderson J, Granell R, Heron J, et al. Associations of wheezing phenotypes in the first 6 years of life with atopy, lung function and airway responsiveness in mid-childhood. *Thorax*. 2008;63:974–980.
3. Savenije OE, Granell R, Caudri D, et al. Comparison of childhood wheezing phenotypes in 2 birth cohorts: ALSPAC and PIAMA. *J Allergy Clin Immunol*. 2011;127:1505 e14–1512.e14.
4. Sears MR, Greene JM, Willan AR, et al. A longitudinal, population-based, cohort study of childhood asthma followed to adulthood. *N Engl J Med*. 2003;349:1414–1422.
5. Jackson DJ, Gangnon RE, Evans MD, et al. Wheezing rhinovirus illnesses in early life predict asthma development in high-risk children. *Am J Respir Crit Care Med*. 2008;178:667–672.
6. Stein RT, Sherrill D, Morgan WJ, et al. Respiratory syncytial virus in early life and risk of wheeze and allergy by age 13 years. *Lancet*. 1999;354:541–545.
7. Henderson J, Hilliard TN, Sherriff A, Stalker D, Al Shammari N, Thomas HM. Hospitalization for RSV bronchiolitis before 12 months of age and subsequent asthma, atopy and wheeze: a longitudinal birth cohort study. *Pediatr Allergy Immunol*. 2005;16:386–392.
8. Holt PG, Sly PD. Viral infections and atopy in asthma pathogenesis: new rationales for asthma prevention and treatment. *Nat Med*. 2012;18:726–735.
9. Simpson A, Tan VY, Winn J, et al. Beyond atopy: multiple patterns of sensitization in relation to asthma in a birth cohort study. *Am J Respir Crit Care Med*. 2010;181:1200–1206.
10. Lazic N, Roberts G, Custovic A, et al. Multiple atopy phenotypes and their associations with asthma: similar findings from two birth cohorts. *Allergy*. 2013;68:764–770.
11. Turner SW, Palmer LJ, Rye PJ, et al. Infants with flow limitation at 4 weeks: outcome at 6 and 11 years. *Am J Respir Crit Care Med*. 2002;165:1294–1298.
12. Bisgaard H, Jensen SM, Bonnelykke K. Interaction between asthma and lung function growth in early life. *Am J Respir Crit Care Med*. 2012;185:1183–1189.
13. Turner S, Fielding S, Mullane D, et al. A longitudinal study of lung function from 1 month to 18 years of age. *Thorax*. 2014;69:1015–1020.
14. Bisgaard H, Loland L, Holst KK, Pipper CB. Prenatal determinants of neonatal lung function in high-risk newborns. *J Allergy Clin Immunol*. 2009;123:651–657. 657.e1–657.e4.
15. Young S, Arnott J, O'Keeffe PT, Le Souef PN, Landau LI. The association between early life lung function and wheezing during the first 2 yrs of life. *Eur Respir J*. 2000;15:151–157.
16. Kerkhof M, Boezen HM, Granell R, et al. Transient early wheeze and lung function in early childhood associated with chronic obstructive pulmonary disease genes. *J Allergy Clin Immunol*. 2014;133:68–76.e1–e4.
17. Stern DA, Morgan WJ, Wright AL, Guerra S, Martinez FD. Poor airway function in early infancy and lung function by age 22 years: a non-selective longitudinal cohort study. *Lancet*. 2007;370:758–764.
18. Mullane D, Turner SW, Cox DW, Goldblatt J, Landau LI, le Souef PN. Reduced infant lung function, active smoking, and wheeze in 18-year-old individuals. *JAMA Pediatr*. 2013;167:368–373.
19. Belsky DW, Sears MR, Hancox RJ, et al. Polygenic risk and the development and course of asthma: an analysis of data from a four-decade longitudinal study. *Lancet Res Med*. 2013;1:453–461.
20. Yamada H, Masuko H, Yatagai Y, et al. Role of lung function genes in the development of asthma. *PLoS One*. 2016;11:e0145832.
21. McGeachie MJ, Yates KP, Zhou X, et al. Genetics and genomics of longitudinal lung function patterns in individuals with asthma. *Am J Respir Crit Care Med*. 2016;194:1465–1474.
22. van der Plaat DA, de Jong K, Lahousse L, et al. Genome-wide association study on the FEV1/FVC ratio in never-smokers identifies HHIP and FAM13A. *J Allergy Clin Immunol*. 2017;139:533–540.
23. Cho SH, Min JY, Kim DY, et al. Association of a PAI-1 gene polymorphism and early life infections with asthma risk, exacerbations, and reduced lung function. *PLoS One*. 2016;11:e0157848.
24. Forno E, Sordillo J, Brehm J, et al. Genome-wide interaction study of dust mite allergen on lung function in children with asthma. *J Allergy Clin Immunol*. 2017. http://dx.doi.org/10.1016/j.jaci.2016.12.967.
25. Patil VK, Holloway JW, Zhang H, et al. Interaction of prenatal maternal smoking, interleukin 13 genetic variants and DNA methylation influencing airflow and airway reactivity. *Clin Epigenetics*. 2013;5:22.
26. Mukherjee N, Lockett GA, Merid SK, et al. DNA methylation and genetic polymorphisms of the Leptin gene interact to influence lung function outcomes and asthma at 18 years of age. *Int J Mol Epidemiol Genet*. 2016;7:1–17.
27. Shorey-Kendrick LE, McEvoy CT, Ferguson B, et al. Vitamin C prevents offspring DNA methylation changes associated with maternal smoking in pregnancy. *Am J Respir Crit Care Med*. 2017. http://dx.doi.org/10.1164/rccm.201610-2141OC.
28. Pauwels RA, Buist AS, Calverley PM, Jenkins CR, Hurd SS. Global strategy for the diagnosis, management, and prevention of chronic obstructive pulmonary disease. NHLBI/WHO Global Initiative for Chronic Obstructive Lung Disease (GOLD) Workshop summary. *Am J Respir Crit Care Med*. 2001;163:1256–1276.
29. Hogg JC, Chu F, Utokaparch S, et al. The nature of small-airway obstruction in chronic obstructive pulmonary disease. *N Engl J Med*. 2004;350:2645–2653.
30. Mannino DM, Doherty DE, Sonia Buist A. Global initiative on obstructive lung disease (GOLD) classification of lung disease and mortality: findings from the atherosclerosis risk in communities (ARIC) study. *Respir Med*. 2006;100:115–122.
31. Eisner MD, Anthonisen N, Coultas D, et al. An official American Thoracic Society public policy statement:

novel risk factors and the global burden of chronic obstructive pulmonary disease. *Am J Respir Crit Care Med.* 2010;182:693–718.

32. Fletcher C, Peto R. The natural history of chronic airflow obstruction. *Br Med J.* 1977;1:1645–1648.

33. Burrows B, Knudson RJ, Lebowitz MD. The relationship of childhood respiratory illness to adult obstructive airway disease. *Am Rev Respir Dis.* 1977;115:751–760.

34. Postma DS, Weiss ST, van den Berge M, Kerstjens HA, Koppelman GH. Revisiting the Dutch hypothesis. *J Allergy Clin Immunol.* 2015;136:521–529.

35. Svanes C, Sunyer J, Plana E, et al. Early life origins of chronic obstructive pulmonary disease. *Thorax.* 2010;65:14–20.

36. Lodge CJ, Lowe AJ, Allen KJ, et al. Childhood wheeze phenotypes show less than expected growth in FEV1 across adolescence. *Am J Respir Crit Care Med.* 2014;189:1351–1358.

37. Tai A, Tran H, Roberts M, Clarke N, Wilson J, Robertson CF. The association between childhood asthma and adult chronic obstructive pulmonary disease. *Thorax.* 2014;69:805–810.

38. Tagiyeva N, Devereux G, Fielding S, Turner S, Douglas G. Outcomes of childhood asthma and wheezy bronchitis. A 50-year cohort study. *Am J Respir Crit Care Med.* 2016;193:23–30.

39. McGeachie MJ, Yates KP, Zhou X, et al. Patterns of growth and decline in lung function in persistent childhood asthma. *N Engl J Med.* 2016;374:1842–1852.

40. Berry CE, Billheimer D, Jenkins IC, et al. A distinct low lung function trajectory from childhood to the fourth decade of life. *Am J Respir Crit Care Med.* 2016;194:607–612.

41. Barker DJ. The fetal and infant origins of adult disease. *BMJ.* 1990;301:1111.

42. Barker DJ, Godfrey KM, Fall C, Osmond C, Winter PD, Shaheen SO. Relation of birth weight and childhood respiratory infection to adult lung function and death from chronic obstructive airways disease. *BMJ.* 1991;303:671–675.

43. Lawlor DA, Ebrahim S, Davey Smith G. Association of birth weight with adult lung function: findings from the British Women's Heart and Health Study and a meta-analysis. *Thorax.* 2005;60:851–858.

44. Stein CE, Kumaran K, Fall CH, Shaheen SO, Osmond C, Barker DJ. Relation of fetal growth to adult lung function in south India. *Thorax.* 1997;52:895–899.

45. Lopuhaa CE, Roseboom TJ, Osmond C, et al. Atopy, lung function, and obstructive airways disease after prenatal exposure to famine. *Thorax.* 2000;55:555–561.

46. Dezateux C, Lum S, Hoo AF, Hawdon J, Costeloe K, Stocks J. Low birth weight for gestation and airway function in infancy: exploring the fetal origins hypothesis. *Thorax.* 2004;59:60–66.

47. Dezateux C, Stocks J, Wade AM, Dundas I, Fletcher ME. Airway function at one year: association with premorbid airway function, wheezing, and maternal smoking. *Thorax.* 2001;56:680–686.

48. Hoo AF, Stocks J, Lum S, et al. Development of lung function in early life: influence of birth weight in infants of nonsmokers. *Am J Respir Crit Care Med.* 2004;170:527–533.

49. Shaheen SO, Sterne JA, Tucker JS, Florey CD. Birth weight, childhood lower respiratory tract infection, and adult lung function. *Thorax.* 1998;53:549–553.

50. Haland G, Carlsen KC, Sandvik L, et al. Reduced lung function at birth and the risk of asthma at 10 years of age. *N Engl J Med.* 2006;355:1682–1689.

51. Postma DS, Rabe KF. The asthma-COPD overlap syndrome. *N Engl J Med.* 2015;373:1241–1249.

52. Gibson PG, McDonald VM. Asthma-COPD overlap 2015: now we are six. *Thorax.* 2015;70:683–691.

53. Rasmussen F, Taylor DR, Flannery EM, et al. Risk factors for airway remodeling in asthma manifested by a low postbronchodilator FEV1/vital capacity ratio: a longitudinal population study from childhood to adulthood. *Am J Respir Crit Care Med.* 2002;165:1480–1488.

54. Tkacova R, Dai DL, Vonk JM, et al. Airway hyperresponsiveness in chronic obstructive pulmonary disease: a marker of asthma-chronic obstructive pulmonary disease overlap syndrome? *J Allergy Clin Immunol.* 2016;138:1571 e10–1579 e10.

55. Kitaguchi Y, Yasuo M, Hanaoka M. Comparison of pulmonary function in patients with COPD, asthma-COPD overlap syndrome, and asthma with airflow limitation. *Int J Chron Obstruct Pulmon Dis.* 2016;11:991–997.

56. Suzuki M, Makita H, Konno S, et al. Asthma-like features and clinical course of chronic obstructive pulmonary disease. An analysis from the Hokkaido COPD cohort study. *Am J Respir Crit Care Med.* 2016;194:1358–1365.

57. Hynes G, Pavord ID. Asthma-like features and chronic obstructive pulmonary disease. *Am J Respir Crit Care Med.* 2016;194:1308–1309.

58. Rogliani P, Ora J, Puxeddu E, Cazzola M. Airflow obstruction: is it asthma or is it COPD? *Int J Chron Obstruct Pulmon Dis.* 2016;11:3007–3013.

59. Bui DS, Burgess JA, Lowe AJ, et al. Childhood lung function predicts adult COPD and asthma-COPD overlap syndrome (ACOS). *Am J Respir Crit Care Med.* 2017;196:39–46.

60. Cazzola M, Rogliani P. Do we really need asthma-chronic obstructive pulmonary disease overlap syndrome? *J Allergy Clin Immunol.* 2016;138:977–983.

61. Barnes PJ. Asthma-COPD overlap. *Chest.* 2016;149:7–8.

62. Stiemsma LT, Arrieta MC, Dimitriu PA, et al. Shifts in *Lachnospira* and *Clostridium* sp. in the 3-month stool microbiome are associated with preschool age asthma. *Clin Sci (Lond).* 2016;130:2199–2207.

63. Quanjer PH, Stanojevic S, Stocks J, et al. Changes in the FEV(1)/FVC ratio during childhood and adolescence: an intercontinental study. *Eur Respir J.* 2010;36:1391–1399.

64. Rosenfeld M, Allen J, Arets BH, et al. An official American Thoracic Society workshop report: optimal lung function tests for monitoring cystic fibrosis, bronchopulmonary dysplasia, and recurrent wheezing in children less than 6 years of age. *Ann Am Thorac Soc.* 2013;10:S1–S11.

65. Subbarao P, Anand SS, Becker AB, et al. The Canadian Healthy Infant Longitudinal Development (CHILD) Study: examining developmental origins of allergy and asthma. *Thorax.* 2015;70:998–1000.

66. Arshad SH, Bateman B, Matthews SM. Primary prevention of asthma and atopy during childhood by allergen avoidance in infancy: a randomised controlled study. *Thorax.* 2003;58:489–493.

67. Chan-Yeung M, Ferguson A, Watson W, et al. The Canadian childhood asthma primary prevention study: outcomes at 7 years of age. *J Allergy Clin Immunol.* 2005;116:49–55.

68. Du Toit G, Roberts G, Sayre PH, et al. Randomized trial of peanut consumption in infants at risk for peanut allergy. *N Engl J Med.* 2015;372:803–813.

69. Fall T, Lundholm C, Ortqvist AK, et al. Early exposure to dogs and farm animals and the risk of childhood asthma. *JAMA Pediatr.* 2015;169:e153219.

70. Ownby DR, Johnson CC. Dogs, cats, and asthma: will we ever really know the true risks and benefits? *J Allergy Clin Immunol.* 2016;138:1591–1592.

71. Perkin MR, Logan K, Marrs T, et al. Enquiring about Tolerance (EAT) study: feasibility of an early allergenic food introduction regimen. *J Allergy Clin Immunol.* 2016;137: 1477 e8–1486 e8.

72. Waalkens HJ, Van Essen-Zandvliet EE, Hughes MD, et al. Cessation of long-term treatment with inhaled corticosteroid (budesonide) in children with asthma results in deterioration. The Dutch CNSLD Study Group. *Am Rev Respir Dis.* 1993;148:1252–1257.

73. Strunk RC, Sternberg AL, Szefler SJ, et al. Long-term budesonide or nedocromil treatment, once discontinued, does not alter the course of mild to moderate asthma in children and adolescents. *J Pediatr.* 2009;154:682–687.

74. McEvoy CT, Schilling D, Clay N, et al. Vitamin C supplementation for pregnant smoking women and pulmonary function in their newborn infants: a randomized clinical trial. *JAMA.* 2014;311:2074–2082.

75. Zosky GR, Hart PH, Whitehouse AJ, et al. Vitamin D deficiency at 16 to 20 weeks' gestation is associated with impaired lung function and asthma at 6 years of age. *Ann Am Thorac Soc.* 2014;11:571–577.

76. Gazibara T, den Dekker HT, de Jongste JC, et al. Associations of maternal and fetal 25-hydroxyvitamin D levels with childhood lung function and asthma: the Generation R Study. *Clin Exp Allergy.* 2016;46:337–346.

77. Lai SH, Liao SL, Tsai MH, et al. Low cord-serum 25-hydroxyvitamin D levels are associated with poor lung function performance and increased respiratory infection in infancy. *PLoS One.* 2017;12:e0173268.

CHAPTER 18

Imaging Procedures and Bronchial Thermoplasty for Asthma Assessment and Intervention

SHWETA SOOD, MD, MS • CHASE HALL, MD • MARIO CASTRO, MD, MPH

ABBREVIATIONS

ADC   Apparent diffusion coefficient
ATS   American Thoracic Society
AWA   Airway wall area
AWT   Airway wall thickness
BT   Bronchial thermoplasty
COPD   Chronic obstructive pulmonary disease
CT   Computed tomography
EBUS   Endobronchial ultrasound
ED   Emergency department
ERS   European Respiratory Society
FDA   U.S. Food and Drug Administration
FEV$_1$ Forced expiratory volume in 1 s
HP MRI   Hyperpolarized MRI
HRCT   High-resolution computed tomography
HU   Hounsfield units
ICS   Inhaled corticosteroids
LA   Lumen area
LABA   Long-acting β-agonists
MDCT   Multidetector CT
OCT   Optical coherence tomography
PEF   Peak expiratory flow
PET   Positron emission tomography
PFT   Pulmonary function testing
qCT   Quantitative CT
QOL   Quality of life
RF   Radiofrequency
TLC   Total lung capacity
X-ray   Radiation

INTRODUCTION

Asthma is characterized by airway epithelial injury, subepithelial fibrosis, excess mucus secretion, airway inflammation, increased airway smooth muscle (ASM) mass, and dysregulated angiogenesis collectively referred to as airway remodeling.[1-3]

Remodeling causes variable airflow obstruction. Airflow obstruction results in reduced lung ventilation, which in turn leads to decreased lung perfusion.[4] Abnormal ventilation and perfusion can lead to air trapping and worsen asthma symptoms. The diagnosis of asthma is based on history, physical examination, pulmonary function tests (PFTs), and bronchoprovocation testing.[5] In the clinical setting, imaging techniques are rapidly evolving to detect remodeling changes and assess response to approved and emerging asthma therapies, such as bronchial thermoplasty (BT).

Historically, asthma severity and the efficacy of asthma treatments have been grossly assessed with subjective assessments and spirometry. However, asthma is a heterogeneous disease because some airways have marked remodeling whereas others have minimal remodeling. Current modalities of assessment cannot detect this heterogeneity or isolate specific lung regions with remodeling or abnormal ventilation. For example, often spirometry can be normal and yet there is known airflow resistance in the small airways.[4] With the development of advanced imaging techniques, distal airway remodeling, air trapping, and alveolar gas exchange can now be evaluated before and after therapeutic interventions. In addition, novel imaging techniques can identify different asthma phenotypes or clusters. By utilizing advanced imaging techniques, asthma diagnosis and therapy can be personalized for each patient.[4] In this chapter, we highlight the strengths and weaknesses of current imaging modalities used to evaluate airway and lung structural and functional defects in asthma patients (Table 18.1). Furthermore, we discuss the role of BT in asthma management and illustrate how imaging modalities may serve to guide BT and serve as biomarkers to predict response to BT.[6]

TABLE 18.1
Summary of Asthma Imaging Techniques

Modality	Structural Assessment	Functional Assessment	Clinical Utility	Disadvantages
CT	Detailed assessment • Airway tree • Vascular tree • Lung parenchyma	• Regional ventilation • Parenchymal perfusion	• Noninvasive measure of airway remodeling • Biomarker to assess response to therapy	• Radiation exposure prohibits serial examinations
MRI	• Lung microstructure using ADC • Combined with CT for detailed structural evaluation	• High spatial resolution evaluation of regional ventilation • Gas exchange	• Biomarker to assess response to therapy • Assessment of ventilation/perfusion ratio	• Less structural detail than CT • Limited to specialized MRI centers
EBUS	• Access airways as small as 4 mm with visualization of multiple layers of airway wall	• None	• Monitor serial airways changes	• Requires bronchoscopy • No functional assessment • Standards not yet established
OCT	• Two-dimensional images of airway wall with spatial resolution of 1–15 µm and penetration of 2–4 mm	• None	• Microscopic view of WT and subepithelial matrix • Monitor serial airway changes	• Requires bronchoscopy • Subject to respiratory cycle movement • Standards not yet established
PET	• Combine with CT for detailed structural evaluation	• Pulmonary inflammation • Ventilation/perfusion	• Response to antiinflammatory therapies • Evaluate inhaled drug delivery	• Limited spatial resolution • Radiation exposure

ADC, apparent diffusion coefficient; *CT*, computed tomography; *EBUS*, endobronchial ultrasound; *MRI*, magnetic resonance imaging; *OCT*, optical coherence tomography; *PET*, positron emission tomography; *WT*, airway wall thickness.
From Trivedi A, Hall C, Hoffman EA, Woods JC, Gierada DS, Castro M. Using imaging as a biomarker for asthma. *J Allergy Clin Immunol.* 2017;139(1):1–10; with permission.

CHEST RADIOGRAPHY

Most asthmatics have normal chest radiographs even during exacerbations.[7,8] Clinically, chest radiographs are not needed routinely but if available can corroborate asthma diagnosis by excluding other pathologies. The most common structural abnormalities seen on asthmatics' chest radiographs include hyperinflation and bronchial wall thickening.[9] Findings such as consolidation, pulmonary edema, pneumothorax, and cardiomegaly can be identified in asthmatics unresponsive to asthma therapy and suggest alternate causes for dyspnea.[10] In general, the decision to obtain a chest radiograph in an asthmatic patient should be guided by the history and physical examination. One study recommended patients with complicated asthma (defined as presenting with fever greater than 100.0°F, heart disease, intravenous drug use, seizures, immunosuppression, other pulmonary comorbidities, or prior thoracic surgery) may benefit the most from chest radiographs in the emergency department (ED).[11]

Chest radiographs have several advantages including portability, relatively low cost, fast examination times, and minimal radiation exposure. However, the major disadvantage is that a simple two-dimensional (2-D) image is captured. Minimal structural data and no functional data can be obtained from chest X-ray. Therefore, more advanced imaging techniques are needed to analyze the focal structural and functional defects that often occur in asthmatic airways.

COMPUTED TOMOGRAPHY SCANS

Throughout the years, there has been a gradual evolution in computed tomography (CT) scan capabilities. Older

CT scans initially employed a single radiation (X-ray) beam that rotated around the patient who sat in the gantry, or the cylindrical tube-shaped CT machine.[12,13] Over time, spiral or helical CT scanners began moving patients through the gantry so that multiple slices could be obtained in a single breath, thus shortening CT scan times and improving spatial resolution. High-resolution computed tomography (HRCT) used multiple detectors and multiple X-ray beam sources and acquired thinner (1–2 mm) slice images in noncontiguous axial planes ~10 mm apart in the lung parenchyma.[1] Pulmonary anatomy up to the secondary pulmonary lobule could be appreciated on HRCT. HRCT can visualize subtle abnormalities such as interlobular thickening, submillimeter nodules, ground-glass opacities, and bronchiectasis better.[14] In recent years, the multidetector row CT (MDCT), also referred to as *volumetric*, obtain contiguous and overlapping axial slices.[15] Most MDCT scans today use 64 or 128 detectors with one or several X-ray beam sources. The use of multiple detectors allows for multiple cross-sectional slices as thin as 0.60–0.75 mm with no interslice gaps to be obtained.[1,15]

The key difference between older CT scans and the latest MDCT is the ability to extract quantitative data from MDCT images. MDCT obtains images of the lung parenchyma continuously with no gaps. Therefore, images can be reconstructed in *x*, *y*, and *z* planes more accurately and depicted as voxels or three-dimensional (3-D) volume elements.[1,2,16,17] Special imaging processing software packages, such as Apollo Workstation (VIDA Diagnostics, Inc.) or Airway Inspector for SLICER (Harvard University), use this data to generate 3-D models.[18] From these models, computer algorithms can acquire quantitative data on airway remodeling and lung density.

Similar to chest radiographs, chest CT scans in asthmatics aid in ruling out other etiologies of dyspnea. This is especially true for difficult-to-treat asthmatics who are unresponsive to traditional therapy and may have comorbidities contributing to their respiratory symptoms. Common CT findings in asthmatics include bronchial wall thickening, air trapping, and bronchiectasis.[2] CT scans can help diagnose diseases that mimic asthma such as intrathoracic or extrathoracic airway obstruction, obliterative bronchiolitis, chronic obstructive pulmonary disease (COPD), congestive heart failure, hypersensitivity pneumonitis, hypereosinophilic syndromes, allergic bronchopulmonary aspergillosis, pulmonary embolism, and eosinophilic granulomatosis with polyangiitis (Churg-Strauss syndrome).[2,19] The ATS/ERS guidelines recommend limiting HRCT imaging to severe asthmatics who have an atypical presentation.[5]

The advantages of all CT scans include improved structural evaluation of all airways compared with chest radiographs. Furthermore, when combined with other imaging techniques such as hyperpolarized gas magnetic resonance imaging (MRI) or xenon enhanced duel energy CT,[20] ventilation abnormalities can be evaluated. However, in contrast to chest radiographs, CT scans expose patients to more radiation, are more time-consuming, are more expensive, and are not portable. As technology evolves, very low-dose CT scan protocols using third-generation CT scanners and iterative reconstruction algorithms are being developed with radiation levels approaching that of a two-view chest radiograph.[21]

In recent years, MDCT images have been used with quantitative software in asthma. It is important for clinicians to be aware of the role of MDCT as a noninvasive biomarker. MDCT and its 3-D reconstructions calculate remodeling changes and lung density alterations via computer algorithms. Remodeling is assessed via airway metrics such as airway wall thickness (WT), airway wall area (WA), airway lumen area (LA), and branch angles. Lung density measurements can be used to evaluate the degree of air trapping and emphysema-like lung. Asthma clusters have also been recently identified by using quantitative CT (qCT) metrics.[22]

Role of Computed Tomography in Assessing Remodeling

Airway remodeling due to inflammation and fibrosis increases WT and WA while simultaneously decreasing airway LA in asthmatics. Previously, remodeling could only be detected on autopsy analysis or bronchial biopsies. WT was noted to be increased 50%–300% of fatal asthma cases and 10%–100% of nonfatal asthmatics.[23] Bronchial biopsies revealed increased airway epithelial layer thickness and lamina reticularis thickness in severe asthma patients compared with normal individuals and patients with chronic bronchitis and mild asthma.[24] However, because asthma is a heterogeneous disease with normal airways interspersed among severely remodeled airways, bronchial biopsies may miss detecting remodeling when samples are inadvertently obtained from nonremodeled lung regions.

MDCT is a noninvasive technique to measure remodeling across all airways and assess the effect of asthma therapies on remodeling. *Aysola* et al. showed a correlation between increased epithelial and lamina reticularis thickness on biopsy samples and WT% and WA% measurements obtained via qCT.[25] Severe asthmatics had thicker epithelial and lamina reticularis on biopsy and higher WT% and WA% on MDCT compared with normal patients and mild asthmatics (Fig. 18.1). This suggested that remodeling changes found on biopsy could be assessed noninvasively with MDCT by measuring WT% and WA%. LA was decreased in patients with severe asthma compared with controls indicating as the airway WT increases it narrows the airway LA and potentially contributes to airflow obstruction.[26] In asthmatics, WA% correlates with duration of asthma and inversely with lower FEV_1 values in a few trials.[22,27,28] The increases in WT and decreases in LA also seem to be diminished in asthmatics more than COPD patients.[29]

Assessing Air Trapping by Measuring Lung Density with Multidetector Computed Tomography

Remodeling causes airflow obstruction that can result in air trapping. Air trapping has been shown to be increased in asthmatic patients compared with healthy subjects and can worsen airway symptoms.[22] It has traditionally been measured with PFT that reveal an elevated residual volume. Now with the emergence of MDCT and quantitative software, small airways and air trapping can be evaluated. CT images are obtained at maximal inhalation (at total lung capacity, TLC) and maximal exhalation (at residual volume). Some institutions obtain images at maximal inhalation and at rest (at functional residual capacity) On CT scans, air trapping due to distal obstruction can result in zones of decreased attenuation called *mosaic attenuation*.[30] Air trapping is defined by voxels that fall below −856 HU at end expiration.[2,17] Alternatively, expiratory to inspiratory mean lung density ratios can also identify regions of air trapping.[31] Patients with asthma have been shown to have increased percentage of lower attenuation areas on MDCT compared with control subjects[32,33] (Fig. 18.2). Furthermore, *Busacker* et al. showed that asthmatics with air trapping (defined as more than 9.66% of their total lung volume at functional residual capacity below −850 HU) were significantly more likely to have a history of asthma related hospitalizations, ICU visits, and/

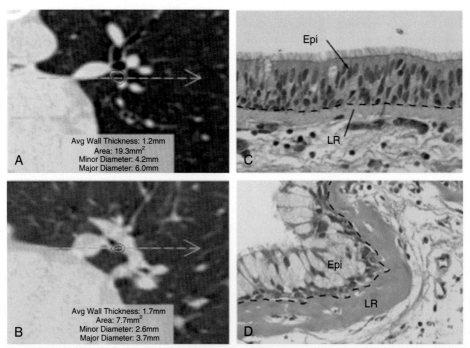

FIG. 18.1 **(A)** Multidetector computed tomography (MDCT) image from a healthy subject. **(B)** MDCT image from a severe asthmatic. **(C)** Corresponding biopsy sample from a healthy subject. **(D)** Corresponding biopsy sample from a severe asthmatic. Note that there is significant narrowing of the airway lumen and increase airway wall thickness and airway wall area in the severe asthmatic (Image **B**), which is also seen on corresponding biopsy sample (Image **D**) compared with healthy subjects (Image **A** and **C**). *Epi*, epithelial layer; *LR*, lamina reticularis; *dashed line* indicates basement membrane. (From Aysola R, et al. Airway remodeling measured by multidetector computed tomography is increased in severe asthma and correlates with pathology. *Chest*. 2008;134(6):1183–1191; with permission.)

or mechanical ventilation.[34] Drug therapies, such as oral and inhaled corticosteroids (ICS) and montelukast, have been shown to improve air trapping in select asthmatics.[4] This suggests that lung density assessment can identify patients at increased risk for complications.

Novel Asthma Phenotypes and Measuring Therapeutic Response via Multidetector Computed Tomography

Several studies have attempted to identify novel asthma phenotypes by utilizing MDCT measurements. For example, *Gupta* et al. described three distinct asthma phenotypes based on clinical and radiologic features.[26] This was one of the first studies to base asthma phenotypes on MDCT measurements. Several studies are currently in progress to evaluate the role of MDCT to characterize phenotypes. *Haldar* et al. found that WT was reduced in subjects treated with mepolizumab compared with patients who were given placebo.[35] Each phenotype may respond to individual asthma therapies in its own unique way and further studies are needed using qCT to assess their impact on airway remodeling.

Limitations of Multidetector Computed Tomography

qCT is currently limited by lack of standardization in obtaining scans using different types of MDCT (4 to 128 detector scanners), dissimilar imaging protocols, and various ways to measure remodeling and lung density. There are no established normal values for airway and lung density measurements, but new standardized protocols are being established.[36,37] Although CT scanners have evolved to visualize small distal airways, it is still difficult to measure airways smaller than 1 mm.[38] Lastly, the radiation dose of CT scanners continues to decrease in newer models but is still significantly higher than digital chest radiography and therefore its application in longitudinal assessments may be limited.

HYPERPOLARIZED MAGNETIC RESONANCE IMAGING

The primary purpose of hyperpolarized MRI (HP MRI) imaging is to evaluate for distal airway abnormalities and ventilation defects. Hyperpolarized gases, such as Helium-3 and Xenon-129, are polarized beyond thermal equilibrium to effectively serve as contrast material filling the airways, terminal bronchioles, and alveoli.[1,39] Helium-3 is confined to the alveolar region. Xenon-129 is mostly confined to the alveoli but about 1/5th of xenon has the capability to cross the alveolar-capillary barrier.[40] This allows Xenon-129 scans to assess both gas exchange and ventilation simultaneously. There has been an increase in xenon-based MRI studies as the demand for Helium-3 (for airport security neutron detectors) exceeded supply (decaying nuclear warheads), causing stricter government allocation regulations for Helium-3.[41] In contrast to Helium-3, Xenon-129 produces lower signal because of its smaller magnetic moment and is more challenging to polarize. Xenon is also routinely inhaled during ventilation-perfusion scans commonly used in clinical

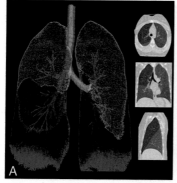
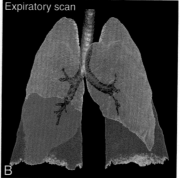

FIG. 18.2 Chest computed tomography (CT) for lung density. **(A)** Three-dimensional volume rendition of the lung, lobes, and bronchial tree detected from a CT image of the fully inflated (total lung capacity) lung of a healthy subject. **(B)** CT scan of the chest showing a similar volume rendition using the expiratory image (in this case functional residual capacity) of a patient with severe asthma. Note the areas of air trapping and pruning of the airways. Image processing was derived by using Apollo software (VIDA Diagnostics, Coralville, Iowa). (From Trivedi A, Hall C, Hoffman EA, Woods JC, Gierada DS, Castro M. Using imaging as a biomarker for asthma. *J Allergy Clin Immunol*. 2017;139(1):1–10; with permission.)

practice; however, Xenon-129 HP MRI images have markedly improved resolution.[41]

During an HP MRI scan, a patient inhales a hyperpolarized gas mixture, a breath hold is performed, and MRI images are obtained. The hyperpolarized gas can be mixed with another inert gas, such as nitrogen, to obtain a prespecified volume for inhalation. Prolonged inhalation of hyperpolarized gas for 10–20 s can lead to transient oxygen desaturations. Once inhaled, a 6- to 15-s breath hold allows the hyperpolarized gas to distribute equally through ventilated airspaces and generate high signal to noise images. Whole lung images are obtained and used to identify ventilation defects. Several methods for quantifying ventilation defects have been described, including manual scoring, pre-determined intensity threshold cutoffs and clustering methods such as K-means or Otsu's method (Fig. 18.3).[2,41a–41e]

Several studies have found that HP MRI identifies regional ventilation defects in asthmatics.[42–44] Asthmatics can have both larger ventilation defects and an increased number of ventilation defects compared with healthy volunteers.[40] Severe asthmatics have larger ventilation defects than mild or moderate asthmatics.[45] The number of ventilation defects is inversely correlated with FEV1 values in some studies.[42,45] Forced expiratory flow (FEF$_{25-75\%}$) values are also decreased in asthmatics with higher amount of ventilation defects.[45] Ventilation defects increase after methacholine challenge testing or exercise in both healthy volunteers and asthmatics.[43,45,46] However, these ventilation defects persist longer in asthmatics compared with controls after methacholine challenge.[47] Furthermore, bronchodilator therapy can result in improvement in ventilation defects in asthmatics.[48] Finally, the integration of MDCT and HP MRI testing in individual patients reveals that regions with impaired ventilation on HP MRI correlate to regions with remodeling on MDCT.[42,48,49]

The major benefit of MRI over other imaging modalities discussed thus far is that there is no radiation risk. Lack of radiation allows for serial imaging to be done to assess disease progression and response to therapy. This is especially vital for monitoring pediatric asthma patients who should not be exposed to excess radiation in childhood. HP MRI elegantly illustrates the heterogeneity of asthma by delineating focal ventilation defects. It may be a useful tool in the future to establish asthma phenotypes based on ventilation defect patterns.

However, the main limitations continue to be the need for experienced staff and expensive equipment (MRI with multinuclear package, polarizer, and a special radiofrequency [RF] coil). Hyperpolarization of gases is a lengthy process and can take up to 12 hours. However, other modalities are being discovered including oxygen-enhanced MR and fluorinated gas MR that do not require special polarization equipment.[50,51] In general, most HP MRI scans are expensive.[39] In addition, MRI alone is not as useful for structural analysis unless coupled to another imaging modality. For example, when combined with MDCT, hyperpolarized MR can provide data on structure (remodeling), function (ventilation defects), and gas exchange defects (Xenon-129 HP MRI).[1] This can be used to isolate distal airways that are most affected by airway remodeling and focus therapies such as BT (discussed below) to these regions.

Hyperpolarized Magnetic Resonance Imaging and Apparent Diffusion Coefficient

All gases diffuse through the tracheobronchial tree at their own rates based on each individual gas' intrinsic physiochemical properties.[52] The walls of the

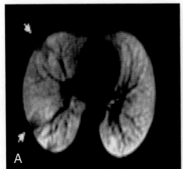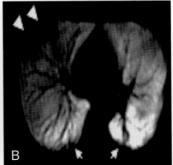

FIG. 18.3 **(A)** Hyperpolarized gas magnetic resonance imaging (HP MRI) images from mild asthmatics showing small ventilation defects (*arrows*). **(B)** HP MRI images from severe asthmatic showing larger ventilation defects (*arrowheads*). (From Castro M, Fain SB, Hoffman EA, et al. Lung imaging in asthmatic patients: the picture is clearer. *J Allergy Clin Immunol*. 2011;128(3):467–478; with permission.)

tracheobronchial tree serve as obstacles to diffusion of these gases. ADC, or apparent diffusion coefficient, is a measure of diffusion of a gas. By using MRI diffusion weighted images, the extent of diffusion can be calculated via computer algorithms and visualized on an ADC map.

Diffusion MRI can measure *short* time scale diffusions over *milliseconds*, which represent diffusion at the alveoli level, with normal ADC values of ~0.2 cm^2/s for healthy lung using Helium-3.[52] Diffusion MRI can also measure *long* time scale diffusion of gases up to 1 s, which represents diffusion at the distal small airways, with normal ADC values ~0.03 cm^2/s in healthy lung.[53] In diseases that destroy airway walls, such as emphysema, ADC increases because gases have fewer barriers and diffuse more easily. This is best appreciated in emphysema as destruction of the alveolar walls results in higher *short* time scale ADC values averaging 0.55 cm^2/s.[52]

In asthma, there is no destruction of the alveolar walls. However, small airway remodeling changes cause air trapping, which can potentially raise ADC values. *Wang* et al. found that normal subjects had low ADC values, asthmatics had specific parenchymal regions with increased ADC values, and COPD patients had diffuse areas of increased ADC values. Furthermore, *long* time ADC values (which measure diffusion of gases through the distal airways rather than alveoli) were significantly higher in asthmatics compared with healthy volunteers.[53] Regional elevations in ADC values occur after methacholine challenge testing in asthmatics.[43] However, there is no correlation between ADC and spirometry testing.[53] It is still unclear if elevations in ADC represent focal areas of air trapping in asthmatics, but this is currently the leading hypothesis.[53]

ENDOBRONCHIAL ULTRASOUND

In endobronchial ultrasound (EBUS), an ultrasonographic probe is advanced through the working channel of a fiberoptic bronchoscope. The probe contains a saline-filled balloon, which when inflated contacts the airway wall and facilitates production of real-time 2-D image using sound waves.[54] EBUS can visualize the three layers of the bronchial wall in distal, noncartilaginous airways.[55] In a small study, the mucosal, submucosal, and smooth muscle layers were significantly thicker in asthmatics compared with controls similar to results from MDCT.[55] Other studies have confirmed airway wall thickness (AWT) is localized to submucosal zones and correlated hypertrophy of these zones to airway hyperresponsiveness.[56] EBUS has several advantages including its ability to produce real-time images and lack of ionizing radiation, which allows for serial imaging over a short period of time. Limitations of EBUS are that it is still a novel technique that requires expert bronchoscopy skills, larger caliber endoscopes capable of housing an ultrasonographic catheter, and sedation as it is a minimally invasive procedure. In asthma, its role is being investigated and validated.

OPTICAL COHERENCE TOMOGRAPHY

As EBUS employs sound wave reverberations to capture images, optical coherence tomography (OCT) uses long-wavelength (near-infrared) light backscatter to provide detail on cellular elements within the airway. An OCT catheter is advanced through bronchoscope and infrared light penetrates the local tissues. Each tissue absorbs and reflects infrared light in a unique pattern based on its intrinsic optical refractive properties.[2,4,57] Two-dimensional in situ and in real-time images are generated of structures that are 2–3 mm in depth and with resolutions of 1–15 μm.[58] In the airway, the thickness of the epithelial layer, basement membrane, and smooth muscle can be measured. Measurements of wall area and lumen area in COPD patients show a strong correlation between MDCT measurements and OCT values.[17] In one study, OCT wall thickness measurements have been shown to improve after BT.[59] OCT has several advantages including its ability to produce real-time images. Unlike sound waves emitted from EBUS, light waves from OCT do not require a liquid interface and create higher resolution pictures than EBUS. Lastly, OCT lacks ionizing radiation and can be used to assess disease progression or response to therapy. Limitations of OCT are similar to EBUS in that it is still a novel technique that requires expert bronchoscopy skills, large caliber endoscopes capable of housing the OCT catheter, sedation, and lacks standardization.

POSITRON EMISSION TOMOGRAPHY

During a positron emission tomography (PET) scan, a radiotracer, such as fluorine-18-fluorodeoxyglucose, is preferentially taken up by metabolically active tissues. Radiotracers emit positrons that are annihilated on interaction with an electron.[4] This annihilation releases photons that can be detected and show preferential uptake of glucose into highly active tissues.[3] These images can be superimposed on CT scans to generate PET-CT images. Nitrogen-13 diffuses from the blood to alveoli in a single breath hold allowing for rapid assessment of perfusion. The volume of nitrogen-13 in the lung is directly proportional to lung perfusion (as long as the patient holds their breath) and ventilation is then measured on exhalation.[4]

In asthma, PET may be helpful in identifying lung inflammation. In a small study with six asthma patients, allergen challenge to the right middle lobe resulted in a localized inflammatory response measured by increased eosinophils in bronchoalveolar lavage and increased thickening of airway walls on MDCT.[60] Furthermore, the right middle lobe showed reduced perfusion and ventilation on PET imaging. This study is interesting and could potentially indicate a role for PET imaging in monitoring patients with eosinophilic asthma who are treated with monoclonal anti-IL-5 antibody.[1] N-13 PET scan provides low-resolution ventilation images compared with other imaging modalities discussed previously.[2]

BRONCHIAL THERMOPLASTY

BT is an intervention for severe asthma patients with uncontrolled symptoms despite combined high-dose ICS and long-acting β-adrenergic agonist bronchodilator (LABA) therapy. ASM hypertrophy and hyperplasia are both increased in fatal asthmatic biopsy specimens and are thought to contribute to remodeling changes and airflow obstruction.[61] BT reduces smooth muscle area, thus minimizing asthma exacerbation rates.[62]

BT is performed using the Alair Bronchial Thermoplasty System comprising the Alair RF Controller and the Alair Catheter.[63] The specialized radiofrequency catheter is advanced through the endoscope into the distal airways. Radiofrequency energy converts into thermal energy with resistance and treats the local bronchial smooth muscle tissue. Airways as small as 3–10 mm can be targeted, but a single session only focuses on treatments to one to two lobes. Usually three sessions are done over 3–6 weeks. Typically, the right lower lobe is treated first, then the left lower lobe, and finally bilateral upper lobes. Historically, the right middle lobe was not treated; however, we (and others) are now treating the right middle lobe at the same session as the right lower lobe.[64] A methodic approach is vital and the physician must move systematically from distal to proximal in each segment to ensure adequate treatment to all accessible lobar segments.

Evidence for Bronchial Thermoplasty

Several clinical studies have evaluated the safety and efficacy of BT in adults (Table 18.2). In 2010, BT was approved by the U.S. Food and Drug Administration (FDA) for adults with severe asthma with uncontrolled

symptoms despite high-dose ICS and LABA. Currently BT has not been studied in children. From a histopathologic standpoint, several studies began to describe reductions in ASM in BT patients. Three months after BT, patients not only reported improved quality of life (QOL) and asthma control but also were found to have decreased ASM area and reductions in subepithelial basement membrane thickening on biopsy.[65] Other studies revealed reductions in ASM mass, airway basement membrane collagen deposition, and inflammatory cytokine production in BT recipients.[66,67]

The largest study of BT was a multicenter, double-blinded, sham-controlled study with 288 adult asthmatics (AIR2). While the BT group received actual BT treatments, the sham group patients underwent bronchoscopy with sham catheters that were indistinguishable from real BT catheters except that no energy was delivered. Nearly 1 year after the treatment sessions were completed, the BT group had a greater improvement in QOL scores compared with the sham group. In addition, the BT group had decreased number of emergency room (ER) visits and less work/school absenteeism compared with the control group. In the first 6 weeks, more patients in the BT group reported increased respiratory-related adverse events, as expected. Patients typically experience increased coughing, wheezing, chest tightness, and dyspnea for 24–48 h after BT but most improve within 1 week.[64] However, up to 1 year later, the BT group had less adverse pulmonary symptoms compared with the sham group.[68] At their 5-year follow-up, the proportion of BT patients with severe exacerbations and ER visits continued to be less than those observed in the 12 months before BT treatment.[69]

A recent study demonstrated peribronchial consolidations or ground-glass opacities within the first 24 hours following BT on CT.[70] These abnormalities sometimes affect an untreated adjacent lobe and resolve or decrease in all patients on follow-up CT 1 month later. These changes may be due to alveolar inflammation and edema secondary to BT thermal therapy. Only 8% of patients had lobar atelectasis on CT scans at 24 h and this resolves by 1 month without bronchoscopic intervention. No patients had evidence of pulmonary infection on CT at 1 month. These studies indicate that a short course of systemic steroids following BT can often help patients recover faster. Finally, both the AIR2 and RISA studies showed that there were no new structural changes on CT scans obtained 5 years after therapy.[62] Thus although BT recipients may have increased pulmonary symptoms and new radiographic findings for several weeks after their BT sessions, these symptoms and imaging abnormalities resolve in a few weeks.

TABLE 18.2
Summary of Bronchial Thermoplasty (BT) Results From Randomized Controlled Trials and Extension Studies

Study	Subjects	Approximate FEV1 values	Results	Conclusions
AIR	• 112 moderate to severe asthmatics • Randomized BT or usual care • Follow-up to 1 year • Age: 39.36 ± 11.18 years	• 72%–76%	• At 12 months, mean rate of mild exacerbation, compared with baseline, reduced in BT group • At 12 months, improved PEF, QOL scores, and less rescue medication use in BT patients (significantly greater than controls) • At 12 months, airway responsiveness and FEV1 similar in both groups • At 6 weeks, increased AE in BT group • At 12 months, AE similar in both groups	• BT causes transient increase in AE at 6 weeks • BT does not cause increased AE or pulmonary decline at 1 year • BT is safe at least at 1 year after therapy
AIR: 5-year follow-up	• 69 asthmatics from AIR • 45/52 BT groups • 24/49 control group • Follow-up to 5 years • Age: 40.0 ± 11.2 years	• 72%–75% • Stable FEV1 values at 5 years	• At 5 years, stable rate of AE in BT group • At 5 years, no increase in hospitalizations or ER visits for BT patients compared with first year after BT • Stable FVC and FEV1 for BT patients over 5 years	• BT is safe and effective at least 5 years after therapy
AIR2	• 288 severe asthmatics • Randomized to BT versus sham-BT therapy • Follow-up to 1 year • Age: 40.7 ± 11.89 years	• 77%–80%	• 6% higher hospitalization rates in BT group in first 6 weeks Between 6 weeks and 52 weeks post-BT • 84% reduction in ER visits for respiratory symptoms in BT group (BT = 0.07 BT vs. sham = 0.43 visits/subject/year) • 73% reduction in hospitalizations for respiratory symptoms in BT group (BT = 2.6% vs. sham = 4.1%) • 66% reduction in absenteeism in BT group (BT = 1.3 vs. sham = 3.9 days/year) • 79% improvement in baseline QOL in BT groups (vs. 64% in sham group) • 32% reduction in severe exacerbations in BT groups (BT = 26.3% vs. sham = 39.8%)	• BT causes transient increase in hospitalizations at 6 weeks • From 6 to 52 weeks, fewer severe exacerbations, ER visits, hospitalizations, and absenteeism for respiratory issues in BT group • BT is safe and effective at least 1 year after therapy

Continued

TABLE 18.2

Summary of Bronchial Thermoplasty (BT) Results From Randomized Controlled Trials and Extension Studies—cont'd

Study	Subjects	Approximate FEV1 values	Results	Conclusions
AIR2: 2-year follow-up	• 166 BT recipients in AIR2 • Follow-up at 2 years • Age: 41.1 ± 11.8 years	• 74.5% • Clinical stability of FEV1 at 2 years	• At 2 years, BT patients had a 23% severe exacerbation rate (2 years earlier, prior to any BT sessions, this same group had a 51% severe exacerbation rate)	• BT is safe and effective at least 2 years after therapy
AIR2: 5-year follow-up	• 162 BT recipients in AIR2 • Follow-up at 5 years • Age: 41.5 ± 11.8 years	• 77%–78% • Clinical stability of FEV1 at 5 years	• At 5 years, 44% average decrease in severe exacerbations • At 5 years, BT patients had no deterioration in FEV1 • At 5 years, BT patients did not have increase in hospitalizations from baseline • At 5 years, HRCT scans did not show any significant structural changes	• A single BT treatment comprising three procedures is safe and provides long-term benefit to at least 5 years
RISA	• 32 severe asthmatics • Randomized to BT or usual care • Age: 39.1 ± 13.0 years	• 63%–66%	• Before 22 weeks, increased hospitalizations in BT groups • At 22 weeks, 14% improvement in FEV1 in BT group. No improvement in FEV1 in control group • At 22 weeks, significant improvement in QOL scores in BT group versus controls • At 22 weeks, significantly less rescue medication use in BT group versus controls	• Transient increase in hospitalizations before 22 weeks • After 22 weeks, marked improvement in FEV1 and QOL scores in BT group • BT may preferentially benefit severe asthmatics with lower FEV1 values than moderate asthmatics
RISA: 5-year follow-up	• 14/15 BT recipients from RISA • Age: 38.6 ± 13.3 years	• 63.5% • Clinical stability in FEV1 at 5 years	• At 5 years, BT patients had stable FEV1 values • At 5 years, BT patients had no increase in hospitalizations compared with the year before BT therapy	• BT is safe and effective for at least 5 years after therapy in severe asthmatics

ER, emergency room; *FEV1*, forced expiratory volume in 1 s; *FVC*, forced vital capacity; *HRCT*, high-resolution computed tomography; *PEF*, peak expiratory flow; *QOL*, quality of life; *AE*, Adverse event.

For the clinician: is bronchial thermoplasty safe and effective for my patient?

The decision to pursue BT for a patient begins with a thorough history, examination, and objective testing. Clinicians should consider BT as a treatment that reduces ASM that complements antiinflammatory therapy with ICS and biologic modifiers. BT should be considered in severe asthma patients that are receiving GINA Step 4 or 5 therapy yet are not achieving asthma control. BT should be avoided in patients who are noncompliant, current tobacco users, during active asthma exacerbations or in patients with prior serious

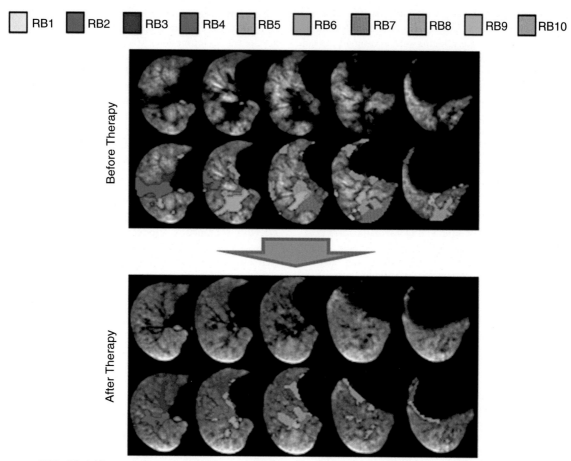

■ RB1 ■ RB2 ■ RB3 ■ RB4 ■ RB5 ■ RB6 ■ RB7 ■ RB8 ■ RB9 ■ RB10

FIG. 18.4 **Top row:** Hyperpolarized gas magnetic resonance imaging (HP MRI) showing defects of the right lung in a severe asthma patient prior to bronchial thermoplasty (BT). Darker regions correspond to regions with focal ventilation defects. **Bottom row:** Ventilation defects with color coded segment labels. Defects are most notable in RB2 (Blue), RB5 (orange), RB6 (green), RB7 (brown), RB10 (purple) for this patient. **Bottom Images:** HP MRI showing defects of the right lung in a severe asthma patient 12 weeks after BT. Note in corresponding regions there is improved ventilation after BT. (From Thomen RP, Sheshadri A, Quirk JD, et al. Regional ventilation changes in severe asthma after bronchial thermoplasty with (3)He MR imaging and CT. *Radiology.* 2015;274(1):250–259; with permission.)

reactions to moderate sedation or anesthesia. Randomized controlled trials have established the safety of BT in individuals with FEV1 values above 50% and less than four exacerbations 1 year before enrollment.[62] However, experienced BT centers have now successfully treated patients with a postbronchodilator FEV1 40% or greater and with more frequent exacerbations (*Hogarth K,* et al. *Castro M. Personal Communication*).

For clinicians, novel imaging techniques have proven useful in evaluating the mechanism of action of BT. Case series utilizing MDCT, HP MRI, and OCT have

noted improvements with select BT recipients. MDCT has found decreased %WA and air trapping in individuals after BT sessions.[71,72] HP MRI also detected regional ventilation changes in patients after BT[73] (Fig. 18.4). *Kirby* et al. used OCT to show reduced AWT in a patient post-BT that persisted for 2 years.[59]

A Cochrane review evaluated three trials with over 400 patients who underwent BT. The authors concluded that BT provides a modest clinical benefit in QOL and decreased asthma exacerbation rates. An increase in adverse events was noted immediately posttreatment, but overall the authors concluded that BT has a reasonable safety profile.[74] A large metaanalysis of 200 moderate to severe asthma patients undergoing BT found there was no significant decline in FEV1 values after 5 years follow-up, suggesting that BT might prevent deterioration of lung function. Furthermore, about 10% patients completely weaned off LABA treatments after BT. These results indicated that not only is BT safe for most patients long term, but it can also stabilize their asthma control and decrease medication use in select patients.[75]

Finally, a study analyzing the cost of BT revealed overall benefits as well. Assessing quality-adjusted life-years (QALY), the study discovered that BT treatment resulted in 6.4 QALY and $7512 in cost compared with 6.2 QALY and $2054 for usual care cost. In addition, there was an expected decrease in ER and hospital costs by about $4600. There was also an expected $3000 savings from reduction in medications. For BT to be cost-effective, a higher probability of asthma exacerbation is required. This highlights the need for BT referral for select patients with severe asthma and uncontrolled symptoms with a history of two or more prior exacerbations requiring systemic corticosteroids.[76]

In conclusion, BT may benefit a specific asthma phenotype with chronic airflow obstruction, bronchial wall thickening, and remodeling on imaging. Patients with severe and uncontrolled symptoms despite medication compliance seem to benefit the most from BT. When the procedure is performed by a physician experienced in bronchoscopy in consultation with an asthma expert, BT is a safe and effective therapy that improves asthma control and QOL while reducing exacerbations. In the future, more studies will evaluate its long-term beneficial effects, and novel imaging techniques may play a role in selecting patients and in guiding therapy.

SUMMARY

Novel lung imaging techniques using qCT, HP MRI, PET, EBUS, and OCT have been developed to assess structural changes, such as airway remodeling, and functional changes, such as air trapping and ventilation defects, in asthma. qCT can generate 3-D models of the tracheobronchial tree and clearly evaluate airway structural changes such as airway remodeling and air trapping. HP MRI can evaluate functional changes in the lung by detecting regional ventilation abnormalities. EBUS and OCT allow for real-time assessment of local

airway structure while PET scans may detect increased regional airway inflammation. A clinician can appreciate the true heterogeneity of airway remodeling in each individual patient, which is not possible with current clinical tests for asthma (such as spirometry or chest X-ray). In the future, these newer imaging techniques should be considered in patients with severe uncontrolled asthma and chronic airflow obstruction or in those with progressive loss of lung function despite therapy with ICS and LABA. Standardization of these techniques in specialized asthma centers will facilitate their application in the future.

Furthermore, these imaging modalities can help better identify asthma phenotypes and response to new therapeutic interventions such as BT. BT is a safe and effective therapeutic intervention to reduce smooth muscle mass in severe uncontrolled asthma when performed by an experienced bronchoscopist in consultation with an asthma expert. HP MRI studies have demonstrated similar ventilation defects in children with asthma; therefore future studies are needed to evaluate the appropriate utilization of BT in children. Ongoing studies are evaluating the predictive value of imaging studies in selecting appropriate patients for BT and in guiding therapy.

FUNDING

The study is supported by the National Heart, Lung, and Blood Institute/National Institutes of Health NIH/NHLBI U10 HL109257 (MC) and NIH/NCATS UL1 TR000448.

REFERENCES

1. Castro M, Fain SB, Hoffman EA, et al. Lung imaging in asthmatic patients: the picture is clearer. *J Allergy Clin Immunol.* 2011;128(3):467–478.
2. Trivedi A, Hall C, Hoffman EA, Woods JC, Gierada DS, Castro M. Using imaging as a biomarker for asthma. *J Allergy Clin Immunol.* 2017;139(1):1–10.
3. Grippi M, Elias J, Fishman J, Pack A, Kotloff R. *Fishman's Pulmonary Diseases and Disorders, 2-Volume Set.* 5th ed. McGraw-Hill Education; 2015.
4. Hartley R, Baldi S, Brightling C, Gupta S. Novel imaging approaches in adult asthma and their clinical potential. *Expert Rev Clin Immunol.* 2015;11(10):1147–1162.
5. Chung KF, Wenzel SE, Brozek JL, et al. International ERS/ATS guidelines on definition, evaluation and treatment of severe asthma. *Eur Respir J.* 2014;43(2):343–373.
6. Szefler SJ, Wenzel S, Brown R, et al. Asthma outcomes: biomarkers. *J Allergy Clin Immunol.* 2012;129(suppl 3):S9–S23.

7. Findley LJ, Sahn SA. The value of chest roentgenograms in acute asthma in adults. *Chest.* 1981;80(5):535–536.

8. Zieverink SE, Patricia Harper A, Holden RW, Kiatte EC, Brittain H. Emergency Room Radiography of Asthma: An Efficacy Study' The chest radiographs of asthmatic patients in an emergency room setting over.

9. Paganin F, Trussard V, Seneterre E, et al. Chest radiography and high resolution computed tomography of the lungs in asthma. *Am Rev Respir Dis.* 1992;146(4):1084–1087.

10. White CS, Cole RP, Lubetsky HW, Austin JH. Acute asthma. Admission chest radiography in hospitalized adult patients. *Chest.* 1991;100(1):14–16.

11. Tsai TW, Gallagher EJ, Lombardi G, Gennis P, Carter W. Guidelines for the selective ordering of admission chest radiography in adult obstructive airway disease. *Ann Emerg Med.* 1993;22(12):1854–1858.

12. Goodman LR, Felson B. *Felson's Principles of Chest Roentgenology.* Saunders Elsevier; 2007.

13. Goldman LW. Principles of CT and CT technology. *J Nucl Med Technol.* 2007;35(3):115–128. quiz 129–130.

14. Kazerooni EA. High-resolution CT of the lungs. *AJR Am J Roentgenol.* 2001;177(3):501–519.

15. Sundaram B, Chughtai AR, Kazerooni EA. Multidetector high-resolution computed tomography of the lungs: protocols and applications. *J Thorac Imaging.* 2010;25(2):125–141.

16. Boone JM. Multidetector CT: opportunities, challenges, and concerns associated with scanners with 64 or more detector rows. *Radiology.* 2006;241(2):334–337.

17. Coxson HO. Lung parenchyma density and airwall thickness in airway diseases. *Breathe.* 2012;9(1):36–45.

18. Grenier PA, Beigelman-Aubry C, Fetita C, Martin-Bouyer Y. Multidetector-row CT of the airways. *Semin Roentgenol.* 2003;38(2):146–157.

19. Richards JC, Lynch D, Koelsch T, Dyer D. Imaging of asthma. *Immunol Allergy Clin North Am.* 2016;36(3):529–545.

20. Kong X, Sheng HX, Lu GM, et al. Xenon-enhanced dual-energy CT lung ventilation imaging: techniques and clinical applications. *AJR Am J Roentgenol.* 2014;202(2):309–317.

21. Newell Jr JD, Fuld MK, Allmendinger T, et al. Very low-dose (0.15 mGy) chest CT protocols using the COPDGene 2 test object and a third-generation dual-source CT scanner with corresponding third-generation iterative reconstruction software. *Invest Radiol.* 2015;50(1):40–45.

22. Gupta S, Hartley R, Khan UT, et al. Quantitative computed tomography-derived clusters: redefining airway remodeling in asthmatic patients. *J Allergy Clin Immunol.* 2014;133(3):729–738.e718.

23. Elias JA, Zhu Z, Chupp G, Homer RJ. Airway remodeling in asthma. *J Clin Invest.* 1999;104(8):1001–1006.

24. Cohen L, E X Tarsi J, et al. Epithelial cell proliferation contributes to airway remodeling in severe asthma. *Am J Respir Crit Care Med.* 2007;176(2):138–145.

25. Aysola RS, Hoffman EA, Gierada D, et al. Airway remodeling measured by multidetector CT is increased in severe asthma and correlates with pathology. *Chest.* 2008;134(6):1183–1191.

26. Gupta S, Siddiqui S, Haldar P, et al. Quantitative analysis of high-resolution computed tomography scans in severe asthma subphenotypes. *Thorax.* 2010;65(9):775–781.

27. Hartley RA, Barker BL, Newby C, et al. Relationship between lung function and quantitative computed tomographic parameters of airway remodeling, air trapping, and emphysema in patients with asthma and chronic obstructive pulmonary disease: a single-center study. *J Allergy Clin Immunol.* 2016;137(5):1413–1422.e1412.

28. Niimi A, Matsumoto H, Amitani R, et al. Airway wall thickness in asthma assessed by computed tomography. Relation to clinical indices. *Am J Respir Crit Care Med.* 2000;162(4 Pt 1):1518–1523.

29. Oguma T, Hirai T, Fukui M, et al. Longitudinal shape irregularity of airway lumen assessed by CT in patients with bronchial asthma and COPD. *Thorax.* 2015;70(8):719–724.

30. Hansell DM, Bankier AA, MacMahon H, McLoud TC, Muller NL, Remy J. Fleischner Society: glossary of terms for thoracic imaging. *Radiology.* 2008;246(3):697–722.

31. Bommart S, Marin G, Bourdin A, et al. Relationship between CT air trapping criteria and lung function in small airway impairment quantification. *BMC Pulm Med.* 2014; 14:29.

32. Lee KY, Park SJ, Kim SR, et al. Low attenuation area is associated with airflow limitation and airway hyperresponsiveness. *J Asthma.* 2008;45(9):774–779.

33. Ueda T, Niimi A, Matsumoto H, et al. Role of small airways in asthma: investigation using high-resolution computed tomography. *J Allergy Clin Immunol.* 2006;118(5):1019–1025.

34. Busacker A, Newell Jr JD, Keefe T, et al. A multivariate analysis of risk factors for the air-trapping asthmatic phenotype as measured by quantitative CT analysis. *Chest.* 2009;135(1):48–56.

35. Haldar P, Brightling CE, Hargadon B, et al. Mepolizumab and exacerbations of refractory eosinophilic asthma. *N Engl J Med.* 2009;360(10):973–984.

36. Choi S, Hoffman EA, Wenzel SE, et al. Quantitative assessment of multiscale structural and functional alterations in asthmatic populations. *J Appl Physiol (1985).* 2015;118(10):1286–1298.

37. Sieren JP, Newell Jr JD, Barr RG, et al. SPIROMICS protocol for multicenter quantitative computed tomography to phenotype the lungs. *Am J Respir Crit Care Med.* 2016;194(7):794–806.

38. Kauczor HU, Wielputz MO, Owsijewitsch M, Ley-Zaporozhan J. Computed tomographic imaging of the airways in COPD and asthma. *J Thorac Imaging.* 2011; 26(4):290–300.

39. Kruger SJ, Nagle SK, Couch MJ, Ohno Y, Albert M, Fain SB. Functional imaging of the lungs with gas agents. *J Magn Reson Imaging.* 2016;43(2):295–315.

40. Fain S, Schiebler ML, McCormack DG, Parraga G. Imaging of lung function using hyperpolarized helium-3 magnetic resonance imaging: review of current and emerging translational methods and applications. *J Magn Reson Imaging.* 2010;32(6):1398–1408.

41. Mugler 3rd JP, Altes TA. Hyperpolarized 129Xe MRI of the human lung. *J Magn Reson Imaging.* 2013;37(2):313–331.

41a. He M, Kaushik SS, Robertson SH, et al. Extending Semi-Automatic Ventilation Defect Analysis for Hyperpolarized 129Xe Ventilation MRI. *Academic radiology.* 2014;21(12): 1530–1541. http://dx.doi.org/10.1016/j.acra.2014.07.017.

41b. Tustison NJ, Avants BB, Flors L, Altes TA, de Lange EE, Mugler JP, Gee JC. Ventilation-based segmentation of the lungs using hyperpolarized 3He MRI. *J Magn Reson Imaging.* 2011;34:831–841. http://dx.doi.org/10.1002/jmri.22738.

41c. Thomen RP, Sheshadri A, Quirk JD, et al. Regional Ventilation Changes in Severe Asthma after Bronchial Thermoplasty with 3He MR Imaging and CT. *Radiology.* 2015;274(1):250–259. http://dx.doi.org/10.1148/radiol.14140080.

41d. Niles DJ, et al. Exercise-induced bronchoconstriction: reproducibility of hyperpolarized 3He MR imaging. *Radiology.* 2013;266:618–625.

41e. Kirby M, et al. Hyperpolarizied 3HE Magnetic Resonance Functional Imaging Semiautomated Segmentation. *Academic Radiology.* 2012;19(2):141–152.

42. Fain SB, Gonzalez-Fernandez G, Peterson ET, et al. Evaluation of structure-function relationships in asthma using multidetector CT and hyperpolarized He-3 MRI. *Acad Radiol.* 2008;15(6):753–762.

43. Costella S, Kirby M, Maksym GN, McCormack DG, Paterson NA, Parraga G. Regional pulmonary response to a methacholine challenge using hyperpolarized (3)He magnetic resonance imaging. *Respirology.* 2012;17(8):1237–1246.

44. Aysola R, de Lange EE, Castro M, Altes TA. Demonstration of the heterogeneous distribution of asthma in the lungs using CT and hyperpolarized helium-3 MRI. *J Magn Reson Imaging.* 2010;32(6):1379–1387.

45. de Lange EE, Altes TA, Patrie JT, et al. Evaluation of asthma with hyperpolarized helium-3 MRI: correlation with clinical severity and spirometry. *Chest.* 2006;130(4):1055–1062.

46. Samee S, Altes T, Powers P, et al. Imaging the lungs in asthmatic patients by using hyperpolarized helium-3 magnetic resonance: assessment of response to methacholine and exercise challenge. *J Allergy Clin Immunol.* 2003;111(6):1205–1211.

47. Tzeng YS, Lutchen K, Albert M. The difference in ventilation heterogeneity between asthmatic and healthy subjects quantified using hyperpolarized 3He MRI. *J Appl Physiol (1985).* 2009;106(3):813–822.

48. Svenningsen S, Kirby M, Starr D, et al. Hyperpolarized (3) He and (129) Xe MRI: differences in asthma before bronchodilation. *J Magn Reson Imaging.* 2013;38(6): 1521–1530.

49. Ash SY, Diaz AA. The role of imaging in the assessment of severe asthma. *Curr Opin Pulm Med.* 2017;23(1):97–102.

50. Chen Q, Jakob PM, Griswold MA, Levin DL, Hatabu H, Edelman RR. Oxygen enhanced MR ventilation imaging of the lung. *Magn Reson Mater Phys Biol Med.* 1998;7(3): 153–161.

51. Couch MJ, Ball IK, Li T, et al. Inert fluorinated gas MRI: a new pulmonary imaging modality. *NMR Biomed.* 2014; 27(12):1525–1534.

52. Yablonskiy DA, Sukstanskii AL, Leawoods JC, et al. Quantitative in vivo assessment of lung microstructure at the alveolar level with hyperpolarized 3He diffusion MRI. *Proc Natl Acad Sci USA.* 2002;99(5):3111–3116.

53. Wang C, Altes TA, Mugler 3rd JP, et al. Assessment of the lung microstructure in patients with asthma using hyperpolarized 3He diffusion MRI at two time scales: comparison with healthy subjects and patients with COPD. *J Magn Reson Imaging.* 2008;28(1):80–88.

54. Shaw TJ, Wakely SL, Peebles CR, et al. Endobronchial ultrasound to assess airway wall thickening: validation in vitro and in vivo. *Eur Respir J.* 2004;23(6):813–817.

55. Soja J, Grzanka P, Sladek K, et al. The use of endobronchial ultrasonography in assessment of bronchial wall remodeling in patients with asthma. *Chest.* 2009;136(3): 797–804.

56. Kita T, Fujimura M, Kurimoto N, et al. Airway wall structure assessed by endobronchial ultrasonography and bronchial hyperresponsiveness in patients with asthma. *J Bronchol Interv Pulmonol.* 2010;17(4):301–306.

57. Hou R, Le T, Murgu SD, Chen Z, Brenner M. Recent advances in optical coherence tomography for the diagnoses of lung disorders. *Expert Rev Respir Med.* 2011;5(5): 711–724.

58. Fujimoto JG, Pitris C, Boppart SA, Brezinski ME. Optical coherence tomography: an emerging technology for biomedical imaging and optical biopsy. *Neoplasia.* 2000;2(1–2): 9–25.

59. Kirby M, Ohtani K, Lopez Lisbona RM, et al. Bronchial thermoplasty in asthma: 2-year follow-up using optical coherence tomography. *Eur Respir J.* 2015;46(3):859–862.

60. Harris RS, Venegas JG, Wongviriyawong C, et al. 18F-FDG uptake rate is a biomarker of eosinophilic inflammation and airway response in asthma. *J Nucl Med.* 2011;52(11):1713–1720.

61. James A, Mauad T, Abramson M, Green F. Airway smooth muscle hypertrophy and hyperplasia in asthma. *Am J Respir Crit Care Med.* 2012;186(6):568. author reply 569.

62. Trivedi A, Pavord ID, Castro M. Bronchial thermoplasty and biological therapy as targeted treatments for severe uncontrolled asthma. *Lancet Respir Med.* 2016;4(7):585–592.

63. Mayse ML, Laviolette M, Rubin AS, et al. Clinical pearls for bronchial thermoplasty. *J Bronchol Interv Pulmonol.* 2007;14(2):115–123.

64. Sheshadri A, Castro M, Chen A. Bronchial thermoplasty: a novel therapy for severe asthma. *Clin Chest Med.* 2013; 34(3):437–444.

65. Pretolani M, Dombret MC, Thabut G, et al. Reduction of airway smooth muscle mass by bronchial thermoplasty in patients with severe asthma. *Am J Respir Crit Care Med.* 2014;190(12):1452–1454.

66. Chakir J, Haj-Salem I, Gras D, et al. Effects of bronchial thermoplasty on airway smooth muscle and collagen deposition in asthma. *Ann Am Thorac Soc.* 2015;12(11): 1612–1618.

67. Denner DR, Doeing DC, Hogarth DK, Dugan K, Naureckas ET, White SR. Airway inflammation after bronchial thermoplasty for severe asthma. *Ann Am Thorac Soc.* 2015; 12(9):1302–1309.

68. Castro M, Rubin AS, Laviolette M, et al. Effectiveness and safety of bronchial thermoplasty in the treatment of severe asthma: a multicenter, randomized, double-blind, sham-controlled clinical trial. *Am J Respir Crit Care Med.* 2010;181(2):116–124.

69. Wechsler ME, Laviolette M, Rubin AS, et al. Bronchial thermoplasty: long-term safety and effectiveness in patients with severe persistent asthma. *J Allergy Clin Immunol.* 2013;132(6):1295–1302.

70. Debray MP, Dombret MC, Pretolani M, et al. Early computed tomography modifications following bronchial thermoplasty in patients with severe asthma. *Eur Respir J.* 2017;49(3).

71. Ishii S, Iikura M, Hojo M, Sugiyama H. Use of 3D-CT airway analysis software to assess a patient with severe persistent bronchial asthma treated with bronchial thermoplasty. *Allergol Int.* 2017;66(3).

72. Sarikonda KSA, Koch T, et al. Predictors of bronchial thermoplasty response in patients with severe refractory asthma. *Am J Respir Crit Care Med.* 2014;189. A2429.

73. Thomen RP, Sheshadri A, Quirk JD, et al. Regional ventilation changes in severe asthma after bronchial thermoplasty with (3)He MR imaging and CT. *Radiology.* 2015;274(1):250–259.

74. Torrego A, Sola I, Munoz AM, et al. Bronchial thermoplasty for moderate or severe persistent asthma in adults. *Cochrane Database Syst Rev.* 2014;(3). http://dx.doi.org/ 10.1002/14651858.CD009910.pub2.

75. Zhou JP, Feng Y, Wang Q, Zhou LN, Wan HY, Li QY. Long-term efficacy and safety of bronchial thermoplasty in patients with moderate-to-severe persistent asthma: a systemic review and meta-analysis. *J Asthma.* 2016;53(1):94–100.

76. Zein JG, Menegay MC, Singer ME, et al. Cost effectiveness of bronchial thermoplasty in patients with severe uncontrolled asthma. *J Asthma.* 2016;53(2):194–200.

CHAPTER 19

Future Directions in Asthma Management

STANLEY J. SZEFLER, MD • FERNANDO HOLGUIN, MD •
MICHAEL E. WECHSLER, MD

WHERE DO WE GO FROM HERE?

We hope that you had the opportunity to read this book "cover-to-cover" to obtain a comprehensive appreciation of the topics included from a population perspective to a systems biology perspective. To move forward in asthma management, there must be a commitment at the individual level to improve the approach to asthma care, as well as a consideration of the spectrum of the issues of the specific population, be it a country, a healthcare system, or a practice setting. There is clearly a role for the asthma specialist to lead this effort in providing up-to-date knowledge regarding cutting-edge research and practice patterns that could alter the paradigm of asthma care.

The primary care physician must coordinate medical teams to be sure that not only asthma but also other medical disorders are managed appropriately. Allied healthcare professionals, such as physician assistants and nurse practitioners, can work as teams to provide asthma education and monitor day-to-day care, such as adherence to medications. It is useful to define metrics to determine if gains are being made in reducing asthma morbidity, such as hospitalizations, urgent care use, and after-hour calls. These efforts will improve not only the quality of life for the patient but also that of the practice setting.

In this multidisciplinary care setting, a population management perspective should be taken to identify those patients who are suffering from frequent asthma exacerbations and/or persistently poorly controlled asthma.[1] Questions should be raised on whether the management plan is adequate or whether the patient may indeed require step-up care to a biologic response modifier that may incur higher costs but balance overall management with reduced asthma exacerbations that require hospitalizations.

To harmonize medical care, there is also a need for standardization of terminology including communication forms, such as asthma action plans for school or for home, and for communication with patients around features of inhaled medication delivery and appropriate times to step up therapy. Avoiding the use of multiple providers, especially those outside the provider's medical system, such as an emergency setting, would help to minimize this confusion.

For children, extending this communication to the school setting and working to harmonize dialogue in the community around asthma care also help to reduce confusion for the patient.[2] Although communication should be fostered within the community, there are information privacy matters that must be addressed in each setting. Hopefully, electronic medical records with appropriate permissions can be used to enhance this level of communication not only among primary care physicians and specialists but also between providers and school nurses. Building up this type of communication at the community level, then at the provider level, and subsequently at a national level could play a role in encouraging more consistent care and reducing overall asthma burden on a global level. Our national societies must play a major role in such activities, with a goal of fostering collaboration across societies to meet patient needs.

PERSONALIZING ASTHMA CARE

Throughout this book, we have emphasized ways that clinicians can begin to look at the unique features of their patients regarding behavior, ability to understand principles of management, overall asthma severity, and risk factors for loss of control and also for adverse effects to medications. Using principles of "big data" can help identify those patients who have frequent exacerbations, have high medication requirements, are poorly adherent with their controller medications, and are high utilizers of rescue therapy that could benefit from a "precision delivery initiative for precision medicine."[3] The Composite Asthma Severity Index can be used to assess an individual's asthma burden by combining information on day-and-night symptoms, exacerbations, treatment step, and pulmonary function.[4,5] Following pulmonary function over time, for example, on an annual basis, including children, will help to identify the patient who is potentially suffering ongoing, irrecoverable loss of pulmonary function and potentially on a pathway for a COPD-like pattern of pulmonary function in adulthood.[6] Questions are being raised on whether asthma exacerbations contribute to irreversible loss in pulmonary function over time. Assessing a patient's risk for an asthma exacerbation, using the asthma exacerbation prediction index, could be useful in designing strategies around prevention of seasonal exacerbations.[7–9] Assessment of this seasonal asthma exacerbation prediction index requires knowledge regarding recent history of an exacerbation, pulmonary function, treatment step, blood eosinophils, and exhaled nitric oxide to determine the potential risk.

Adherence monitoring tools are now available that can provide information on day-to-day use of asthma controller medications as well as rescue medications.[10–12] This does require an additional level of coordination to have a team member check on the adherence level and make appropriate calls. In addition, these monitoring tools also have reminder systems for those patients who need such reminders to take their routine medications. If a patient is identified as being poorly adherent, then support systems with the family involving shared decision-making or perhaps even administering medications in school for children could be used to facilitate medication adherence.[13,14]

If indeed the patient demonstrates adequate adherence and is doing everything possible to control his/her asthmatic condition including environmental control measures, this would help to justify the use of the more expensive biologic response modifiers, such as anti-IgE or anti-IL-5 therapies, assuming they meet the necessary biomarker criteria. These therapies, and others that are emerging (e.g., anti IL-4/13), are all predicated on the notion that different asthma patients may have different mechanisms at play that result in the common phenotype we recognize as asthma. An important goal in the coming years will be to not only work with physicians to help identify which biomarkers are associated with specific subtypes of asthma in a given patient but also to tie those biomarkers to specific therapies and to work over the next several years to identify newer biomarkers (even novel molecular and genetic biomarkers) and newer therapies to truly deliver personalized therapy to our patients.

COORDINATING ASTHMA RESEARCH

Once this key information is accumulated, databases can be developed to identify those patients at risk for asthma exacerbations, asthma progression, and adverse adult respiratory outcomes. These strategies could then prompt a more proactive approach in developing individualized asthma strategies (for example, intermittent inhaled steroid therapy for those who do not require daily therapy or stepping-up therapy to biologic response modifiers for those refractory to conventional treatment, perhaps even on a seasonal basis).[9,15] These challenging patients could also be more easily identified for conducting clinical research on the evaluation of biomarkers associated with progression, as well as changes in pulmonary physiology and biomarkers associated with various interventions, especially the new therapies, where little is known about their effect on the natural history of asthma. That way a more coordinated approach to asthma research can be developed based on various phenotypes and endotypes, similar to that developed in the area of cancer management.

With an organized system, such as that described, there is a greater potential to discover new biomarkers and new treatment strategies similar to the experience with cystic fibrosis.[16–18] It will be important to coordinate that development to meet regulatory requirements for the application of new biomarkers. In addition, multiple racial and ethnic populations can be evaluated in a systematic way to identify unique genetic features of response to medications or pathways of disease development. It is also important to incorporate a measure of social determinants of health to address issues that may impact overall asthma care in those suffering health disparities.[19,20]

Ultimately, we would like to move from a strategy of preventing asthma exacerbations to one that prevents asthma progression and finally to a strategy of preventing disease onset, as described in this set of topic reviews. That will require a very careful level of coordinated care and knowledge assimilation. This information could also be useful in developing housing, school, and living conditions that minimize the factors that contribute to airway inflammation and the prevalence and severity of asthma. Perhaps, looking at respiratory disease as a composite of various respiratory disorders including what we now call asthma and COPD will yield better insights into disease management by coordinating data regarding prevalence, severity, and regional areas of unusually high prevalence throughout the lifespan.

To accomplish these goals, systems of collaboration among medical care systems, government agencies, pharmaceutic industry, and clinicians will be needed. A carefully coordinated system would not only lead to improved strategies for care but could also lead to new insights for medication development. We are currently undergoing an unprecedented era of the introduction of new medications in various categories. Understanding the successes and failures of these strategies is key to developing these new insights.

CONCLUSIONS

To date, we have depended on asthma guidelines, either in the form of local or national guidelines or global strategies to coordinate our knowledge around asthma. However, new information is coming so rapidly that even periodic updates to the guidelines cannot keep up with these rapid developments and applications to practice. Novel mechanisms may be needed to make this new information available to clinicians who are dedicated to moving asthma care to an individualized level. In addition, new mechanisms must be developed to convey this information to clinicians so that they can apply it on site for individual patients. If all of these factors evolve, we should be able to see a new era in disease management that would hopefully lead to better outcomes and reduced morbidity and mortality related to respiratory disease.

REFERENCES

1. Chipps BE, Zeiger RS, Borish L, et al. Key findings and clinical implications from the epidemiology and natural history of asthma; outcomes and treatment regimens (TENOR) study. *J Allergy Clin Immunol*. 2012;130:332–342.
2. Lemanske RF, Kakumanu S, Shanovich K, et al. Creation and implementation of SAMPRO™: a school-based asthma management program. *J Allergy Clin Immunol*. 2016;138:711–723.
3. Parikh RB, Schwartz JS, Navathe AS. Beyond genes and molecules – a precision delivery initiative for precision medicine. *N Engl J Med*. 2017;376:1609–1612.
4. Wildfire JJ, Gergen PJ, Sorkness CA, et al. Development and validation of the composite asthma severity index – an outcome measure for use in children and adolescents. *J Allergy Clin Immunol*. 2012;129:694–701.
5. Krouse RZ, Sorkness CA, Wildfire JJ, et al. Minimally important differences and risk levels for the composite asthma severity index. *J Allergy Clin Immunol*. 2017;139:1052–1055.
6. McGeachie MJ, Yates KP, Zhou X, et al. Patterns of growth and decline in lung function in persistent childhood asthma. *N Engl J Med*. 2016;374:1842–1852.
7. Teach SJ, Gergen PJ, Szefler SJ, et al. Seasonal risk factors for asthma exacerbations among inner city children. *J Allergy Clin Immunol*. 2015;135:1465–1473.
8. Hoch HE, Calatroni A, West JB, et al. Can we predict fall asthma exacerbations? Validation of the seasonal asthma exacerbation index. *J Allergy Clin Immunol*. 2017. http://dx.doi.org/10.1016/j.jaci.2017.01.026. pii: S0091-6749(17)30318-4. PMID: 28238748. [Epub ahead of print].
9. Teach SJ, Gill MA, Togias A, et al. Preseasonal treatment with either omalizumab or an inhaled corticosteroid boost to prevent fall asthma exacerbations. *J Allergy Clin Immunol*. 2015;136:1476–1485.
10. Merchant RK, Inamdar R, Quade RC. Effectiveness of population health management using the propeller health asthma platform: a randomized clinical trial. *J Allergy Clin Immunol Pract*. 2016;4:455–463.
11. Chan AHY, Stewart AW, Harrison J, Black PN, Mitchell EA, Foster JM. Electronic adherence monitoring device performance and patient acceptability: a randomized clinical trial. *Expert Rev Med Devices*. 2017;14:401–411.
12. Souverein PC, Koster ES, Colice G, et al. Inhaled corticosteroid adherence patterns in a longitudinal asthma cohort. *J Allergy Clin Immunol Pract*. 2017;5:448–456.
13. Wilson SR, Strub P, Buist S, et al. Shared treatment decision making improves adherence and outcomes in poorly controlled asthma. *Am J Respir Crit Care Med*. 2010;181:566–577.
14. Halterman JS, Szilagyi PG, Fisher SG, et al. Randomized, controlled trial to improve care for urban children with asthma. *Arch Pediatr Adolesc Med*. 2011;163:262–268.
15. Hoch HE, Szefler SJ. Intermittent steroid inhalation for the treatment of childhood asthma. *Expert Rev Clin Immunol*. 2016:183–194.
16. James BC. The cystic fibrosis improvement story: we count our successes in lives. *BMJ Qual Saf*. 2014;23:268–271.
17. Stolz DA, Meyerholz Welsh MJ. Origins of cystic fibrosis lung disease. *N Engl J Med*. 2015;372:351–362.
18. Ramsey BW, Nepom GT, Lonial S. Academic, foundation, and industry collaboration in finding new therapies. *N Engl J Med*. 2017;376:1762–1769.
19. Adler NE, Glymour MM, Fielding J. Addressing social determinants of health and health inequalities. *JAMA*. 2016;316(16):1641–1642.
20. Fuchs VR. Social determinants of health: caveats and nuances. *JAMA*. 2017;317:25–26.

Index

A

ABPM. *See* Allergic bronchopulmonary mycoses (ABPM)
ACOS. *See* Asthma-COPD overlap syndrome (ACOS)
ACQ. *See* Asthma Control Questionnaire (ACQ)
ACRN. *See* Asthma Clinical Research Network (ACRN)
ACT. *See* Asthma Control Test (ACT)
Acute severe RSV bronchiolitis, 175–176
Adherence
  conceptual approach, asthma medication, 135t
  inhaled corticosteroids and importance, 132–137
  monitoring tools, 208
  strategies, adherence improvement, 135t
ADRB2, 101, 153
  polymorphisms, 127
β-2 Adrenergic receptor, 127
  agonists, 102t
    inhaled, 101–104
    pharmacogenetic studies, 101–102
Adult asthmatics (AIR2), 28, 198
Adult endpoints, 72–73
Advocacy, 119–120
AERD. *See* Aspirin-exacerbated respiratory disease (AERD)
β-Agonist response, 102–103
Air, 117–118
AIR. *See* Asthma Intervention Research (AIR)
AIR2. *See* Adult asthmatics (AIR2)
Airborne PM, 117
Airflow limitation, 37
Airway
  biomarkers, 43
  microbiome
    asthma phenotypic features and, 163–164
    influence on medication responses in asthma, 164–166
  remodeling, 27, 191
Airway Inspector for SLICER, 193
Airway lumen area (LA), 193
Airway smooth muscle (ASM), 191
  cells, 100–101
Airway wall area (WA), 193
Airway wall thickness (AWT), 193, 197

Airways Disease Endotyping for Personalized Therapeutics study, 157–158
Alair Bronchial Thermoplasty System, 198
Alkaline phosphatase, tissue-nonspecific isozyme (ALPL), 90
Allergen
  environmental control, 115t
  mouse, 114–116
  sensitization reduction, 186
Allergic bronchopulmonary mycoses (ABPM), 124–125
Allergic/allergy
  inflammation, 52
  program strategy, 4–6
    contact-person network, 5
    measuring outcomes, 5–6
    primary prevention, 6b
    secondary and tertiary prevention, 6b
  sensitization, 113
ALOX5 variation, 105
ALPL. *See* Alkaline phosphatase, tissue-nonspecific isozyme (ALPL)
American Thoracic Society (ATS), 19, 35, 49
Anaphylaxis, 25
Anti-IL-4. *See* Antiinterleukin-4 (Anti-IL-4)
Anti-IL-4Rα therapy, 50
Anticholinergics, 21–22
Antiinterleukin-4 (Anti-IL-4), 26–27
  dupilumab, 26–27
  lebrikizumab, 26
  tralokinumab, 26
Antiinterleukin-5 (Anti-IL-5), 20, 23–26
  benralizumab, 25–26
  mepolizumab, 23–24
  reslizumab, 24–25
Antiinterleukin-13 (Anti-IL-13), 26–27
Apollo Workstation, 193
Apparent diffusion coefficient (ADC), 196–197
AQLQ. *See* Asthma Quality-of-Life Questionnaire (AQLQ)
ARG1. *See* Arginase-1 (ARG1)
Arg16 homozygotes, 101
Arginase-1 (ARG1), 103
Arginase-2 (ARG2), 103
Arginases, 103
L-Arginine, 103

ASM. *See* Airway smooth muscle (ASM)
Aspirin-exacerbated respiratory disease (AERD), 123, 125
Association, 132
Asthma, 59, 87, 97, 118–119, 143, 176, 179, 191
  asthma-chronic obstructive pulmonary disease overlap syndrome, 185
  control, 34
  early detection and progression prevention, 185–187
    characteristics prevalence, 186f
    lifestyle factors, 188
    loss of function, children, 187
    pharmacologic management, 186–187
    allergen sensitization reduction, 186
  functionally defined chronic obstructive pulmonary disease, 183–184
  microbial environment affect asthma development, 162–163
  microbiome impact, asthma phenotype and medication response, 163–166
  progression to chronic obstructive pulmonary disease, 182–183
  relapse predictor, inhaled glucocorticoid reduction, 53
  severity, 34, 191
  systems biology, 151–152
  therapy, 123
    phenotype determinants, 124t
Asthma care
  Children's Hospital Colorado (CHCO), 16f
  personalizing, 207–208
  providers, 145
  school as important component, 143
  systematic approach
    Children's Hospital Colorado (CHCO), 15–17
    children population management, 11–15
Asthma Clinical Research Network (ACRN), 101
Asthma Control Questionnaire (ACQ), 21, 37, 164
Asthma Control Test (ACT), 131

Note: Page numbers followed by "f" indicate figures, "t" indicate tables and "b" indicate boxes.

Asthma exacerbations, 129
  environmental exposures and
    exacerbation risk, 132
  fraction of exhaled nitric oxide
    (FeNO), 53
  prediction, 129–132, 130t
    index, 207–208
  prevention, 132–137
    immunomodulatory biologic
      therapies, 135–136
    inhaled corticosteroids and
      adherence importance, 132–137
    interventions, 134t
    medication adherence and
      control, 135t
    Seasonal Exacerbation Predictive
      index, 133f, 134t
    severity reduction, 136–137
    strategies, adherence
      improvement, 135t
    triggers reduction, 136
  severity characteristics, 130t
Asthma genotypes, 126–127
Asthma Intervention Research (AIR),
  27
Asthma management, future directions
  in, 207
  asthma research coordination,
    208–209
  personalizing asthma care, 207–208
Asthma phenotypes, 19, 37–38, 40,
  123, 131
  determinants, asthma therapy, 124t
  eosinophilic and early-onset asthma
    phenotype, 124–125
  noneosinophilic asthma, 125–127
  severe eosinophilic asthma
    phenotypes, 125
  therapeutic decision-making
    guidance, 123–124
Asthma prevention
  environmental and host factors, 171
  factors, 172f
  fish oil supplementation, 173–174
  microbiome modification, 174–175
  respiratory tract infections, 175–176
  vitamin D supplementation,
    171–173
Asthma program strategy, 2–4
  asthma emergency visits and
    hospital days, Finland, 4f
  burden decreased, 2–3
  costs, 3–4
  early detection, timely treatment, 2
  epidemic remained, 4
  paradigm change, 2
  strategic planning, implementation
    and evaluation, 3f
  total asthma costs, Finland, 5f
Asthma Quality-of-Life Questionnaire
  (AQLQ), 22
Asthma Therapy Assessment
  Questionnaire (ATAQ), 131

Asthma-COPD overlap syndrome
  (ACOS), 182–183, 185
Asthmatics, 124–125
ATAQ. *See* Asthma Therapy Assessment
  Questionnaire (ATAQ)
ATS. *See* American Thoracic Society
  (ATS)
ATS/ERS guidelines, 193
AWT. *See* Airway wall thickness (AWT)
Azithromycin for Prevention of
  Exacerbations in Severe Asthma Trial
  (AZISAST), 126, 29

B
Bacteria, 174
BAL. *See* Bronchoalveolar lavage (BAL)
BALF. *See* Bronchoalveolar lavage fluid
  (BALF)
"Bandwidth" of system, 13
BARD. *See* Best African American
  Response to Asthma Drugs (BARD)
BARGE trial. *See* Beta Agonists
  Response by Genotype trial
  (BARGE trial)
Barker hypothesis, 184–185
Baseline asthma care process data, 14
Baseline health data collection,
  14–15
Bayesian analysis, 104
BDP. *See* Beclomethasone dipropionate
  (BDP)
BDR. *See* Bronchodilator response
  (BDR)
Beclomethasone dipropionate (BDP),
  54
Benralizumab, 25–26, 63
Best African American Response to
  Asthma Drugs (BARD), 126–127
Beta Agonists Response by Genotype
  trial (BARGE trial), 101
Better Evaluation Tools, 71
BHR. *See* Bronchial
  hyperresponsiveness (BHR)
"Big data" principles, 207–208
Bioinformatics, 154
Biologic candidate gene studies,
  glucocorticoid response, 98–99
Biologic pathway candidate gene
  studies, β-agonist response, 102–103
Biologic therapies, 63–65
  development, 106
Biomarker(s), 50, 55, 69, 92. *See also*
  Pediatric biomarkers
  in asthma, 87–88
    management, 88–89
  drug development, 71–74
  monitoring, 70
  orphans, 69
  predictive, 70
  qualification, 74–84
Blood
  eosinophilia, 87
  eosinophils, 61–62, 88

Branch angles, 193
Bronchial hyperresponsiveness (BHR),
  50, 131
Bronchial thermoplasty (BT), 20,
  27–28, 42–43, 191, 198–202. *See
  also* Imaging procedures
  evidence for, 198–202
  randomized controlled trials and
    extension studies, 199t–200t
Bronchial wash, 61
Bronchoalveolar lavage (BAL), 20,
  89–90
Bronchoalveolar lavage fluid (BALF),
  153
  eosinophil counts, 61
Bronchodilator response (BDR), 52
Bronchoscopy with biopsy, 60
BT. *See* Bronchial thermoplasty (BT)

C
C-C Motif Chemokine Ligand 5
  (CCL5), 42
C-X-C motif. *See* Chemokine motif
  (C-X-C motif)
C-X-C Motif Chemokine Ligand 1
  (CXCL1), 42
*CA*10 variant, 98–99
CAAPA. *See* Consortium on Asthma
  in African Ancestry Populations
  (CAAPA)
CACT. *See* Childhood Asthma Control
  Test (CACT)
CAMP. *See* Childhood Asthma
  Management Program (CAMP)
Candidate gene studies, 97–99
  leukotriene biosynthetic and
    signaling pathways, 104–105
Carboxypeptidase A3 (CPA3), 90
Causation, 132
CC-chemokine ligands, 152
CCL5. *See* C-C Motif Chemokine
  Ligand 5 (CCL5)
Centers for Disease Control and
  Prevention (CDC), 117
CF. *See* Cystic fibrosis (CF)
CFTR gene, 83
Charcot-Leyden crystal protein (CLC),
  63, 90
CHCO. *See* Children's Hospital
  Colorado of Asthma Care (CHCO)
Chemokine ligands, 152
Chemokine motif (C-X-C motif), 90
Chemokine motif receptor 2 (CXCR2),
  90
Chest radiography, 192
Childhood
  asthma, 52–53, 113
  wheezing, 179
Childhood Asthma Control Test
  (CACT), 37, 52–53
Childhood Asthma Management
  Program (CAMP), 92–93, 99–100,
  131

Children, 113
    early intervention strategies
        asthma development factors, 172f
        fish oil supplementation,
            173–174
        microbiome modification,
            174–175
        respiratory tract infections,
            175–176
        vitamin D supplementation,
            171–173
    preschool, 38
Children's Hospital Colorado of
    Asthma Care (CHCO), 15–17, 16f
Chlamydophila pneumoniae, 28
Chronic bronchitis, 182
Chronic obstructive pulmonary disease
    (COPD), 42, 165, 179, 182, 193
    asthma evolution, 183–184
    asthma progression, 182–183
    asthma-COPD overlap syndrome,
        185
    COPD–like asthma, 181
    historical concepts, 183
    low lung function and, 180
    neonatal contribution, 184–185
Churg-Strauss syndrome, 193
Clarithromycin, 126
CLC. *See* Charcot-Leyden crystal
    protein (CLC)
Clinical endpoints, drug development,
    71–72
Cochrane review, 174, 201–202
Community health workers, 114
Community-based caregivers, 11
Composite exacerbation, 132
Computed tomography scans (CT
    scans), 192–195, 192t
    for lung density, 195f
    multidetector computed
        tomography (MDCT)
        air trapping assess, lung density
            measurement, 194–195
        limitations, 195
        novel asthma phenotypes
            and therapeutic response
            measurement, 195
    remodeling, 193–194
Conditional Gaussian Bayesian
    Network, 154–155
Consortium on Asthma in African
    Ancestry Populations (CAAPA), 107,
    155
Contact-person network, 5
COPD. *See* Chronic obstructive
    pulmonary disease (COPD)
Corticosteroids, 62, 165–166
Corticotropin-releasing hormone
    receptor 1 gene (*CRHR*1 gene), 98
Corticotropin-releasing hormone
    receptor 2 (*CRHR*2), 102–103
CPA3. *See* Carboxypeptidase A3
    (CPA3)

*CRHR*1 gene. *See* Corticotropin-
    releasing hormone receptor 1 gene
    (*CRHR*1 gene)
*CRHR*2. *See* Corticotropin-releasing
    hormone receptor 2 (*CRHR*2)
CRISPLD2, 100–101
CRTh2 antagonists, 27
CT scans. *See* Computed tomography
    scans (CT scans)
*CTNNA*3 variation, 98–99
CXCL1. *See* C-X-C Motif Chemokine
    Ligand 1 (CXCL1)
CXCR2. *See* Chemokine motif receptor
    2 (CXCR2)
CYP3A4, 98
Cysteinyl leukotriene receptor 1
    antagonists, 104
Cystic fibrosis (CF), 165

D
Deoxyribonuclease I-like 3
    (DNASE1L3), 90
Developmental Origins of Health
    and Disease (DOHaD). *See* Barker
    hypothesis
DHA. *See* Docosahexaenoic acid
    (DHA)
"Difficult-to-treat" asthma, 19, 35
DNA methylation, 181–182
DNASE1L3. *See* Deoxyribonuclease
    I-like 3 (DNASE1L3)
Docosahexaenoic acid (DHA),
    173–174
DREAM trial, 23–24
Drug development, 69–74
Dupilumab, 26–27, 55, 88–89

E
Early intervention strategies, children
    asthma development factors, 172f
    fish oil supplementation, 173–174
    microbiome modification, 174–175
    respiratory tract infections, 175–176
    vitamin D supplementation,
        171–173
Early-onset asthma phenotype,
    124–125
EBC. *See* Exhaled breath condensate
    (EBC)
EBUS. *See* Endobronchial ultrasound
    (EBUS)
ED. *See* Emergency department (ED)
EDN. *See* Eosinophil-derived
    neurotoxin (EDN)
Effective gene-environment interaction,
    4
Efficacy endpoints, drug development,
    71–72
Eicosapentaenoic acid (EPA),
    173–174
Electronic health record (EHR),
    14–15
Electronic medical record (EMR), 108

ELF. *See* Epithelial lining fluid (ELF)
Emergency department (ED), 11, 132,
    192
Emergency room (ER), 198
EMR. *See* Electronic medical record
    (EMR)
Endobronchial ultrasound (EBUS),
    192t, 197
Endotypes, 89, 151–152
Environmental assessment
    advocacy, 119–120
    assessment and implementation
        air, 117–118
        home, 114–116
        school, 116–117
    GIS, 118
    public health, 119
Environmental control, 113
    of allergens and mold, 115t
    implementation, 113–114
Environmental exposures, 132
Environmental intervention studies,
    116
Environmental tobacco smoke (ETS),
    117–118
Eosinophil peroxidase (EPX), 59
Eosinophil-derived neurotoxin (EDN),
    59
Eosinophil-predominant type 2
    inflammatory phenotype, 40–42
Eosinophil(s), 59
    bioactivity, 59–60
    biologic therapies, 63–65
    depletion, 61–62
    diurnal variation, 61, 62f
    eosinophilic asthma
        characteristics, 60
        treatment algorithm, 63f
    factors, eosinophil measurement, 61
    eosinophilia measurement, 60–61
    response to steroids, 62–63
    therapy and therapeutic response,
        61–65
Eosinophilia, 55, 60
    measurement, 60–61
Eosinophilic asthma, 124t
    anti-IL-4, 23–26
    anti-IL-5, 23–26
        mepolizumab, 23–24
        reslizumab, 24–25
        benralizumab, 25–26
    anti-IL-13, 23–26
    bronchial thermoplasty, 27–28
    characteristics, 60
    CRTh2 antagonists, 27
    macrolide antibiotics, 28–29
    treatment, 64t
        algorithm, 63f
Eosinophilic inflammation, 60
Eosinophilic phenotype, 124–125
EPA. *See* Eicosapentaenoic acid (EPA);
    U.S. Environmental Protection
    Agency (EPA)

Epigenomics, 152–153
Epithelial damage, 59–60
Epithelial lining fluid (ELF), 153
EPR. *See* Expert Report Panel (EPR)
EPR-3. *See* Expert Panel Report 3 (EPR-3)
EPX. *See* Eosinophil peroxidase (EPX)
eQTL. *See* Expression quantitative trait loci (eQTL)
ER. *See* Emergency room (ER)
ERS. *See* European Respiratory Society (ERS)
ERS/ATS. *See* European Respiratory Society and American Thoracic Society (ERS/ATS)
Ethnic-specific loci, pharmacogenetic studies, 104
ETS. *See* Environmental tobacco smoke (ETS)
European Respiratory Society (ERS), 35
European Respiratory Society and American Thoracic Society (ERS/ATS), 19
Evidence-based NAEPP Expert Panel Report 3 guidelines, 119
Exacerbation
  predictors, 131–132
  risk, 132
  severity reduction, 136–137
  triggers reduction, 136
Exhaled breath condensate (EBC), 153
Exhaled nitric oxide testing. *See* Fraction of exhaled nitric oxide (FeNO)
Expert Panel Report 3 (EPR-3), 19
Expert Report Panel (EPR), 125
Exposure risk, 113–114
Expression quantitative trait loci (eQTL), 100–101
External stimuli, 152–153

F
FDA. *See* U.S. Food and Drug Administration (FDA)
FEF. *See* Forced expiratory flow (FEF)
FeNO. *See* Fraction of exhaled nitric oxide (FeNO)
FEV1. *See* Forced expiratory volume in 1s (FEV1)
FEV1/FVC ratio. *See* Forced expiratory volume in 1s/forced vital capacity ratio (FEV1/FVC ratio)
Filha. *See* Finnish Lung Health Association (Filha)
Finnish Allergy Programme, 4, 5b
Finnish Asthma Program, 2, 2b, 11
Finnish healthcare system, 1
Finnish Lung Health Association (Filha), 4
Fish oil supplementation, 173–174

Fluticasone propionate (FP), 54
Forced expiratory flow (FEF), 131
Forced expiratory volume in 1s (FEV1), 19–20, 37, 99–100, 155, 163, 182–185
Forced expiratory volume in 1s/forced vital capacity ratio (FEV1/FVC ratio), 131, 185–186
FP. *See* Fluticasone propionate (FP)
Fraction of exhaled nitric oxide (FeNO), 50–52, 28, 49–50, 51f, 131, 157–158
  asthma exacerbations, 53
  asthma relapse predictor, inhaled glucocorticoid reduction, 53
  asthma severity and control measure, 52–53
  diagnostic test, asthma, 50–52
  interleukin-4 and interleukin-13-mediated inflammation, 50
  severe asthma, 54
  measurement and production, 49–50
  nonadherence, inhaled glucocorticoid therapy, 53–54
  response to
    biologic agents, 55
    glucocorticoid therapy, 54–55
  and wheezing phenotypes, 52

G
GC therapy. *See* Glucocorticoid therapy (GC therapy)
17q21 Gene locus, 153
Gene-gene interactions, 104
General practitioner services (GP services), 1
Genetic profiles, precision medicine, 104
Genetic risk score (GRS), 180–181
Genome-wide association studies (GWAS), 97–101, 100f, 103–104, 152
Genomics, 152
  analytical methods, 100–101
Geographic information system (GIS), 118
Geographic region of care, 13
GINA. *See* Global Initiative for Asthma (GINA)
GIS. *See* Geographic information system (GIS)
GLCCI1. *See* Glucocorticoid-induced transcript-1 gene (*GLCCI1*)
Global Asthma Network, 2
Global Initiative for Asthma (GINA), 125, 19
  guidelines, 129
  report, 39
Glucocorticoid therapy (GC therapy), 49
Glucocorticoid-induced transcript-1 gene (*GLCCI1*), 99–100

Gly[16] homozygotes, 101
Gly[16]Arg variant, 102
Gold Standard/International Guidelines treatment, 35–37, 39–40
GP services. *See* General practitioner services (GP services)
Green housing, 118
GRS. *See* Genetic risk score (GRS)
Guided self-management, 2
GWAS. *See* Genome-wide association studies (GWAS)

H
HAT activity. *See* Histone acetyl transferase activity (HAT activity)
Health payment reform, 119
Healthcare
  providers, 120
  system, 11
Heat-shock protein gene (*HSPA8*), 103
Helper-inducer T-lymphocytes type 2 phenotype (Th2 phenotype), 152–153
HEPA. *See* High-efficiency particulate arrestance (HEPA)
HFA. *See* Hydrofluoroalkane (HFA)
High-efficiency particulate arrestance (HEPA), 113
High-resolution computed tomography (HRCT), 192–193
High-throughput sequencing technologies, 152
Histone acetyl transferase activity (HAT activity), 152–153
Home, 114–116
Host-derived nutrients, 161–162
HP MRI. *See* Hyperpolarized magnetic resonance imaging (HP MRI)
HRCT. *See* High-resolution computed tomography (HRCT)
HSPA8. *See* Heat-shock protein gene (*HSPA8*)
Human-associated microbes, 161
Hydrofluoroalkane (HFA), 35–37
25-Hydroxyvitamin D_3 (25OHD), 171–172
Hygiene hypothesis, 161
Hyperpolarized magnetic resonance imaging (HP MRI), 195–197
  and apparent diffusion coefficient, 196–197
  mild asthmatics, 196f
  severe asthma patient, lung defects, 201f

I
ICSs. *See* Inhaled corticosteroids (ICSs)
ICU. *See* Intensive care unit (ICU)
IgE. *See* Immunoglobulin E (IgE)
IL. *See* Interleukin (IL)
IL-4 receptor α-subunit (IL-4Rα), 26, 50

Imaging procedures, 192t. *See also*
    Bronchial thermoplasty (BT)
  chest radiography, 192
  computed tomography (CT) scans,
    192–195
  endobronchial ultrasound (EBUS),
    197
  hyperpolarized magnetic resonance
    imaging (HP MRI), 195–197
  optical coherence tomography
    (OCT), 197
  positron emission tomography
    (PET), 197–198
Immunoglobulin E (IgE), 40–41,
  59–60, 64, 98–99, 113, 154
Immunomodulatory biologic
  therapies, 135–136
Immunosuppressants, 40
Indoor allergen exposure, 114–116
Induced-exacerbations, 53
Inducible nitric oxide synthase (iNOS),
  50
Inflammatory biomarkers, 131
Inhaled corticosteroids (ICSs), 19,
  35–37, 61, 97–101, 132, 163,
  194–195
  adherence importance, 132–137
  biologic candidate gene studies,
    glucocorticoid response,
    98–99
  genome-wide association studies
    and integrative genomics,
    99–101
  pharmacogenetic candidate genes,
    99t
Inhaled GC/LABA therapy, 53
Inhaled glucocorticoids
  asthma relapse predictor, 53
  nonadherence predictor, 53–54
Inhaled β2-adrenergic receptor
  agonists, 101–104
  β-agonist response, biologic
    pathway candidate gene studies,
    102–103
  pharmacogenetic studies
    β2-adrenergic receptor gene,
      101–102
    β-agonists, 101
Inner-city homes, 114–116
iNOS. *See* Inducible nitric oxide
  synthase (iNOS)
Integrated pest management (IPM),
  113–116
Integrative genomics, 99–101,
  103–104
Intensive care unit (ICU), 54
Interleukin (IL), 59, 106
  IL-4, 50
  IL-5, 88
  IL-17 receptor A, 42
IPM. *See* Integrated pest management
  (IPM)
Ivacaftor, 83

L
LA. *See* Airway lumen area (LA)
LABA. *See* Long-acting β-agonist
  (LABA)
LAMA. *See* Long-acting muscarinic
  antagonists (LAMA)
LARGE. *See* Long-Acting β-Agonist
  Response by Genotype (LARGE)
LAVOLTA I, 26
LAVOLTA II, 26
LCPUFAs. *See* Long-chain
  polyunsaturated fatty acids
  (LCPUFAs)
LD. *See* Linkage disequilibrium (LD)
Lebrikizumab, 26, 41–42, 55, 88–89
Leukotriene modifiers (LTMs), 97,
  104–106
  candidate genes studies, leukotriene
    biosynthetic and signaling
    pathways, 104–105
  genome-wide association studies,
    Zileuton response, 106
  leukotriene modifying drugs, 104
  pharmacogenetic candidate genes,
    105t
  retrospective pharmacogenetic
    analysis, leukotriene pathway
    genes, 105f
Leukotriene receptor antagonist
  (LTRA), 35–37, 40
Lifestyle factors, 188
5-Lipooxygenase (5-LO), 104
Linkage disequilibrium (LD), 97
Long-acting muscarinic antagonists
  (LAMA), 125–126
Long-acting β-agonist (LABA), 20,
  35–37, 97, 101
  add-on therapy, 40
  bronchodilator therapy, 198
  therapy, 134
Long-Acting β-Agonist Response by
  Genotype (LARGE), 101–102
Long-chain polyunsaturated fatty acids
  (LCPUFAs), 173–174
Low lung function, 179–180, 184–185
Lower respiratory tract infections
  (LRTIs), 29
LTMs. *See* Leukotriene modifiers
  (LTMs)
LTRA. *See* Leukotriene receptor
  antagonist (LTRA)
Lung function
  genetic, gene-environment, and
    epigenetic effects, 180–182
  trajectories, 184f
  and wheezing syndromes, 179–180,
    180f
Lung protection strategies, 186

M
Macrolide antibiotics, 28–29
Magnetic resonance imaging (MRI),
  192t, 193

Major basic protein (MBP), 59
Mass spectrometry (MS), 153
Mass spectrometry-based 'omics', 153
MBP. *See* Major basic protein (MBP)
MDCT. *See* Multidetector computed
  tomography (MDCT)
Mechanisms of the Development of
  ALLergy (MeDALL), 154
  allergen-chip, 155
  study, 155
MeDALL. *See* Mechanisms of the
  Development of ALLergy (MeDALL)
Mepolizumab, 23–24, 55, 63
Messenger RNAs (mRNA), 153
Metabolomics, 153–154
Microbiome, 161–162
  future directions, 166–167
  impact on asthma, 163–166
    airway microbiome influence,
      medication responses, 164–166
    bronchial bacterial microbiota
      composition, 165f
    phenotypic features and airway
      microbiome, 163–164
  microbial environment, asthma
    development, 162–163
  modification, 174–175
Microliter (μL), 60
6-Min walk test (6MWT), 72–73
Mold, environmental control of, 115t
Molecular analyses, 92
Molecular phenotyping, severe asthma,
  90
Monitoring biomarker, 70
Montelukast, 194–195
Mortality, 72–73
Mosaic attenuation, 194–195
Mouse allergen, 114–116
MRI. *See* Magnetic resonance imaging
  (MRI)
mRNA. *See* Messenger RNAs
  (mRNA)
MS. *See* Mass spectrometry (MS)
Multidetector computed tomography
  (MDCT), 192–194, 194f
  air trapping assess, lung density
    measurement, 194–195
  limitations, 195
  novel asthma phenotypes
    and therapeutic response
    measurement, 195
Muscarinic cholinergic receptors, 103
6MWT. *See* 6-Min walk test (6MWT)
Mycoplasma pneumoniae, 28

N
N-6 polyunsaturated fatty acids,
  173–174
NACP. *See* National Asthma Control
  Program (NACP)
NAEPP. *See* National Asthma
  Education and Prevention Program
  (NAEPP)

National Asthma Control Program (NACP), 119

National Asthma Education and Prevention Panel. *See* National Asthma Education and Prevention Program (NAEPP)

National Asthma Education and Prevention Program (NAEPP), 38–39, 113

National Cooperative Inner-City Asthma Study, 114–116

National Heart, Lung, and Blood Institute (NHLBI), 19

National Institute of Allergy and Infectious Disease (NIAID), 116

National Institutes of Health (NIH), 60, 116

Negative predictive value (NPV), 53–54

Network of Asthma Care (NOAC), 11
  examples, United States, 12t
  NOAC 3.0, 12f

Network of care leaders, priorities and abilities, 11–13

Neutrophil-predominant inflammatory phenotype, 40, 42

Neutrophilic airway inflammation, 125–126

Next-generation sequencing (NGS). *See* High-throughput sequencing technologies

NGO. *See* Nongovernmental organization (NGO)

NHLBI. *See* National Heart, Lung, and Blood Institute (NHLBI)

NIAID. *See* National Institute of Allergy and Infectious Disease (NIAID)

NIH. *See* National Institutes of Health (NIH)

NIH Human Microbiome Project, 161

NIH/NIAID SICAS Intervention Study, 116–117

Nitrogen dioxide (NO_2), 117

NOAC. *See* Network of Asthma Care (NOAC)

Non-CF-related patients, 165

Noneosinophilic asthma, 29, 124t, 125–127
  obesity asthma phenotype, 126
  race and ethnicity, 126–127

Noneosinophilic phenotypes, 125–126

Nongovernmental organization (NGO), 4

"Not-well-controlled" status, 37

Novel inhaled corticosteroid pharmacogenetic loci, 99–101

Novel β-agonist pharmacogenetic loci, 103–104

NPV. *See* Negative predictive value (NPV)

O

Obesity asthma phenotype, 126

Obesity-related asthma, 125–126

Objective endpoints, 72

OCS. *See* Oral corticosteroid (OCS)

OCT. *See* Optical coherence tomography (OCT)

25OHD. *See* 25-Hydroxyvitamin D_3 (25OHD)

OM-85 BV, 176

Omalizumab, 22–23, 55, 64–65

"One-disease one-treatment" concept, 123

"One-size-fits-all" treatment approach, 40

Optical coherence tomography (OCT), 192t, 197

Oral corticosteroid (OCS), 24

Outdoor allergen exposures, 118

P

PAI-1. *See* Plasminogen activator inhibitor-1 (PAI-1)

Particulate matter (PM), 116–117

Patient-Centered Outcomes Research Institute, 119–120

PCR. *See* Polymerase chain reaction (PCR)

Peak expiratory flow rate (PEFR), 101

Pediatric "network of care", 11

Pediatric asthma, 69, 71, 92

Pediatric biomarkers
  categories and definitions, 69–71, 70f
  endpoints and biomarkers, drug development, 71–74
    adult *vs.* pediatric endpoints, 72–73
    pediatric asthma research, 74
    pediatric endpoints, 73–74, 73f
    primary and secondary endpoints, 72
  pediatric endpoints breakdown, 74f
  qualification, 74–84
    biomarker acceptance pathways, 83f
    codevelopment process, therapeutic product, 84
    endpoints, 76t–82t
    Food and Drug Administration (FDA) experience, 74–84
    regulatory history, biomarker qualification, 71
    surrogate endpoints, 71

Pediatric endpoints, 72–73
  in asthma research, 74
  breakdown, 74f
  drug development, 73–74, 73f
  outcome, 75f

PEFR. *See* Peak expiratory flow rate (PEFR)

Periostin, 88–89

Peripheral blood eosinophil counts, 61

Personalized medicine, 29, 43, 87, 158

Personalizing asthma care, 207–208

Personalizing asthma therapy, 87
  biomarkers, 87–89, 92
    unmet needs, 89
  endotyping and biomarker discovery, 89f
  molecular phenotyping, 90
  pediatric considerations, 92–93
  personalized medicine, 87
  U-BIOPRED omics analysis, 90–92
  unbiased classification, clinical, physiologic, and inflammatory features, 89–90

PET. *See* Positron emission tomography (PET)

PFTs. *See* Pulmonary function tests (PFTs)

PGD2, 27

Pharmacodynamic endpoints, 98

Pharmacogenetics, 97
  β2-adrenergic receptor gene, 101–102
  profiles, 108
    components, 108
    electronic medical record expansion, 108

Pharmacogenomics and applications, asthma management
  biologic therapies development, 106
  gene-gene interactions and genetic profiles, precision medicine, 104
  genetic variants, 103f
  genome-wide association studies and integrative genomics, 103–104
  inhaled β2-adrenergic receptor agonists, 101–104
  inhaled corticosteroid (ICS), 98–101
  leukotriene modifiers, 104–106
  limitations, 106–107
    asthma subgroup, outcome evaluation, 107
    ethnically diverse cohorts, 106–107
    exacerbation frequency, 107f
    loci replication inability, 106
  pharmacogenetic profiles, 108
    components, 108
    electronic medical record expansion, 108
  pharmacogenetic studies, in asthma, 97
    human genetic variation, 97–98
    multiethnic cohorts, 104

Pharmacologic management, 186–187

Phenotypes
  of asthma, 87
  phenotype-directed treatment strategies, 40–42
    for children, severe asthma, 41f
    eosinophil-predominant type 2 inflammatory phenotype, 40–42
    neutrophil-predominant inflammatory phenotype, 42

Phosphodiesterase 4 (PDE$_4$), 42
PIAMA cohort study, 143
Pipeline problem, 71
Pitrakinra, 106
Plasminogen activator inhibitor-1 (PAI-1), 181
PM. *See* Particulate matter (PM)
Point mutations. *See* Single nucleotide polymorphisms (SNPs)
"Point-of-care" biomarkers, 92
Polymerase chain reaction (PCR), 28
Population health management
  children with asthma, 11–15
    baseline health data collection, 14–15
    geographic region of care, 13
    key metrics, asthma care, 15t
    key stakeholders identification and assessing needs, 13
    priorities and abilities, network of care leaders, 11–13
    set priorities, 13–14
    target population identification, 13
    team building and steering committee, 14
    team education, 15
  Children's Hospital Colorado, 15–17
Population management model, 8f, 8b, 11
  allergy program strategy, 4–6
  asthma program strategy, 2–4
  direct healthcare cost distribution, 7f
  Finnish healthcare system, 1
  generic template, public health program, 9f
  prevalence and need, 1–2
Positive predictive value (PPV), 50–51
Positron emission tomography (PET), 192t, 197–198
Postbronchodilator peak expiratory flow rates, 20
PPV. *See* Positive predictive value (PPV)
Precision medicine, 33, 63
  components, pharmacogenetic profiles, 108
Predictive biomarkers, 70, 87–88
Predictive enrichment biomarkers, 83
Preschool children, 38
Primary endpoint, 29
  in drug development, 72
Primary prevention, 171
Private health insurance, 1
Prognostic biomarkers, 87–88
Protein kinase C theta (*PRKCQ*), 103–104
Proteomics, 153
Pseudomonas aeruginosa, 165
Public health, 119
  agencies, 119
Pulmonary function, 207–208
Pulmonary function tests (PFTs), 43, 191

Q
Quality of life (QOL), 53, 198
Quality-adjusted life-years (QALY), 202
Quantitative CT (qCT), 193, 195
Quick-relief inhalers, 145–146

R
Radiofrequency coil (RF coil), 196
Radiotracers, 197–198
RANTES. *See* Regulated on activation, normal T cell expressed and Secreted (RANTES)
Reactive airway disease, 14
"Reasonably likely" surrogate endpoint, 71–72
Regulated on activation, normal T cell expressed and Secreted (RANTES), 152
Relative risk (RR), 53
Research in Severe Asthma (RISA), 27
Reslizumab, 24–25, 63
Respiratory syncytial virus (RSV), 174, 179
Respiratory tract illnesses (RTIs), 53
Respiratory tract infections, 175–176
RF coil. *See* Radiofrequency coil (RF coil)
Rhinovirus, 174
RISA. *See* Research in Severe Asthma (RISA)
RNA sequencing (RNA-Seq), 100–101, 153
RR. *See* Relative risk (RR)
RSV. *See* Respiratory syncytial virus (RSV)
RTIs. *See* Respiratory tract illnesses (RTIs)

S
SABA. *See* Short-acting bronchodilators (SABA)
Salmeterol Asthma Multicenter Research Trial (SMART), 127, 101
SAMPRO. *See* School-based Asthma Management Programs (SAMPRO)
SARP. *See* Severe Asthma Research Program (SARP)
SBHCs. *See* School-based health centers (SBHCs)
SCFAs. *See* Short-chain fatty acids (SCFAs)
School, 116–117
  programs, 14
School Inner-City Asthma Study (SICAS), 116–117
School-based Asthma Management Programs (SAMPRO), 144
School-based health centers (SBHCs), 117
School-centered asthma programs, 14

asthma management plans, 143–144
school, family, and provider communication and coordination, 144
asthma care component, 143
supportive and asthma friendly schools
  programs and resources, 144, 145b
clinicians care, 145–148
SCs. *See* Subject clusters (SCs)
Seasonal Asthma Exacerbation Index, 132
Seasonal Exacerbation Predictive index, 133f, 134t
Secondary endpoints, drug development, 72
Severe asthma management and prevention, children, 33–37
  disorders, 36t
  early identification, 38–39
  emerging treatments, 42–43
  factors, 34f
  future directions and needs, 43
  high-dose inhaled corticosteroid treatment, 36t
  key features, 37–38
  low-dose inhaled corticosteroid treatment, 39t
  medications, 39–40
  phenotype-directed treatment strategies, 40–42
  phenotypes, 38f
  priority research questions, 43t
  three-stage approach, 35f
Severe asthma management, adults, 19. *See also* Population health management
  eosinophilic asthma and biologics, 23–29
  epidemiology, 20
  key features, assessment and pathophysiology, 20
  treatment, 20–23
    advanced, new, and emerging asthma therapies, 21t–22t
    anticholinergics, 21–22
    omalizumab, 22–23
    traditional asthma therapies, 21t
Severe Asthma Research Program (SARP), 124–125, 92–93
Severe eosinophilic asthma phenotypes, 89, 125
Short-acting bronchodilators (SABA), 20–21, 101, 131
  β-agonists, 97
  prescription dispensing, 131
Short-chain fatty acids (SCFAs), 162
SICAS. *See* School Inner-City Asthma Study (SICAS)
SII. *See* Social Insurance Institution (SII)

Single nucleotide polymorphisms
(SNPs), 97, 180–181
SMART. *See* Salmeterol Asthma
Multicenter Research Trial (SMART);
Specific, Measurable, Attainable and,
Realistic, and Time-limited goal
(SMART)
Snips. *See* Single nucleotide
polymorphisms (SNPs)
SNPs. *See* Single nucleotide
polymorphisms (SNPs)
Social Insurance Institution (SII), 1
Specific, Measurable, Attainable and,
Realistic, and Time-limited goal
(SMART), 13–14
Spectral clustering, 92–93
Spiriva Respimat, 21
Spirometry, 38–39
Sputum eosinophils, 50, 60–62
Sputum transcriptomics, 90
Squamous cells, 60–61
Statistical cluster analyses,
37–38
Steering committee, 14
Step Up asthma program, 14
Subject clusters (SCs), 54
Subjective end-points, 72
Suboptimal control, 52–53
Supportive and asthma friendly
schools
programs and resources, 144,
145b
clinicians care, 145–148
checklist, summer back to school
follow-up visit, 147t
local schools engagement,
146–148
exposures to triggers, school
setting, 146
schedule summer visit, child/
youth, 145–146
Surrogate endpoints, 71
Surrogate measure, 71–72
Systemic corticosteroids. *See* Inhaled
corticosteroids (ICSs)
Systems biology, 104, 151–152
asthma research result, 159f
limitations and future projections,
155–158
multiple cohorts/biofluids,
156t–157t
researchers tools, 152–154
bioinformatics, 154
epigenomics, 152–153
genomics, 152
high-throughput sequencing
technologies, 152

Systems biology (*Continued*)
mass spectrometry-based 'omics',
153
metabolomics, 153–154
proteomics, 153
transcriptomics, 153
treatment options and efficacy,
154–155

T
T gene, 100
T-helper type 2 cells (Th2 cells), 50,
90–91, 163
molecular phenotype, 89–90
receptor, 42
T2-high asthma, 88
TACs. *See* Transcriptome-associated
clusters (TACs)
TARC. *See* Thymus and activation-
regulated chemokine (TARC)
Team building, 14
Team education, 15
Telithromycin, Chlamydophila, and
Asthma trial (TELICAST), 28
Test for Respiratory and Asthma
Control in Kids (TRACK), 38–39
TGF-β, 26
Th2 cells. *See* T-helper type 2 cells (Th2
cells)
Th2 phenotype. *See* Helper-inducer
T-lymphocytes type 2 phenotype
(Th2 phenotype)
Th2-mediated asthma, 50
Therapeutic decision-making,
123–124
Third-hand smoke exposure (THS
exposure), 118
Thr^{164}Ile, 102
THS exposure. *See* Third-hand smoke
exposure (THS exposure)
Thymus and activation-regulated
chemokine (TARC), 55
Tiotropium, 42
TLC. *See* Total lung capacity (TLC)
TNF. *See* Tumor necrosis factor (TNF)
Tobacco smoke exposure, 136
TopMed Program. *See* Trans-Omics
for Precision Medicine Program
(TopMed Program)
Total lung capacity (TLC), 49–50,
194–195
Total serum IgE level, 88
TRACK. *See* Test for Respiratory and
Asthma Control in Kids (TRACK)
Tralokinumab, 26
Trans-Omics for Precision Medicine
Program (TopMed Program), 107

Transcriptome-associated clusters
(TACs), 90–91, 91t
Transcriptomics, 153
Triple Aim, 11
Tumor necrosis factor (TNF), 20
Type 2-"low" inflammatory profile
asthma, 163
Type-2/type-2-helper inflammatory
pathway (T2/Th2 inflammatory
pathway), 59

U
U-BIOPRED omics analysis, 90–92
U.S. Environmental Protection Agency
(EPA), 117
U.S. Food and Drug Administration
(FDA), 21, 70, 101, 198
biomarker qualification program,
83
guidance, 71
Unbiased approach, 89
clinical, physiologic, and
inflammatory features, 89–90
US National Institutes of Health
National Heart, Lung, and Blood
Institute Expert Panel Report (NIH
NHLBI Expert Panel Report), 129

V
Viral infections, 179
Vitamin D in Asthma (VIDA), 125
Vitamin D supplementation,
171–173
Volatile organic compounds (VOCs), 92
Volumetric CT. *See* Multidetector
computed tomography (MDCT)

W
WA. *See* Airway wall area (WA)
Weighted Gene Co-expression Network
Analysis (WGCNA), 90
Wheezing, 179
childhood, 179
phenotypes, 52
syndromes, 179–180
World Health Organization (WHO),
19, 34–35

X
Xenon, 195–196
Xenon-129, 195–196
Xolair Persistency of Response After
Long-Term Therapy (XPORT),
22–23

Z
Zileuton response, 106